FEVER

Fever

Editor

James M. Lipton, Ph.D.

Professor
Departments of Physiology and Neurology
University of Texas Health Science Center at Dallas
Dallas, Texas

Raven Press ▪ New York

Raven Press, 1140 Avenue of the Americas, New York, New York 10036

Made in the United States of America

Great care has been taken to maintain the accuracy of the information contained in the volume. However, Raven Press cannot be held responsible for errors or for any consequences arising from the use of the information contained herein.

Library of Congress Cataloging in Publication Data

International Symposium of Fever, Dallas, 1979.
  Fever.

  Based on proceedings of the International
Symposium on Fever, held in Dallas, Tex., Apr. 11–
12, 1979, sponsored by the University of Texas
Health Science Center at Dallas and McNeil
Consumer Products Co.
  Includes bibliographies and index.
  1. Fever—Congresses. I. Lipton, James M.
II. University of Texas Health Science Center at
Dallas. III. McNeil Consumer Products Co.
IV. Title.
RB129.I57 1979   616'.047   78–65832
ISBN 0–89004–451–1

Preface

The association between fever and disease has been recognized for 2,500 years, and fever phenomena are of paramount importance in modern clinical medicine. Yet there has been no single source to which students, researchers, and health care professionals could turn for a statement on the current level of understanding of fever. The febrile response has been studied broadly in recent years, using approaches ranging from molecular probes through clinical studies. The resulting data and theories are scattered in the literature and are generally known only to the fever specialist. To meet the need for a modern source book on fever, experts from several countries were brought together to discuss aspects of the pyrogenic reaction. The aims of the conference on which this volume is based were to evaluate existing concepts of fever, to examine recent research findings and to publish a book on fever that is useful to students and professionals in the life sciences generally and to basic and clinical scientists who are fever specialists.

James M. Lipton, Ph.D.

Acknowledgments

The conference on which this volume is based, the International Symposium on Fever, was held in Dallas, Texas, April 11–12, 1979. The symposium was sponsored by the University of Texas Health Science Center at Dallas and co-sponsored by McNeil Consumer Products Co. Funds for partial support of the meeting were generously supplied by the following:

Bureau of Drugs, FDA

Burroughs Wellcome Co.

Coca Cola Bottling Works, Inc., Dallas

Fogarty International Center, NIH

Hoffmann-LaRoche Inc.

International Business Machines Corporation

Merck Sharp & Dohme Postgraduate Program

McNeil Laboratories

National Institute of Allergy and Infectious Diseases, NIH

Naval Medical Research and Development Command, NNMC

Omega Engineering, Inc.

A. H. Robins Company

Smith Kline & French Laboratories

Southwest Airlines

I thank Mrs. Sandra Parker for her tireless assistance in the planning and execution of the symposium and the book. The assistance of students in my laboratory is gratefully acknowledged. Special thanks to Carol.

Contents

Contributors

Elisha Atkins
Department of Internal Medicine
Yale University School of Medicine
New Haven, Connecticut 06510

Christopher C. Barney
Department of Physiology
University of Florida College of Medicine
Gainesville, Florida 32610

William R. Beisel
U.S. Army Medical Research Institute of
Infectious Diseases
Fort Detrick
Frederick, Maryland 21701

Harry A. Bernheim
Department of Internal Medicine
Yale University School of Medicine
New Haven, Connecticut 06510

Clark M. Blatteis
Department of Physiology and Biophysics
University of Tennessee Center for the
Health Sciences
Memphis, Tennessee 38163

John Bligh
Institute of Arctic Biology
University of Alaska
Fairbanks, Alaska 99701

M. Cabanac
Claude Bernard University
South Lyon Faculty of Medicine
Laboratory of Physiology
Oullins, France

Martha E. Casterlin
Marine Biology Program
Center for the Life Sciences
University of New England
Biddeford, Maine 04005

Wesley G. Clark
Department of Pharmacology
University of Texas Health Science Center
at Dallas
Dallas, Texas 75235

Keith E. Cooper
Division of Medical Physiology
Faculty of Medicine
University of Calgary
Calgary, Alberta T2N 1N4, Canada

Jerry B. Covert
Department of Biology
Pennsylvania State University
Hazleton, Pennsylvania 18201

William I. Cranston
Department of Medicine
St. Thomas' Hospital Medical School
London SE1, England

N. J. Dawson
National Institute for Medical Research
London NW7 1AA, England

Charles A. Dinarello
Department of Medicine
Division of Experimental Medicine
Tufts-New England Medical Center
Boston, Massachusetts 02111

G. W. Duff
Department of Medicine
St. Thomas' Hospital Medical School
London SE1, England

L. Francis
Department of Internal Medicine
Yale University School of Medicine
New Haven, Connecticut 06510

Melvin J. Fregly
Department of Physiology
University of Florida College of Medicine
Gainesville, Florida 32616

Zbigniew Górka
Institute of Pharmacology
Polish Academy of Sciences
31–519 Cracow, Poland

J. Hattingh
Department of General Physiology
University of Witwatersrand
Johannesburg 2001, South Africa

Richard F. Hellon
National Institute for Medical Research
London NW7 1AA, England

O. Kadlecová
Institute of Pharmacology
Czechoslovak Academy of Sciences
120 00 Prague 2, Czechoslovakia

Richard F. Kampschmidt
Biomedical Division
The Samuel Roberts Noble Foundation,
* Inc.*
Ardmore, Oklahoma 73401

Norman W. Kasting
Division of Medical Physiology
Faculty of Medicine
University of Calgary
Calgary, Alberta T2N 1N4, Canada

Michael J. Katovich
Department of Physiology
University of Florida College of Medicine
Gainesville, Florida 32610

Naomi Kleitman
Departments of Psychology, Physiology,
* and Biophysics*
University of Illinois
Champaign, Illinois 61820

Matthew J. Kluger
Department of Physiology
University of Michigan Medical School
Ann Arbor, Michigan 48104

Helen Laburn
Department of Physiology
University of Witwatersrand Medical
* School*
Johannesburg 2001, South Africa

James M. Lipton
Departments of Physiology and Neurology
University of Texas Health Science Center
* at Dallas*
Dallas, Texas 75235

Karl Mašek
Institute of Pharmacology
Czechoslovak Academy of Sciences
120 00 Prague 2, Czechoslovakia

B. Massonnet
Claude Bernard University
South Lyon Faculty of Medicine
Laboratory of Physiology
Oullins, France

Anthony S. Milton
Department of Pharmacology
Marischal College
University of Aberdeen
Aberdeen AB9 1AS, Scotland

Duncan Mitchell
Department of Physiology
University of Witwatersrand Medical
* School*
Johannesburg 2001, South Africa

Robert D. Myers
Departments of Psychiatry and Pharma-
* cology*
University of North Carolina School of
* Medicine*
Chapel Hill, North Carolina 27514

P. Petrovický
Institute of Anatomy
Charles University Medical School
120 00 Prague 2, Czechoslovakia

M. Pont
North Lyon Faculty of Medicine
Department of Internal Medicine
69373 Lyon 2, France

William W. Reynolds
Marine Biology Program
Center for the Life Sciences
University of New England
Biddeford, Maine 04005

Barbara A. Rothenburg
Department of Physiology
University of Michigan Medical School
Ann Arbor, Michigan 48104

Thomas A. Rudy
School of Pharmacy
University of Wisconsin
Madison, Wisconsin 53706

W. D. Ruwe
Departments of Psychiatry and Pharma-
cology
University of North Carolina School of
Medicine
Chapel Hill, North Carolina 27514

Evelyn Satinoff
Departments of Psychology, Physiology,
and Biophysics
University of Illinois
Champaign, Illinois 61820

Eugene P. Schoener
Department of Pharmacology
Wayne State University School of Med-
icine
Detroit, Michigan 48201

Harvey B. Simon
Infectious Disease Unit
Department of Medicine
Massachusetts General Hospital
Boston, Massachusetts 02114

Philip Z. Sobocinski
U.S. Army Medical Research Institute of
Infectious Diseases
Fort Detrick
Frederick, Maryland 21701

Jacek A. Spławiński
Department of Pharmacology
Copernicus Medical Academy
31–531 Cracow, Poland

Y. Townsend
Department of Medicine
St. Thomas' Hospital Medical School
London SE1, England

Paul E. Tyler
Department of Physiology
University of Florida College of Medicine
Gainesville, Florida 32610

Adelbert S. J. P. A. M. van Miert
Institute of Veterinary Pharmacology and
Toxicology
Faculty of Veterinary Medicine
The State University
3572 BP Utrecht, The Netherlands

Warren L. Veale
Division of Medical Physiology
Faculty of Medicine
University of Calgary
Calgary, Alberta T2N 1N4, Canada

Barbara Wojtaszek
Department of Pharmacology
Copernicus Medical Academy
31–531 Cracow, Poland

Sheldon M. Wolff
Department of Medicine
Tufts University School of Medicine
New England Medical Center Hospital
Boston, Massachusetts 02111

Sumner J. Yaffe
University of Pennsylvania
Children's Hospital of Philadelphia
Philadelphia, Pennsylvania 19104

Charles W. Young
Memorial Sloan-Kettering Cancer Center
New York, New York 10021

Elżbieta Zacny
Institute of Pharmacology
Polish Academy of Sciences
31–519 Cracow, Poland

Fever, edited by James M. Lipton.
Raven Press, New York © 1980.

Endogenous Pyrogens

Charles A. Dinarello

*Department of Medicine, Division of Experimental Medicine, Tufts-New England Medical
Center, Boston, Massachusetts 02111*

The demonstration that the host produces its own pyrogenic substance is one of the most important discoveries in two centuries of fever research. Although this finding was foretold by Menkin in 1943 (26), it was the meticulous work of Beeson and Bennett (6) in eliminating the ubiquitous bacterial endotoxin from pyrogenic granulocytic extracts which led to the description and early characterization of endogenous pyrogen (EP). Subsequent research has supported and broadened the original concept; for example, EP was demonstrated in plasma during experimental fevers caused by typhoid vaccine (3), viruses (2), and antigens (22). EP was also shown to be produced by human peripheral leukocytes *in vitro,* and, moreover, EP from human cells caused rapid onset of fever when injected into human subjects (13). In 1958, some 10 years after Beeson's first paper, Wood (34) summarized the knowledge of host-produced pyrogen: "Endogenous pyrogen derived from polymorphonuclear leukocytes has a central role in the pathogenesis of a number of forms of experimental fever."

Some knowledge of the sources, production, and physical nature of EP has been attained since the early research, but much still eludes us today. At first it seemed that EPs were all similar in that there was little or no species, order, or even class specificity (7,15). However, with the production of antibody against human pyrogen (18) and with continued chemical characterization (14,17), it became clear that EPs are antigenically distinct and of molecular heterogeneity. Today the pathogenesis of fever can be divided into three areas of study: (a) the production of EP from host cells; (b) the chemical characteristics of EPs which are related to their ability to cause fever; and (c) the neurotransmitter, neuronal, and other hypothalamic changes involved in raising body temperature above normal levels. A primary question in modern fever research is what characteristic of the molecular structure or physical nature of the EP molecule enables it to influence the activity of thermoregulatory neurons?

PRODUCTION OF EP

Although peritoneal exudate granulocytes and peripheral blood neutrophils were the first cells shown to produce EP *in vitro,* other cell sources are now recognized. These include blood monocytes (10), eosinophils (27), alveolar macrophages (4), peritoneal exudate macrophages (21), and fixed tissue macrophages such as splenic sinusoidal cells and hepatic Kupffer cells (16). The mechanisms by which exogenous pyrogens are able to activate the leukocyte remain unknown, and the multiplicity and varied nature of exogenous pyrogens suggest that more than a single mechanism exists. Since cells that are capable of producing EP also have membrane receptors for immunoglobulins and complement, these and other membrane receptors may contribute to the activation process. Lymphokines, although they have not yet been characterized, are able to activate the EP-producing cells and function as endogenous stimulators of EP (1,5).

Given the direct (28) as well as indirect (3) evidence that EP is a newly synthesized molecule, it seems appropriate to propose that the production of EP complies with expected mechanisms for gene expression. Following activation by exogenous pyrogens, the steps of de-repression, new messenger RNA synthesis, and translation of new protein take place in the formation of EP as they do in other inducible proteins. The transcription of DNA into new mRNA for EP synthesis is rapidly curtailed before significant amounts of EP are produced (8), but how this is controlled is poorly understood. However, this de-induction step is apparently impaired in certain tumor lines which produce EP without de-repression (9). What post-translational events take place after EP is synthesized is still conjectural at this time, but evidence exists that perhaps post-translational aggregation does occur. In deciphering the physical requirement of the EP molecule necessary to produce fever, post-translational changes may be important for biological activity.

CHEMICAL CHARACTERISTICS OF EP

Molecular Heterogeneity

Figure 1A is a typical chromatograph of human EP produced by peripheral blood leukocytes. The leukocytes were prepared by dextran sedimentation of whole blood and were composed of about 75% neutrophils and 5% monocytes (the remaining 20% consisted of lymphocytes which do not make EP). The single peak of pyrogenic activity elutes from this Sephadex G-50 column (105 × 5.6 cm) at about 15,000 daltons (17). This same elution pattern has been shown by other investigators for rabbit (24,29) and human leukocyte supernates (11) which contained primarily neutrophils.

Figure 1B is a chromatograph with two peaks of pyrogenic activity: one peak occurs at 15,000 and a second at about 40,000 daltons. The EP applied to this column was made from human leukocyte suspensions which contained mostly monocytes. There are several cellular differences between monocytes and neutrophils, and when cultured *in vitro* neutrophil and monocyte cultures have significantly different pH and enzyme content. For example, neutrophil supernates are more acidic and contain more protein per unit of EP activity (17). The 40,000 dalton pyrogen which is present in monocyte cultures may

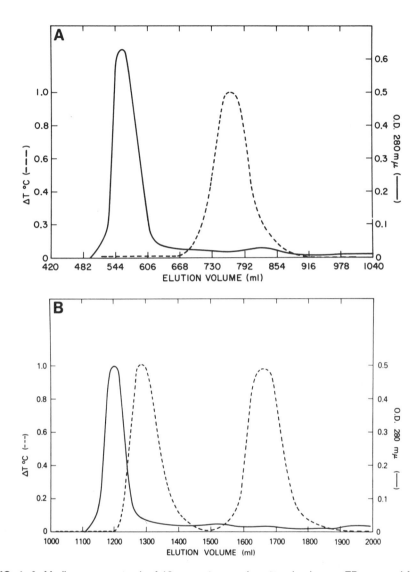

FIG. 1. A: Median pyrogen peak of 13 separate experiments using human EP prepared from neutrophils. Sephadex G-50 (105 × 3.8 cm, 0.85% NaCl, pH 6.8). Fraction size, 13.0 ml; each fraction was divided and injected into 3 rabbits. **B:** Median pyrogen peak of 4 separate experiments using human EP prepared from monocytes. Sephadex G-50 (165 × 5.6 cm, 0.85% phosphate-buffered saline, pH 7.4). Fraction size, 6.5 ml; each fraction was divided and injected into 3 rabbits. (From Dinarello et al., ref. 17, with permission).

represent post-translational changes occurring in monocytes themselves or in the less acidic conditions of the monocyte supernate. However, both molecular species are found in monocyte supernates.

The demonstration of molecular heterogeneity of EPs is not new. Table 1

TABLE 1. *Physical characteristics of endogenous pyrogens*

Cell source	Molecular weight	pH	Reference
Human blood leukocytes (75% neutrophils, 5% monocytes)	15,000	6.9	17
Human blood leukocytes	13,700	—	11
Human blood leukocytes (5% neutrophils, 30% monocytes)	40,000; 15,000	5.1; 6.9	17
Rabbit peritoneal granulocytes	14,000	7.3	24,29,31
Rabbit peritoneal macrophages	14,000	5.1	12
Rabbit Kupffer cells	40,000; 15,000	—	20
Rabbit febrile plasma	50,000	—	33
Rabbit febrile serum	45,000	—	32
Mouse lymphoma	60,000; 30,000	—	9

lists the findings of several investigators who have observed pyrogenic activity corresponding to molecules larger than 15,000 daltons. The mononuclear cells seem to correlate with finding a larger molecular weight pyrogen. An interesting finding is that EP isolated from plasma of febrile rabbits consistently has a larger molecular weight moiety than rabbit EP produced *in vitro,* which repeatedly chromatographs at 14,000 daltons. One may speculate that the naturally occurring EP is a large molecular weight species or that EP produced *in vivo* by intravenous bolus injection of an exogenous pyrogen is a product of fixed macrophagic cells. However, we observed this molecular heterogeneity during the purification and radiolabeling of the 15,000 dalton human EP.

Following concentration of EP produced by human monocytes *in vitro,* the crude supernate was passed over an immunoadsorbent of anti-human EP covalently bound to Sepharose. Pyrogen was eluted with citric acid and chromatographed over Sephadex G-50. Only the 15,000 dalton pyrogen was isolated and this materal gave a single staining band on SDS polyacrylamide gels. The 15,000 dalton EP was then labeled with ^{125}I using a N-hydroxysuccinimide ester of phenylpropionic acid without loss of biological activity. This material was further chromatographed over Sephadex G-15 and DEAE-cellulose. The eluted pyrogen caused fever in rabbits, appeared as a single band on isoelectric focusing, and eluted as a homogenous peak on high-pressure liquid chromatography (19).

Figure 2 represents labeled human EP during high-pressure liquid chromatography (HPLC) in a gradient of acetonitrile. A single peak of radioactivity occurs at a concentration of 20% acetonitrile and 80% aqueous buffer. Although to date no one has purified enough EP to allow a complete amino acid sequence, we feel that HPLC is sufficient evidence for homogeneity of the labeled preparation. However, if this preparation of purified labeled pyrogen is allowed to stay at pH 8.1 at 4°C for a few days, another peak of radioactivity appears at

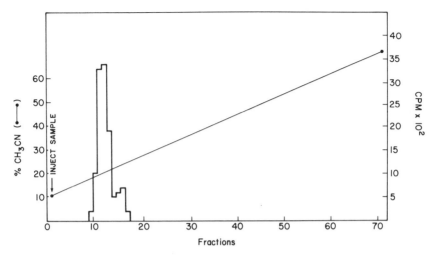

FIG. 2. High-pressure liquid chromatography of ^{125}I-human EP (μ Bondapak C_{18} column; 7 mm × 30 cm; gradient of CH_3CN and 0.01 in KH_2PO_4, pH 7.8; Waters Associates, Milford, Mass.). Each fraction (2 ml) was counted in a Beckman 3000 gamma counter.

pH of 5.2 when subjected to isoelectric focusing in polyacrylamide disc gels. The amount of radioactivity focusing at pH 5.2 increases with storage time.

Figure 3 represents the same chromatographic conditions as shown in Fig. 1B. However, in this case, radiolabeled EP has been applied which was stored in Tris buffer, 0.01 M, pH 8.1, for 7 days. Two peaks of radioactivity appear again: one at 15,000 and the other at above 40,000 daltons. As shown in Fig. 4, more precise molecular weight determinations using Sephadex G-75, 159 cm, revealed that the molecular weights are 15,000 and about 45,000 daltons. Thus the large molecule appears to be a trimer of the 15,000 dalton pyrogen.

When labeled EP was chromatographed on Sepharose in the presence of dissociating conditions such as 6 M guanidine HCl, the 45,000 dalton molecule disappeared and all the radioactivity was found in the 15,000 dalton peak (Fig. 5). This is further evidence to support the concept that the large molecular weight species of human EP is a molecular aggregate.

Several issues remain unresolved. First, we do not know whether aggregation takes place *in vivo,* and hence we do not know whether the aggregate form of EP is the active form. Labeled EP injected intravenously into the rabbit is rapidly broken down into small, dialyzable units. This has been observed by other investigators using biologically active pyrogen during *in situ* hepatic perfusion studies (25).

However, EP synthesized *in vivo* following the injection of viruses into rabbits seems to be similar to our 45,000 dalton aggregate (32,33). In addition, under the more physiologic conditions of monocyte cultures the original demonstration of a large molecular weight EP *in vitro* was observed. Whether the molecular

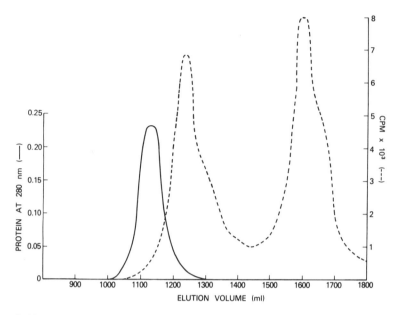

FIG. 3. Gel filtration of ^{125}I-labeled human EP over Sephadex G-50 (same column and conditions as shown in Fig. 1B).

aggregation takes place within the monocytes themselves as a post-translational event, or under the conditions of monocyte culture supernate, or *in vivo* after its injection remains for future experimentation.

Molecular Properties Necessary for Fever Production

In addition to investigation concerning the molecular weight of active EPs, other areas of research have focused on defining the physical requirements within the molecule necessary to produce fever. Because of the large quantity and variety of proteins present in crude leukocyte supernates containing EP, it is necessary to use semipurified preparations in carrying out such experiments. Even then, one cannot rule out the presence of interfering substances. Using crude and semipurified 14,000 dalton rabbit EP, several investigators have demonstrated that oxidation of sulfhydryl groups in alkaline conditions or by irreversible oxidizing agents renders the EP nonpyrogenic (11,23,24,29,31). This dependency on reduced sulfhydryl groups suggests that secondary or tertiary structure of rabbit pyrogen is essential for its biological activity or that a reduced sulfhydryl group participates in the active site. On the other hand, both crude and semipurified 15,000 dalton human EP is unaffected by these oxidizing conditions, even at 37°C (Fig. 5). Thus the ability of human EP to produce fever in the rabbit either does not involve reduced sulfhydryl groups or its active site is unaffected by such oxidations. In addition, we have been unable to show

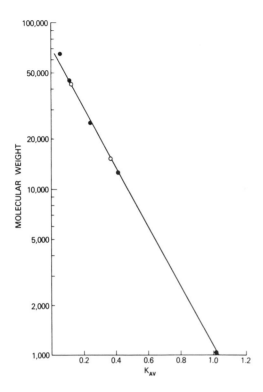

FIG. 4. Gel filtration of ^{125}I-labeled human EP over Sephadex G-75 superfine (159 × 2 cm, 0.85% NaCl, pH 6.8). *Solid circles* represent standards with molecular weights 60,000, 45,000, 24,000, 13,000, and 1,000; *open circles* represent the two radioactive peaks.

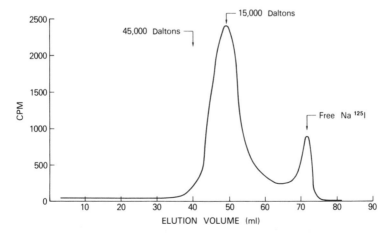

FIG. 5. Gel filtration of ^{125}I-labeled human EP over Sepharose-CL-6B in 6 M guanidine HCl (60 × 3 cm). The position of the 45,000 eluting protein was determined using ovalbumin.

an essential carbohydrate moiety for human EP. Neuroaminidase obtained from influenza viruses had no effect on EP, suggesting that sialic acid residues are absent (17). Also, Con A attached to Sepharose does not bind the biological activity of human EP *(unpublished observations)*. Finally, that a lipid moiety is essential to the action of EP also seems doubtful (24).

These experiments present a dilemma in forming a unifying concept of the mechanism through which EP causes fever. Like the insulins which are biologically active in several species but still retain antigenic specificity, it seems likely that EPs cause fever in many species because they share the same active site and that this active site excites the same processes in all species. EP is a polypeptide the active site of which has yet to be determined. Hopefully, this path of research will help uncover the precise molecular requirements for the ability of EP to set off the hypothalamic events that lead to fever.

ACKNOWLEDGMENT

This research is supported by NIH Grant RO1 AI 15614–01 and by the Posner and Ziskind Funds, New England Medical Center.

REFERENCES

1. Atkins, E., and Francis, L. (1978): Pathogenesis of fever in delayed hypersensitivity: Factors influencing release of pyrogen-inducing lymphokines. *Infect. Immun.,* 21:806–812.
2. Atkins, E., and Huang, W. D. (1958): Studies on the pathogenesis of fever with influenzal viruses. I. The appearance of an endogenous pyrogen in the blood following intravenous infection of virus. *J. Exp. Med.,* 107:383–435.
3. Atkins, E., and Wood, W. B., Jr. (1955): Studies on the pathogenesis of fever. I. The presence of transferable pyrogen in the blood stream following the injection of typhoid vaccine. *J. Exp. Med.,* 101:519–528.
4. Atkins, E., Bodel, P., and Francis, L. (1967): Release of an endogenous pyrogen *in vitro* from rabbit mononuclear cells. *J. Exp. Med.,* 126:357–386.
5. Atkins, E., Francis, L., and Bernheim, H. A. (1978): Pathogenesis of fever in delayed hypersensitivity: Role of monocytes. *Infect. Immun.,* 21:813–820.
6. Bennett, I. L., Jr., and Beeson, P. B. (1953): Studies on the pathogenesis of fever. II. Characteristics of fever-producing substance from polymorphonuclear leukocytes and from the sterile exudates. *J. Exp. Med.,* 98:493–508.
7. Bernheim, H. A., and Kluger, M. J. (1977): Endogenous pyrogen-like substance produced by reptiles. *J. Physiol.,* 267:659–666.
8. Bodel, P. (1974): Studies on the mechanism of endogenous pyrogen production. II. Role of cell products in the regulation of pyrogen release from blood leukocytes. *Infect. Immun.,* 10:451–457.
9. Bodel, P. (1978): Spontaneous production by mouse histiocytic and myelomonocytic tumor cell lines *in vitro. J. Exp. Med.,* 147:1503–1516.
10. Bodel, P., and Atkins, E. (1967): Release of endogenous pyrogen by human monocytes. *N. Engl. J. Med.,* 276:1002–1008.
11. Bodel, P. T., Wechsler, A., and Atkins, E. A. (1969): Comparison of endogenous pyrogens from human and rabbit leukocytes utilizing Sephadex filtration. *Yale J. Biol. Med.,* 41:376–387.
12. Cebula, T. A., Hanson, D. F., Moore, D. M., and Murphy, P. A. (1979): Synthesis of four endogenous pyrogens by rabbit macrophages. *J. Lab. Clin. Med. (in press).*
13. Cranston, W. I., Goodale, F., Jr., Snell, E. S., and Wendt, F. (1956): The role of leukocytes in the initial action of bacterial pyrogens in man. *Clin. Sci.,* 15:219–226.

14. Dinarello, C. A., and Wolff, S. M. (1977): Partial purification of human leukocytic pyrogen. *Inflammation,* 2:179–189.
15. Dinarello, C. A., and Wolff, S. M. (1978): Pathogenesis of fever in man. *N. Engl. J. Med.,* 298:607–612.
16. Dinarello, C. A., Bodel, P., and Atkins, E. (1968): The role of the liver in the production of fever and in pyrogenic tolerance. *Trans. Assoc. Am. Physicians,* 81:334–344.
17. Dinarello, C. A., Goldin, N. P., and Wolff, S. M. (1974): Demonstration and characterization of two distinct human leukocytic pyrogens. *J. Exp. Med.,* 139:1369–1381.
18. Dinarello, C. A., Renfer, L., and Wolff, S. M. (1977): The production of antibody against human leukocytic pyrogen. *J. Clin. Invest.,* 60:465–472.
19. Dinarello, C. A., Renfer, L., and Wolff, S. M. (1977): Human leukocytic pyrogen: Purification and development of a radioimmunoassay. *Proc. Natl. Sci. U.S.A.,* 74:4624–4627.
20. Haeseler, F., Bodel, P., and Atkins, E. (1977): Characteristics of pyrogen production by isolated rabbit Kupffer cells *in vitro. J. Reticuloendothel. Soc.,* 22:569–581.
21. Hahn, H. H., Char, D. C., Postel, W. B., and Wood, W. B., Jr. (1967): Studies on the pathogenesis of fever. XV. The production of endogenous pyrogen by peritoneal macrophages. *J. Exp. Med.,* 126:385–394.
22. Hall, C. H., Jr., and Atkins, E. (1959): Studies on tuberculin fever. I. The mechanism of fever in tuberculin hypersensitivity. *J. Exp. Med.,* 109:339–359.
23. Kaiser, H. K., and Wood, W. B., Jr. (1962): Studies on the pathogenesis of fever. X. The effect of certain enzyme inhibitors on the production and activity of leukocyte pyrogen. *J. Exp. Med.,* 115:37–47.
24. Kozak, M. S., Hahn, H. H., Lennarz, W. J., and Wood, W. B., Jr. (1968): Studies on the pathogenesis of fever. XVI. Purification and further chemical characterization of granulocytic pyrogen. *J. Exp. Med.,* 127:341–357.
25. Lorber, D., Tenenbaum, M., Thurston, S., Gander, G. W., and Goodale, F. (1971): The fate of circulating leukocytic pyrogen in the rabbit. *Proc. Soc. Exp. Biol. Med.,* 137:896–901.
26. Menkin, V. (1943): Chemical basis of injury in inflammation. *Arch. Pathol.,* 36:269–288.
27. Mickenberg, I. D., Root, R. K., and Wolff, S. M. (1972): Bactericidal and metabolic properties of human eosinophils. *Blood,* 39:67–80.
28. Moore, D. M., Murphy, P. A., Chesney, J. P., and Wood, W. B., Jr. (1973): Synthesis of endogenous pyrogen by rabbit leukocytes. *J. Exp. Med.,* 157:1263–1274.
29. Murphy, P. A., Chesney, J., and Wood, W. B., Jr. (1974): Further purification of rabbit leukocyte pyrogen. *J. Lab. Clin. Med.,* 83:310–322.
30. Nordlund, J. J., Root, R. K., and Wolff, S. M. (1970): Studies on the origin of human leukocytic pyrogen. *J. Exp. Med.,* 131:727–743.
31. Rafter, G. W., Cheuk, S. F., Krause, D. W., and Wood, W. B., Jr. (1966): Studies on the pathogenesis of fever. XIV. Further observations on the chemistry of leukocytic pyrogen. *J. Exp. Med.,* 123:433–444.
32. Rieck, T., and Kohlhage, H. (1970: Behaviour of different endogenous pyrogens in a biogel column. *Life Sci.,* 9:985–989.
33. Siegert, R., Pollmann, W., and Shu, H. L. (1966): Zur chemischen Natur des endogenen, durch Myxoviren induzierten Pyrogens. *Z. Naturforsch.,* 226:320–323.
34. Wood, W. B., Jr. (1958): Studies on the cause of fever. *N. Engl. J. Med.,* 258:1023–1027.

Fever, edited by James M. Lipton.
Raven Press, New York © 1980.

Hypersensitivity Fever: Cell-Mediated and Antibody-Mediated Mechanisms

H. A. Bernheim, L. Francis, and E. Atkins

*Department of Internal Medicine, Yale University School of Medicine,
New Haven, Connecticut 06510*

Although fever has been associated with hypersensitivity reactions since early in this century (1), the mechanisms by which immune processes produce fever have only recently begun to be understood. Injection of heterologous serum proteins such as human or bovine serum albumin and bovine gamma globulin or various microbial antigens will produce fever in sensitized animals (2,3). Depending on the techniques of sensitization, these febrile responses may be due to cell-mediated immunity (CMI) or humoral (antibody-mediated) immunity (HI). In cell-mediated immunity, fever appears to be mediated by one or more soluble products of sensitized lymphocytes (lymphokines), which activate phagocytic cells to release endogenous pyrogen (EP), the low molecular weight (13 $\times$ 10^3 daltons) protein that, in turn, acts (directly or indirectly) on the thermoregulatory centers in the brain to cause elevated body temperature (4–6). In humoral immunity, on the other hand, the activators of cells releasing EP appear to be antigen–antibody (Ag-Ab) complexes, with or without complement (7,8).

Fevers induced by i.v. injection of Ag in hypersensitive hosts differ from those produced by i.v. injection of EP in their longer latency and duration (9), and, at least in some instances of delayed hypersensitivity (DH), the height of fever is correlated with the degree of dermal sensitivity (6). Recent work in our laboratory has concentrated on determining the probable steps involved in EP production in both cellular and Ab-mediated immunity.

FEVERS ASSOCIATED WITH CELL-MEDIATED IMMUNITY

Figure 1 shows the steps we believe are involved in the production of EP during fever in CMI. An Ag (e.g., ovalbumin) first reacts with a sensitized lymphocyte. This combination then produces a nonpyrogenic soluble factor (i.e., a lymphokine), which, in turn, stimulates effector cells to release EP. Using a model of CMI in rabbits sensitized by foot pad inoculation with one of several protein Ags in complete Freund adjuvant (CFA), we have shown that sensitized draining lymph node (DLN) lymphocytes incubated with specific antigen will

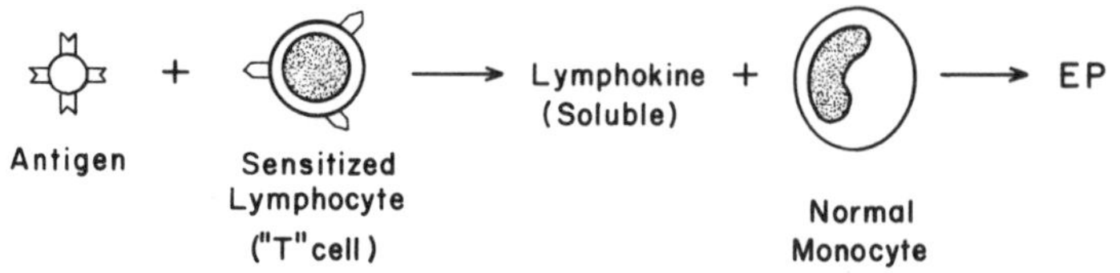

FIG. 1. Postulated pathway for the production of endogenous pyrogen activating factor (EPAF). For details see text.

activate co-cultured normal monocytes to release EP (Table 1). When sensitized monocytes (separated by Ficoll-Hypaque gradient centrifugation and layered on plastic dishes) are incubated with antigen alone they do not release EP, suggesting that lymphocytes are essential mediators of this reaction and that the reaction of Ag and cytophilic Ab on the surface of monocytes is not the main mechanism by which EP is released. Supernatants of sensitized DLN cells incubated for 18 hr with Ag will also activate normal monocytes to produce significant amounts of EP (Table 2) indicating that a soluble factor is released by sensitized lymphocytes in the presence of Ag. The term we have coined for this substance is endogenous pyrogen-activating factor (EPAF). Since Ag added to supernatants of DLN cells incubated alone does not activate normal monocytes, it seems likely that the factor in these supernatants is indeed a lymphokine (LK) rather than a complex of Ag-Ab released by DLN cells into these supernatants.

The physicochemical properties of this LK are not known, although it seems to have an essential protein moiety. Whether EPAF is identical with any of the LKs previously described such as macrophage or leukocyte (granulocyte) inhibiting factors (MIF and LIF) (10–13) remains to be determined, although its selective activity on monocytes rather than granulocytes would indicate a more likely relationship to MIF than to LIF. The steps involved in the activation of effector cells to release EP by EPAF are unknown but presumably involve

TABLE 1. *Role of specific Ags (OA or HSA) in EP production by monocytes incubated 18 hr in vitro with sensitized DLN cells*

			Mean temp change (°C)			
					+DLN cells	
DLN cells from donor sensitized to:	Normal monocytes	No. of recipients	+OA	+HSA	+HSA	+OA
HSA[a]	1×10^7	6	—	0.10	*0.45[c]*	0.19
OA[b]	1×10^7	6	0.15	—	0.28	*0.55[c]*

[a] Immunized 11–19 days earlier.
[b] Immunized 8–12 days earlier.
[c] In this and following tables, all italicized values are significantly different ($p < 0.01$).

TABLE 2. *Role of a lymphokine (released by sensitized DLN cells incubated with homologous Ag) in EP production by monocytes*

DLN cells from donor sensitized to:	Normal monocytes	No. of recipients	Mean temp change (°C)			18 hr sups of DLN cells + homologous AG without monocytes
			+18 hr sup of DLN cells			
			−AG	+HSA	+OA	
HSA[a]	1×10^7	6	0.15	*0.47*	0.18	(0.21)
OA[b]	1×10^7	6	0.05	0.13	*0.44*	(0.14)

[a] Immunized 11–19 days earlier.
[b] Immunized 8–14 days earlier.

de novo protein synthesis as has been described following phagocytosis of bacteria such as *Staphylococcus albus in vitro* (14,15).

In CMI significant amounts of EP are generated by monocytes only when they are incubated with homologous Ag and sensitized DLN cells, or with supernatants of DLN cells previously incubated with homologous Ag. Heterologous Ag (e.g., human serum albumin, HSA) fails to activate ovalbumin (OA)-sensitized DLN cells to release LK and vice versa (6). In this regard, EPAF is similar to other LK which are released by Ag and specifically sensitized lymphocytes only (12,13).

The effector (i.e., EP-producing) cell in this reaction appears to be the monocyte rather than the granulocyte (Table 3). PMNs isolated from Ficoll-Hypaque density gradients were not activated by either suspensions of sensitized DLN cells and Ag or supernatants of previously incubated cells and Ag. Although PMNs isolated by these techniques were somewhat less reactive in terms of EP production than are monocytes to nonspecific stimuli, such as phagocytosis, the difference was slight and did not seem sufficient to account for the apparent lack of reactivity of the PMNs to the LK.

TABLE 3. *Comparison of EP production by normal monocytes and PMNs incubated 18 hr in vitro with or without Ag (OA) and sensitized DLN cells[a] (or their supernatants)*

Effector cells	No. of recipients	Mean temp change (°C) with effector cells +					
		+OA	DLN −OA	Cells +OA	18 hr sups of DLN cells		+Staph
					−OA	+OA	
Monocytes (1×10^7)	6	0.19	0.14	*0.58*	0.13	*0.51*	*0.82*
PMNs (2.5×10^7)	6	0.17	0.10	0.18	0.09	0.19	*0.64*

[a] At 8–14 days after immunization.

The apparent selective action of EPAF on monocytes may be merely a matter of dose, since its effect is a weak one, stimulating monocytes to produce amounts of EP that are only severalfold above background for the fever assay. When more concentrated and purified material becomes available, higher doses of EPAF should be tested with PMNs to see if the difference in the choice of effector cells is absolute. Few known stimuli for EP production activate either PMNs or monocytes alone, although evidence suggests that certain steroid hormones, which appear to activate only human (as opposed to rabbit) leukocytes, have their main, if not only, EP-inducing action on monocytes rather than on PMNs (16).

Peritoneal exudate (PE) cells derived from guinea pigs sensitized to OA or bovine gamma globulin (BGG) release EP when incubated with specific Ag *in vitro* (Table 4) (17; *unpublished observations*). These PE cells contain both effector cells (PMNs and monocytes) and sensitized lymphocytes. The reaction is specific and does not occur with heterologous Ag. Normal guinea pig PE cells or relatively pure populations of granulocytes or monocytes derived from them will also release EP when they are incubated with sensitized DLN cells and specific Ag. In guinea pigs as well as in rabbits, therefore, Ag appears to stimulate specifically sensitized lymphocytes to activate phagocytic cells to release EP. However, unlike our findings with rabbits, crude supernatants from guinea pig DLN cells incubated with Ag appear to have little if any detectable ability to activate effector cells to release EP. Possibly, more concentrated materials will have clear-cut activity. Alternatively, release of EP may involve a cell-to-cell interaction between sensitized lymphocytes and effector cells.

Uhr and Brandriss (18) and Salvin (19) have shown that when guinea pigs with CMI to various protein Ags are desensitized with a single injection of Ag, they have little or no febrile response to reinjection of Ag. We have recently shown *(unpublished work)* that DLN cells taken from desensitized guinea pigs and incubated with specific Ag do not activate normal phagocytes to release as much EP as do DLN cells taken from sensitized animals. Whether deletion or inactivation of sensitized cells or, conversely, activation of suppressor T cells

TABLE 4. *EP production by sensitized guinea pig PE cells*[a] *incubated* in vitro *with specific or nonspecific antigen*

			Mean temp change (°C)[c]			
Cell source	Donor sensitized to:	No. of recipients	Control	+OA	+BGG	+Staph
Sensitized PE cells						
(2.5 × 10⁷/dose)[b]	OA[a]	24	0.28	*0.84*	0.37	*1.85*
	BGG[a]	12	0.22	0.24	*0.86*	*1.82*

[a] Immunized 11 days earlier.
[b] Differential: mono., 50%; PMN, 30%; lymph., 20%.
[c] In this and Table 5, temperature change is sum of 2 successive 18-hr incubations.

is responsible for modifying production of EP in these experiments has not yet been determined.

T and B Cells

Modern immunology has divided lymphocytes into two categories. Both originate from stem cells in the bone marrow. One type eventually circulates to the thymus where it is "processed" and emerges as a thymic or T cell; the other lymphocyte type is probably processed in the bone marrow (in man) and emerges as a B cell. T cells are the lymphocytes generally associated with cellular immunity and LK production, whereas B cells are associated with humoral immunity and Ab production (20). This division, however, is not absolute, as B calls can produce at least some lymphokines (21) and T cells can contribute as helper cells to humoral immunity (22,23).

To determine whether T or B cells were responsible for the production of EPAF, guinea pigs were immunized to OA. When they were skin test positive they were sacrificed and their draining lymph nodes (popliteal and axillary) were removed and the lymphocytes separated. In addition, the thymus glands were removed and the thymic cells isolated. Mixtures of sensitized T and B cells were then passed through a nylon wool column, which selectively removed macrophages, B cells, and presumably "sticky" T cells and allowed a relatively pure population of T cells to pass through. The nonadherent, adherent, and thymic cells were then mixed with specific Ag and effector cells. The 18-hr supernatants of these cell mixtures were then assayed for EP content by injection into rabbits.

From Table 5 it can be seen that thymocytes do not release EPAF. Presumably these cells are immature and are not yet capable of responding to Ag. However, when nylon wool-nonadherent cells from DLN were incubated with Ag and effector cells, there was a significant release of EP. When analyzed by rosetting with rabbit red blood cells and immunofluorescent Ab, these cells appeared to be predominantly T cells. Nylon wool-adherent cells (consisting of approximately equal numbers of T and B cells) also stimulated effector cells to release significant amounts of EP. These results indicate that T (or null) cells are capable of releasing LK independently of B cells. However, since this method does not provide a relatively pure population of B cells, we do not know whether these cells can also produce LK. More specific purification procedures will have to be done before further conclusions can be drawn.

Summary

When incubated with specific Ag, sensitized DLN cells from rabbits are capable of producing a soluble pyrogen-activating factor, EPAF, which has the ability to stimulate monocytes to release EP. Ag-Ab complexes do not appear to play

TABLE 5. *EP production by normal guinea pig PE cells incubated* in vitro *with various populations of sensitized lymphocytes ± antigen*[a]

Cell mixture	Added sensitized cells				ΔT (°C)	
	% T cells	% B cells	% other cells	T cells $\times 10^7$	Control	OA[b]
PE cells alone	—	—	—	—	0.22[b]	0.20
PE cells + thymocytes (2×10^8)	94	4	2	19	0.25	0.23
PE cells + unfractionated DLN cells (2×10^8)	59	34	7	12	0.29	*0.74*
PE cells + nylon-nonadherent DLN cells (3×10^7)	60	8	22	1.8	0.18	*0.87*
PE cells + nylon-adherent DLN cells (5×10^7)	33	32	35	1.7	0.32	*0.66*
PE cells + staph						*1.54*

[a] Results of 3 experiments (6 recipients).
[b] See Table 1.

a role in this process. Under the same conditions, DLN cells from sensitized guinea pigs will also stimulate effector cells, granulocytes as well as monocytes, to release EP. Clear evidence for a soluble LK has not been obtained in the guinea pig model. T (or null) lymphocytes appear to be responsible for these immunological phenomena, although pure preparations of B cells have not yet been tested in this system.

FEVERS ASSOCIATED WITH HUMORAL (Ab-MEDIATED) IMMUNITY

In diseases characterized by certain forms of Ab-mediated immunity (e.g., serum sickness), fever is probably due to the reaction of circulating Ag-Ab complexes with appropriate effector cells resulting in the release of EP. Sensitized rabbits will become febrile after injection of specific Ag (2). In addition, after passive transfer of specifically immune serum, normal animals will respond with fever to intravenously injected Ag (24). There is also a positive correlation between Ab titers in actively sensitized animals and the febrile response to Ag (3). Finally, Ag-Ab complexes produced *in vitro* will cause fever when given intravenously to normal recipients (9). These results all clearly indicate humoral, not cell-mediated, mechanisms.

When sensitized rabbits are injected with a specific Ag, such as HSA, two distinct pyrogenic agents appear sequentially in their sera (9). Five minutes after challenge with Ag, the serum from donor animals contains an agent that produces a fever in normal rabbits after a moderate latent period similar to that produced in rabbits injected with Ag-Ab complexes. Repeated injection of this pyrogen rapidly induces a state of pyrogenic tolerance in normal recipients. Serum removed 2 hr after injection, on the other hand, contains a pyrogen which produces a fever identical to that of EP (i.e., brief, monophasic response) and does not induce tolerance on repeated injections. Unlike "2-hr" serum, "5-min" serum does not produce fever in normal rabbits made tolerant (unresponsive) to Ag-Ab complexes by previous injection of these complexes. The early appearing pyrogen thus seems to be Ag-Ab complexes, whereas the later appearing pyrogen is EP presumably mobilized by host cells activated by the complexes. These observations suggest, therefore, that fever produced by Ag in animals with Ab-mediated immunity is due to the initial interaction of the Ag with specific Ab to form Ag-Ab complexes which then activate cells of the host to release EP.

In earlier work, Atkins and co-workers (4) failed to stimulate rabbit peripheral blood leukocytes (largely granulocytes) to release EP when incubated with either precipitated or soluble complexes of BGG-DNP and Ab. When Chusid and Atkins (25) incubated leukocytes with antiserum and Ag (penicilloyl protein conjugates), EP was released *in vitro*. However, the exact Ag moiety and the effector cells were not identified. More recently, in our laboratory, a medical student, Bruce Markle, and Phyllis Bodel carried out a series of experiments to determine whether a protein Ag (BGG) and its antiserum are capable of stimulating human layered monocytes to release EP (B. M. Markle, M.D. thesis).

Rabbits were first sensitized by injecting 1.25 mg of BGG in CFA into each footpad. Booster injections of 1 mg of BGG were given intravenously 4 weeks later. Seven to ten days later, the animals were bled by cardiac puncture. The antiserum was then mixed with increasing amounts of BGG. The point of equivalence (where the maximum amount of Ag + Ab are precipitated and the supernatant fluid is free of both Ag and Ab) was determined with a spectrophotometer at a wavelength of 280 nm (Fig. 2). At either side of the equivalence point there is a mixture of both soluble and insoluble complexes as well as free Ag or Ab. Complexes of Ag-Ab were prepared in 10× and 50× excess and 10× Ab excess (expressed in terms of the amount by weight of Ag combined with Ab at equivalence). When human monocytes layered on plastic tissue culture flasks were incubated with Ag-Ab complexes in 10× Ag or Ab excess, these cells produced large amounts of EP (Fig. 3). Layered monocytes incubated with precipitated complexes [or with Ag or Ab alone (not shown)] did not release EP.

Monocytes incubated with complexes in 50× Ag excess released little EP in contrast to those cells incubated with 10× Ag or Ab excess (Fig. 3). These results may be due to the macromolecular composition of immune complexes formed at different levels of Ab and Ag excess. In any given reaction mixture of Ag and Ab, whether *in vitro* (26) or *in vivo* (27), various sizes of immune complexes form. In zones of progressively higher Ag excess, there is an increase in the ratio of small to large complexes (26). Small complexes do not attach readily to phagocytic cells, and in addition they markedly inhibit the attachment of larger complexes (28). Activation of monocytes to release EP during HI may be dependent on the attachment of immune complexes to the Fc receptors

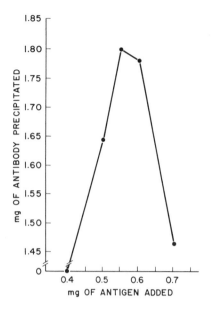

FIG. 2. Quantitative precipitation of BGG and rabbit antiserum. Maximum precipitation (equivalence point) occurs when 0.6 mg of BGG (0.6 ml of a 1 mg/ml solution) is added to 1 ml of a 1:4 dilution of rabbit antiserum.

of the monocytes. The increased number of small complexes in $50\times$ Ag excess may prevent any large complexes present from attaching to monocytes and stimulating monocytes to release EP. In addition, BGG is itself an immunoglobulin and as such has an Fc component. In $50\times$ Ag excess, the large amounts of free BGG may competitively inhibit the interaction between monocytes and large immune complexes, preventing the release of EP.[1]

Precipitated complexes did not stimulate monocytes to produce pyrogen, even though the monocytes were degranulated and appeared to have phagocytized the complexes. Apparently, phagocytosis of complexes, as with latex beads (30), is not itself a sufficient stimulus for EP production. The failure of precipitated complexes to activate monocytes may be due to noncovalent binding between Fc regions on the Ab molecules which would prevent the attachment of the precipitated complexes to Fc receptors on the monocytes.

In fevers mediated by Ag-Ab complexes, only certain classes of Abs appear to be involved. Jandl and Tomlinson (31) observed that hemolysis due to anti-D antibodies in humans produced significantly higher fevers than did hemolysis due to anti-A or anti-B antisera. The anti-D Abs were from the IgG class whereas anti-A and anti-B antibodies were IgM molecules (32). Later, Mott

---

[1] Monocytes incubated with BGG (Ag) and normal serum frequently released EP, although generally less than did immune complexes. It appears likely that this nonspecific activation was due to aggregated BGG. Since aggregated immunoglobulins are capable of stimulating human neutrophils to produce superoxide anions and H_2O_2 (29) and, indeed, are used as a model for activation of cells by complexes, they may also be able to activate phagocytes to release EP. In future experiments this phenomenon can be avoided by high-speed centrifugation to remove aggregates or by using an Ag which is not itself an Ab (e.g., OA) in preparing immune complexes.

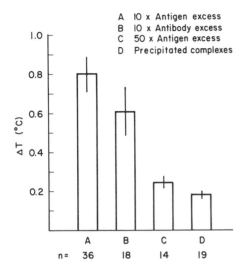

A   10 x Antigen excess
B   10 x Antibody excess
C   50 x Antigen excess
D   Precipitated complexes

FIG. 3. Monocyte pyrogen production in response to soluble and precipitated immune complexes of different Ab:Ag ratios (± SEM).

and Wolff (3) demonstrated that passive transfer of febrile reactivity to injected HSA in normal rabbits was successful only with fractions of serum which were shown by immunoelectrophoresis to contain predominantly 7S (IgG) globulins. Fractions rich in 19S (IgM) macroglobulins produced no significant febrile reactivity to antigen in the passively sensitized host. Of these two classes of immunoglobulins it seems, then, that only IgG is involved in the production of fever during states of HI. Whether this is true for the *in vitro* activation of monocytes by immune complexes has not been determined.

The role of complement in fevers during HI is uncertain. In our *in vitro* system, complement seems to be essential since complexes (both 10× Ag and Ab excess) incubated with heat-inactivated serum did not activate monocytes to release EP. In *in vivo* situations, however, the role of complement is less clear. Relatively large immune complexes (3× Ab excess or less) but not smaller complexes (10× Ag excess or greater) produce fevers when injected into decomplemented rabbits (7,8). Moreover, the febrile response of either actively or passively sensitized rabbits to intravenously injected Ag is unaltered after decomplementation (8). In light of these observations and the fact that both large as well as small complexes form after injection of Ag into sensitized hosts (27), it seems likely that large complexes can act independently of complement to activate phagocytes to release EP in HI, whereas small complexes (10× Ag excess or greater) may require complement to induce EP release.

Summary

Fever during states of humoral immunity (HI) appears to be due to the activation of phagocytes to release EP by soluble Ag-Ab complexes. From both *in vivo* and *in vitro* experiments, it appears that these complexes must be above a certain size and consist of antibodies of the IgG (versus IgM) class. Under the conditions of these *in vitro* experiments, complement appeared to be essential for activation of cells to produce EP. However, its role in the production of fever by antigen *in vivo* has not been clearly established.

REFERENCES

1. Von Pirquet, C. E. (1911): Allergy. *Arch. Intern. Med.*, 7:259–288; 383–436.
2. Farr, R. S., Campbell, D. H., Clark, S. L., Jr., and Proffitt, J. E. (1954): The febrile response of sensitized rabbits to the intravenous injection of antigen. *Anat. Rec.*, 118:385 (abstr.).
3. Mott, P. D., and Wolff, S. M. (1966): The association of fever and antibody response in rabbits immunized with human serum albumin. *J. Clin. Invest.*, 45:372–379.
4. Atkins, E., Feldman, J. D., Francis, L., and Hursch, E. (1972): Studies on the mechanism of fever accompanying delayed hypersensitivity. The role of the sensitized lymphocyte. *J. Exp. Med.*, 135:1113–1132.
5. Atkins, E., and Francis, L. (1978): Pathogenesis of fever in delayed hypersensitivity: Factors influencing release of pyrogen-reducing lymphokines. *Infect. Immun.*, 21:806–812.
6. Atkins, E., Francis, L., and Bernheim, H. A. (1978): Pathogenesis of fever in delayed hypersensitivity: Role of monocytes. *Infect. Immun.*, 21:813–820.
7. Mickenberg, I. D., Snyderman, R., Root, R. K., Mergenhagen, S. E., and Wolff, S. M. (1970): Immune fever in the rabbit: Responses of the hematologic and complement systems. *J. Immunol.*, 107:1457–1465.
8. Mickenberg, I. D., Snyderman, R., Root, R. K., Mergenhagen, S. E., and Wolff, S. M. (1970): The relationship of complement consumption to immune fever. *J. Immunol.*, 107:1466–1476.
9. Root, R. K., and Wolff, S. M. (1968): Pathogenetic mechanisms in experimental immune fever. *J. Exp. Med.*, 128:309–323.
10. David, J. R. (1966): Delayed hypersensitivity in vitro. Its mediation by cell-free substances formed by lymphoid cell–antigen interaction. *Proc. Natl. Acad. Sci. U.S.A.*, 56:72–77.
11. Bloom, B. R., and Bennett, B. (1966): Mechanism of a reaction in vitro associated with delayed-type hypersensitivity. *Science*, 153:80–82.
12. Rocklin, R. E., Remold, H. G., and David, J. R. (1972): Characterization of human migration inhibitory factor (MIF) from antigen stimulated lymphocytes. *Cell. Immunol.*, 5:436–445.
13. Rocklin, R. E. (1974): Products of activated lymphocytes: Leukocyte inhibitory factor (LIF) distinct from migration inhibitory factor (MIF). *J. Immunol.*, 112:1461–1466.
14. Bodel, P. (1970): Studies on the mechanism of endogenous pyrogen production. I. Investigation of new protein synthesis in stimulated human blood leucocytes. *Yale J. Biol. Med.*, 43:145–163.
15. Nordlund, J. J., Root, R. K., and Wolff, S. M. (1970): Studies on the origin of human leukocytic pyrogen. *J. Exp. Med.*, 131:727–743.
16. Bodel, P., and Dillard, M. (1968): Studies on steroid fever. I. Production of leukocyte pyrogen in vitro by etiocholanolone. *J. Clin. Invest.*, 47:107–117.
17. Chao, P. L., Francis, L., and Atkins, E. (1977): The release of an endogenous pyrogen from guinea pig leukocytes in vitro. A new model for investigating the role of lymphocytes in fevers induced by antigen in hosts with delayed hypersensitivity. *J. Exp. Med.*, 145:1288–1298.
18. Uhr, J. W., and Brandriss, M. W. (1958): Delayed hypersensitivity. IV. Systemic reactivity of guinea pigs sensitized to protein antigens. *J. Exp. Med.*, 108:905–924.
19. Salvin, S. B. (1962): Specificity of allergic reactions. V. Observations on the systemic delayed reaction in guinea pigs sensitized to purified protein-conjugates. *J. Immunol.*, 89:910–919.
20. Hood, L. E., Weissman, I. L., and Wood, W. B. (1978): *Immunology.* Benjamin/Cummings, Menlo Park, Calif.
21. Rocklin, R. E., MacDermott, R. P., Chess, L., Schlossman, S. F., and David, J. R. (1974): Studies on mediator production by highly purified human T and B lymphocytes. *J. Exp. Med.*, 140:1303–1316.
22. Claman, H. N., and Chaperon, E. A. (1969): Immunologic complementation between thymus and marrow cells. A model for the two-cell theory of immunocompetence. *Transplant. Rev.*, 1:92–113.

23. Cantor, H., and Boyse, E. A. (1975): Functional subclasses of T lymphocytes bearing different Ly antigens. I. The generation of functionally distinct T-cell subclasses in a differentiative process independent of antigen. *J. Exp. Med.,* 141:1376–1389.

24. Grey, H. M., Briggs, W., and Farr, R. S. (1961): The passive transfer of sensitivity to antigen-induced fevers. *J. Clin. Invest.,* 40:703–706.

25. Chusid, M. J., and Atkins, E. (1972): Studies on the mechanism of penicillin-induced fever. *J. Exp. Med.,* 136:227–240.

26. Arend, W. P., Teller, P. C., and Mannik, M. (1972): Molecular composition and sedimentation characteristics of soluble antigen-antibody complexes. *Biochem.,* 11:4063–4072.

27. Francis, G. E., Hawkins, J. D., and Wormall, A. (1957): The fate of some intravenously injected native proteins in normal and immune rabbits. *Biochem. J.,* 65:560–569.

28. Phillips-Quaglioto, J. M., Levine, B. B., Quaglioto, F., and Uhr, J. W. (1971): Mechanism underlying binding of immune complexes to macrophages. *J. Exp. Med.,* 133:589–601.

29. Johnston, R. B., and Lehmeyer, J. E. (1976): Elaboration of toxic oxygen by-products by neutrophils in a model of immune complex disease. *J. Clin. Invest.,* 57:836–841.

30. Berlin, R. D., and Wood, W. B., Jr. (1964): Studies on the pathogenesis of fever. XIII. The effect of phagocytosis on the release of endogenous pyrogen by polymorphonuclear leukocytes. *J. Exp. Med.,* 119:715–726.

31. Jandl, J. H., and Tomlinson, A. S. (1958): The destruction of red cells by antibodies in man. II. Pyrogenic, leukocytic and dermal responses to immune hemolysis. *J. Clin. Invest.,* 37:1202–1228.

32. LoBuglio, A. F., Cobron, R. S., and Jandl, J. H. (1967): Red cells coated with immunoglobulin G: Binding and sphering by mononuclear cells in man. *Science,* 158:1582–1585.

Fever, edited by James M. Lipton.
Raven Press, New York © 1980.

Albumin Fever

*D. Mitchell, *Helen Laburn, and **J. Hattingh

*Department of Physiology, University of the Witwatersrand Medical School; and
**Department of General Physiology, University of the Witwatersrand,
Johannesburg 2001, South Africa

The elevation of body temperature in most fevers, although perhaps not all
(15), is caused by the action of endogenous pyrogen on neurons of the anterior
hypothalamus. Endogenous pyrogen is a protein or family of proteins (3) that
arise from phagocytic cells under the influence of endotoxin or other agents
(9,14). The biochemical purification of endogenous pyrogen is difficult, and the
amino acid composition is not known.

Crude endogenous pyrogen can be prepared in the laboratory by incubation
of suitable phagocytic cells with endotoxin. We use a simple method which
employs whole blood (3). Fresh whole blood is incubated for 1 hr at 37°C in
the presence of endotoxin, usually lipopolysaccharide extracted from *Salmonella
typhosa* in a concentration of 30 μg/100 ml of blood. After 1 hr the cells are
separated by centrifugation and washed three times in 5% dextrose saline solution. They are then suspended in 5% dextrose saline and incubated for a further
4 hr. The cells are then separated by centrifugation and discarded; the supernatant contains endogenous pyrogen.

The supernatant, however, contains more than endogenous pyrogen. We discovered that the supernatant obtained after incubation of either bovine cells
or rabbit cells with endotoxin contained several other proteins, particularly albumin. Dinarello and Wolff (5) observed previously that incubation of human
leucocytes with *Staphylococcus* produced an albumin as well as endogenous
pyrogen. Indeed, considerably more albumin than endogenous pyrogen was present in their supernatant.

What is the significance of the presence of albumin in crude preparations
of endogenous pyrogen? One possibility is that the albumin is simply an unrelated
by-product of the incubation process. We pursued an alternative possibility,
namely, that albumin is somehow intrinsically involved in the generation of
endogenous pyrogen. There have been reports in the recent literature of fevers
associated with albumin. Therapeutic injection of normal human serum albumin
in patients sometimes results in fever (22). Indeed, 0.75% of all batches of
human serum albumin manufactured in the United States between 1970 and
1974 were implicated in febrile reactions in patients (19). The likely origin of
the febrile reaction in patients after albumin injection was contamination of

23

the albumin with endotoxin (2). We wished to investigate the possibility that albumin *per se* is pyrogenic. We attempted, therefore, to prepare albumin free of endotoxin contamination.

DECONTAMINATION OF ALBUMIN

The removal of pyrogen from solution is an everyday problem for the manufacturers of blood products and other substances destined for human injection. The endotoxins are lipopolysaccharides with molecular weights of about one million (14); albumin is a protein of molecular weight 67,000 or 68,000. At first sight, therefore, separation of albumin from endotoxin by ultrafiltration would not appear difficult.

However, we were unable to separate albumin from endotoxin using ultrafiltration. A 1 μg/ml solution of *S. typhosa* endotoxin in saline was tested for pyrogenicity in rabbits. Then 2 ml of the solution was injected, via an ear marginal vein, into conscious rabbits restrained in conventional stocks. Rectal temperatures were monitored using indwelling thermistor probes. Passing the solution through membrane filters which retained molecules of nominal molecular weight down to 50,000 failed to remove the pyrogenic moiety. Membrane filters with a nominal molecular weight retention of 50,000 will also retain albumin, and so cannot be used to separate albumin from endotoxin.

Although endotoxin has a molecular weight of one million or more, pyrogenic fragments of the molecule appear to pass through a filter which retains molecules of a much lower weight. Lipopolysaccharides exist in solution in various states of aggregation and fragmentation which depend on the chemical nature of the solution (20). Fragmentation occurs by the readily reversable breakage of noncovalent bonds, and fragments with molecular weights between 10,000 and 20,000 may be formed. Removal of all the pyrogenic fragments of endotoxin from solution therefore requires ultrafiltration through a molecular filter which retains a molecular weight of about 10,000 (4,10,20). Endogenous pyrogen has a weight in excess of 10,000; therefore, as in the case of albumin, it is impossible to separate endogenous pyrogen from endotoxin by ultrafiltration.

Chromatography offers another possible method of separating endotoxin from albumin (and endogenous pyrogen). We passed commercial bovine serum albumin repeatedly through Sephadex G-150 columns at pH 7.5. Characterization of the purified product by 5% polyacrylamide gel electrophoresis and by crossed immunoelectrophoresis against anti-whole bovine serum revealed that all proteins other than albumin were removed from the solution. However, even if the solution was free of extraneous proteins, it was still possible that it was contaminated with endotoxin (12).

We were unable, therefore, to produce an albumin solution which we were sure was free of endotoxin. We had to resort to other methods to demonstrate that any febrile reactions to albumin injection were not the consequence of endotoxin contamination.

ALBUMIN FEVER

Figure 1 shows the mean rectal temperature changes in three groups of four naive conscious rabbits for the 160 min after injection of three pyrogens (8). For each rabbit we calculated the change of rectal temperature from that prevailing at the time of injection and expressed this change as a percentage of the maximum change for that rabbit in the 160-min period. The data points in Fig. 1, then, represent the means and standard errors of the percentage changes. The method of presenting the data in this figure normalizes the amplitude of the fever following injection of the various pyrogens and allows examination of the time course of the fever.

One group of rabbits was given 2 µg of endotoxin from *S. typhosa,* one group received 2 ml of rabbit endogenous pyrogen prepared from homologous blood by the method described above, and the third group was injected with 10 mg of commercial bovine serum albumin (BDH) in saline solution. In all three groups, fever ensued with a remarkably similar time course; in all cases rectal temperatures were elevated significantly in 20 min or less following injection.

The commercial bovine serum albumin contained monomeric albumin together with its dimers, trimers, and higher polymers. Purification by repeated passage through Sephadex G-150 columns permitted elimination of the trimers and higher polymers, and reduction of the dimer concentration to less than 3% of the total albumin. Figure 2 shows the rectal temperature changes in conscious rabbits after injection of various doses of this purified bovine serum albumin, virtually monomeric (8). The data are expressed as the mean elevation of rectal temperature above that prevailing at the time of injection, measured 70 min

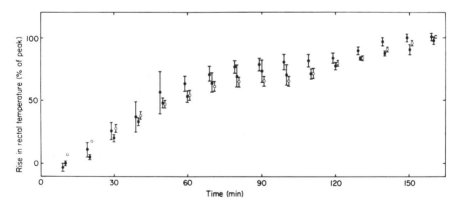

FIG. 1. Changes in rectal temperature in 3 groups of 4 rabbits, following intravenous injections at time zero. Each point represents the mean ± SE of the individual changes calculated as the percentages of the maximum change for each rabbit. *(Solid circles)* Bovine serum albumin, 10 mg; *(open circles) S. typhosa* endotoxin, 2 µg; *(squares)* rabbit endogenous pyrogen, 2 ml. (From Hattingh et al., ref. 8, with permission.)

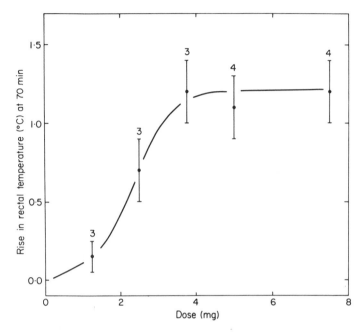

FIG. 2. Rise in rectal temperature (mean ± SE) in groups of rabbits, measured 70 min after intravenous injection of decontaminated bovine serum albumin in different doses. Numbers above each point specify the numbers of animals in each group. (From Hattingh et al., ref. 8, with permission.)

after injection. The time of measurement corresponds to the beginning of a transient plateau in the time course of the fever (Fig. 1).

Inspection of Fig. 2 shows that the injection of 2 ml of bovine serum albumin into naive conscious rabbits produced a significant increase in rectal temperature, and that a maximum fever of about 1.2°C was produced at doses of albumin of 4 mg and higher. Since each rabbit would have had about 8 g of serum albumin in the vascular space, the intravenous injection of 2 mg of bovine serum albumin represents a dilution of the rabbit's own albumin by about 0.03%.

It remained for us to show that the fevers which followed injection of bovine serum albumin into rabbits were not due to endotoxin contamination of the bovine serum albumin. This we did in two ways (8). The first made use of the fact that lipopolysaccharides are relatively stable in solution at a temperature of 70°C, whereas albumin is not (21). If the fever were due to endotoxin contamination, then heating the solution to be injected should have had little effect on the fever. In fact, heating the solution for 1 hr at 70°C removed its pyrogenicity entirely, which strongly suggests that the pyrogenic action was associated with the protein and not with any lipopolysaccharide which may have been present.

The second line of evidence involved the febrile response of rabbits to repeated injection of the albumin. Repeated daily injections of endotoxin into rabbits results in the development of tolerance: successive fevers decrease in magnitude (1,18). We injected 2 μg of *S. typhosa* endotoxin intravenously into four rabbits on 5 successive days. The magnitude of the fever measured 150 min after injection diminished by half between the first and the fifth injection. When 20 mg of decontaminated monomeric bovine serum albumin was injected on 5 consecutive days, there was no difference in the magnitude of the fever. In fact, the rate of rise of rectal temperature increased with successive injections. Thus, repeated injection of the albumin did not induce tolerance, as would have been the case if the fever were due to endotoxin contamination.

We concluded, therefore, that intravenous injection of decontaminated bovine serum albumin into rabbits produced a dose-dependent fever. The quantities of albumin required amounted to less than 0.1% of the circulating albumin of the rabbit. The time course of the albumin fever could not be distinguished from the time courses of endogenous pyrogen fever and endotoxin fever. Finally, even though commercial albumin may be contaminated with bacterial endotoxin, the fever which followed our injections of decontaminated albumin was not due to residual endotoxin contamination.

DISCUSSION

Having discovered, unexpectedly, that bovine serum albumin is intrinsically pyrogenic when injected into naive rabbits, we are faced with the problem of establishing the nature of albumin fever and particularly the relationship between albumin and endogenous pyrogen. The release of endogenous pyrogen from phagocytic cells is normally consequent to the action on those cells of one of several different kinds of exogenous pyrogens. Among these exogenous pyrogens are endotoxin, Gram-positive bacteria, viruses, protozoa, and unidentified products of neoplasia and necrosis (9). It may be that bovine serum albumin simply constitutes another exogenous pyrogen in rabbits, and therefore acts in series with endogenous pyrogen. However, there are also several other intriguing possibilities. Fever production seems to depend on the synthesis of at least one protein in addition to endogenous pyrogen (16,17). It may be possible, therefore, that albumin acts in series with endogenous pyrogen, but not as an exogenous pyrogen. It is also possible that albumin acts in parallel with endogenous pyrogen; it has been suggested that there are pathways for the development of fever which do not involve endogenous pyrogen (15).

It is highly unlikely that the pyrogenic action of albumin results from the binding of endogenous pyrogen to albumin. Endogenous pyrogen appears to be a mixture of two proteins, both pyrogenic, with the major component being a protein of molecular weight 15,000 and the minor component a protein of molecular weight 38,000 (6,7). A complex consisting of endogenous pyrogen bound to albumin would therefore exhibit a molecular weight easily distinguishable from that of albumin alone.

Albumin acts as a carrier not only for other proteins, but also for fatty acids. It is possible that our bovine serum albumin, even when decontaminated, retained bound to it arachidonic acid or dihomogammalinolenic acid. These fatty acids are the precursors of the prostaglandins, and their breakdown to prostaglandin and related products leads to the development of fever (21). It seems doubtful, however, that sufficient pyrogenic fatty acid could have been bound to the albumin to cause the fevers we observed when just 2 mg of albumin was injected intravenously. Prostaglandin has a short half-life in blood.

Although it is unlikely, therefore, that the pyrogenic action of albumin results from endogenous pyrogen or a prostaglandin precursor bound to the albumin, it remains possible that endogenous pyrogen is actually a component of albumin. We have some preliminary evidence that bovine serum albumin simply left to stand in a cell-free solution releases a smaller protein which is also pyrogenic in rabbits.

Apart from the question of the relationship between albumin and endogenous pyrogen, our observations open several other avenues of possible research. One such avenue concerns the origin of the albumin which originally led us to investigate the possible pyrogenic properties of albumin. The albumin appeared during the incubation of a suspension of blood cells in dextrose saline. The cells had been washed thoroughly in dextrose saline, and we ascertained that the final wash was free of albumin. Nevertheless, 4 hr later the solution in which the cells were suspended contained high levels of albumin. Dinarello and Wolff (5) have also recorded, without comment, the appearance of albumin during the manufacture of human endogenous pyrogen from leukocytes. It is possible that the albumin is serum albumin that has adhered to the cells and become dislodged during the incubation. However, it is also possible that the albumin is of intracellular origin. Albumin bound to the cytoplasmic surface of the cell membrane has been detected in lymphocytes (13), but not yet in other leukocytes. Finally, although small quantities of bovine serum albumin are pyrogenic in rabbits, rabbit albumin is clearly not markedly pyrogenic in rabbits. What is the difference between bovine serum albumin and rabbit serum albumin which makes the bovine serum albumin so pyrogenic in naive rabbits? Are there circumstances in which rabbit serum could become pyrogenic in rabbits?

ACKNOWLEDGMENTS

We thank R. C. Cantrill and F. P. Ross for their help and advice and the South African Medical Research Council, South African Council for Scientific and Industrial Research, Medical Faculty Research Endowment Fund, and Senate of the University of the Witwatersrand for financial support.

REFERENCES

1. Beeson, P. B. (1947): Tolerance to bacterial pyrogens. II. Role of the reticulo-endothelial system. *J. Exp. Med.,* 86:39–44.

2. Bito, L. Z. (1977): Inflammatory effects of endotoxin-like contaminants in commonly used protein preparations. *Science,* 196:83–85.
3. Borsook, D., Laburn, H., and Mitchell, D. (1978): The febrile responses in rabbits and rats to leucocyte pyrogens of different species. *J. Physiol. (Lond.),* 279:113–120.
4. Cradock, J. C., Guder, L. A., Francis, D. L., and Morgan, S. L. (1978): Reduction of pyrogens— Application of molecular filtration. *J. Pharm. Pharmacol.,* 30:198–199.
5. Dinarello, C. A., and Wolff, S. M. (1978): The production of antibody against human leukocytic pyrogen. *J. Clin Invest.,* 60:456–472.
6. Dinarello, C. A., and Wolff, S. M. (1978): Pathogenesis of fever in man. *N. Engl. J. Med.,* 298:607–612.
7. Haeseler, F., Bodel, P., and Atkins, E. (1977): Characteristics of pyrogen production by isolated rabbit Kupffer cells *in vitro. J. Reticuloendothel. Soc.,* 22:569–581.
8. Hattingh, J., Laburn, H., and Mitchell, D. (1979): Fever induced in rabbits by intravenous injection of bovine serum albumin. *J. Physiol. (Lond.),* 290:69–77.
9. Hellon, R. F. (1975): Monoamines, pyrogens and cations: Their actions on central control of body temperature. *Pharmacol. Rev.,* 26:289–321.
10. Henderson, L. W., and Beans, E. (1978): Successful production of sterile pyrogen-free electrolyte solution by ultrafiltration. *Kidney Int.,* 14:522–525.
11. Laburn, H., Mitchell, D., and Rosendorff, C. (1977): Effects of prostaglandin antagonism on sodium arachidonate fever in rabbits. *J. Physiol. (Lond.),* 267:559–570.
12. Murphy, P. A., and Levin, J. (1977): Separation of endogenous pyrogen from endotoxin. *Proc. Soc. Exp. Biol. Med.,* 25:491A.
13. Owen, M. J., Barber, B. H., Faulkes, R. A., and Crumpton, M. J. (1978): Albumin is associated with the inner surface of the lymphocyte plasma membrane. *Biochem. Soc. Trans.,* 6:920–922.
14. Rosendorff, C. (1976): Neurochemistry of fever. *S. Afr. J. Med. Sci.,* 41:23–48.
15. Schlievert, P. M., and Watson, D. W. (1978): Group A streptococcal pyrogenic exotoxin: Pyrogenicity, alteration of blood-brain barrier, and separation of sites for pyrogenicity and enhancement of lethal endotoxin shock. *Infect. Immun.,* 21:753–763.
16. Siegert, R., Philipp-Dormston, W. K., Radsak, K., and Menzel, H. (1975): Inhibition of Newcastle disease virus-induced fever in rabbits by cycloheximide. *Arch. Virol.,* 48:367–373.
17. Siegert, R., Philipp-Dormston, W. K., Radsak, K., and Menzel, H. (1976): Mechanism of fever induction in rabbits. *Infect Immun.,* 14:1130–1137.
18. Snell, E. S., and Atkins, E. (1965): The presence of endogenous pyrogen in normal rabbit tissues. *J. Exp. Med.,* 121:1019–1038.
19. Steere, A. C., Rifaat, M. K., Seligmann, E. B., Hochstein, H. D., Friedland, G., Dasse, P. Wustrack, K. O., Axnick, K. J., and Barker, L. F. (1978): Pyrogen reactions associated with the infusion of normal serum albumin (human). *Transfusion,* 18:102–107.
20. Sweadner, K. J., Forte, M., and Nelson, L. L. (1977): Filtration removal of endotoxin (pyrogens) in solution in different states of aggregation. *Appl. Environ. Microbiol.,* 34:382–385.
21. Work, E. (1971): Production, chemistry and properties of bacterial pyrogens and endotoxins. In: *Pyrogens and Fever,* edited by G. E. W. Wolstenholme and J. Birch, pp. 23–45. Churchill-Livingstone, Edinburgh.
22. Wye, E. J., and Kim, M. K. (1977): Processes to increase the yields of normal serum albumin. *Vox Sang.,* 32:182–184.

Fever, edited by James M. Lipton.
Raven Press, New York © 1980.

Fever, Trace Metals, and Disease

Matthew J. Kluger and Barbara A. Rothenburg

*Department of Physiology, University of Michigan Medical School,
Ann Arbor, Michigan 48109*

Until the latter part of the 19th century, it was generally believed that fever was a response of the infected individual which had some useful function. The belief that fever was beneficial probably had its origins in the humoral theory of disease. According to this theory, disease occurred when one of the four bodily humors was produced in excess. Once this happened the body's defenses came into play, as demonstrated by the patient's raised body temperature, resulting in the excess humor being "cooked" and separated and eventually eliminated (see ref. 19 for more detail). The humoral theory of disease greatly simplified early medical practice since the physician could utilize two basic types of therapy. One involved drugs, which either raised body temperature or helped to "evacuate" the humor (such as diuretics, emetics, sudorifics, purgatives), and the other involved such physical means as external warming or bloodletting (17,38).

This view of fever persisted from the time of Hippocrates to the advent of the industrial synthesis of antipyretic drugs in the 19th century. Whether there is any direct connection between the availability of drugs which could lower fevers and the belief that moderate fevers were harmful is open to debate. Nevertheless, by the end of the 19th century the view that fever was beneficial was changing (25).

In 1960 Bennett and Nicastri (3) reviewed the question of whether fevers were beneficial and were unable to conclude whether fever was a host defense response or a harmful side effect of disease. In the last decade, however, there have been considerable data which shed more light on the question of the function of fever. These have involved three types of evidence, all of which support an adaptive role for fever.

The first type of evidence is based on the phylogeny of fever. An elevation in the thermoregulatory set-point in response to pathogenic microorganisms, endogenous pyrogen-like substances, and other inducers of fever in mammals has been demonstrated in vertebrates from fishes to mammals (see reviews in refs. 18 and 19). The long evolutionary history for fever, an energetically costly process, argues in favor of fever having some beneficial role in disease.

The second type of evidence in support of an adaptive role for fever is based on experiments involving the effects of body temperature on morbidity and mortality rates. Experiments involving fish (11), reptiles (6, 20), and mammals

(10,22,28,33,34) support the hypothesis that fever is a host defense response to both bacterial and viral infections.

The third group of experiments were designed to look at various components of the host defense system in order to determine whether such processes as antibody production and white blood cell function are sensitive to the changes in temperature normally encountered during infection. These investigations have revealed that elevations in temperature of as little as 2°C increase such processes as lymphocyte transformation (1,31), polymorphonuclear granulocyte mobility (4,7,29,30), and the intracellular killing by white blood cells of some species of engulfed pathogens (12,32).

FEVER AND CHANGES IN TRACE METALS—A POSSIBLE SYNERGISM

Another aspect of the host defense response to infection which has received considerable attention in the last several years is that of "nutritional immunity." It is known that during infections with many types of pathogens the plasma concentrations of several trace metals change (see reviews in refs. 2, 8, and 36). For example, when rabbits are infected with live pathogenic bacteria the plasma concentrations of iron and zinc fall and that of copper rises (Fig. 1). Similar findings occur in human patients during most viral and bacterial infections. Kochan (23), Weinberg (36,37), and others have suggested that the changes in concentration of some of these trace metals (most notably iron) could act to reduce the growth of the pathogens, hence the term "nutritional immunity." In support of this hypothesis are the data from Bullen's group which showed that the injection of Fe^{3+} into mice or guinea pigs increased the virulence of many species of bacteria (see review in 9). Similar results have been found in bacterially infected lizards (14). In addition, Murray et al. (27) have shown that the incidence of infection increased significantly in iron-deficient Somali nomads when they were treated with iron supplements in the form of ferrous sulfate.

A potentially important link between changes in trace metals and a rise in body temperature acting together as a coordinated host defense response was suggested by Garibaldi (13). In that study it was found that the biosynthesis of iron transport compounds (siderophores) by *Salmonella typhimurium* was decreased as temperature was raised in the normal physiological range. These bacteria grew well at 36.9°C when the growth medium was supplemented with 0.03 μg Fe/ml, but this same level of iron supplement led to no growth at 40.3°C. Only by adding an iron transport compound or considerably more iron (3.0 μg/ml) to the growth medium would the bacteria grow at 40.3°C. Garibaldi went on to show that even when the bacteria grew well at 40.3°C they still failed to produce large amounts of these iron transport compounds. As a result he suggested that "one role that fever may play in the defensive process . . . is to raise the temperature to the critical point which prevents

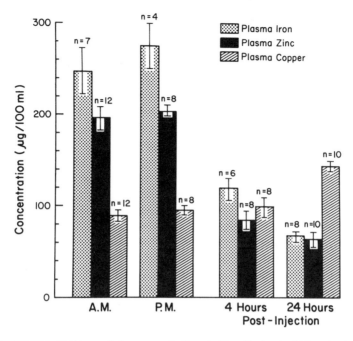

FIG. 1. Plasma iron, copper, and zinc concentrations in New Zealand rabbits prior to (at 1000 and 1400 hr) and following injection with live pathogenic bacteria (1 ml of 1 × 10¹⁰ cells/ml of *Pasteurella multocida*).

the biosynthesis of iron transport compounds which may be a mandatory requirement if the invading microorganism is to establish itself in the host." Kochan (24) found similar results with *Escherichia coli.* The amount of siderophore produced by *E. coli* (called enterochelin in this species) was greater at 26°C than at 33 or 37°C, and at 41 and 44°C virtually no enterochelin was produced.

In both Garibaldi's and Kochan's studies, the temperature at which these organisms were grown was not related to the normal febrile temperature of an infected host. In an attempt to determine whether during infection the normally observed changes in both trace metals and body temperature were involved synergistically to decrease the growth of pathogenic microorganisms, we initiated studies using the desert iguana *(Dipsosaurus dorsalis)* and the laboratory rabbit *(Oryctolagus cuniculus).*

In the first experiments lizards were injected with either dead or live pathogenic bacteria *(Aeromonas hydrophila),* and the plasma concentrations of iron were determined (14). The plasma levels of iron fell regardless of whether the lizards were held at temperatures corresponding to an afebrile temperature (38.5°C) or a febrile one (41.5°C) (5,35). When the bacteria were grown *in vitro* at the normal uninfected levels of iron, the growth rates were similar at the febrile and afebrile temperatures. However, when the bacteria were grown in either a reduced iron medium or one containing an iron-binding agent (desferioxamine β methane sulfate), the growth rate was considerably lower at the febrile temperature. As a result, it was suggested that the fall in plasma iron, coupled with an elevation in body temperature, is a host defense mechanism which acts by severely restricting the amount of iron available to the pathogenic microorganisms.

In a subsequent series of experiments it was shown that there was a positive correlation between the fever developed in rabbits infected with *Pasteurella multocida* and their resultant survival rates for fevers of up to 2.25°C (22). This corresponded to temperatures of about 39.50 to 41.75°C. To determine whether the fall which is observed in plasma iron concentration might partially explain the enhanced survival rate at the elevated temperatures, *P. multocida* was grown in artificial broth media at a concentration of iron corresponding to the normal level (266 μg Fe/100 ml) and to those corresponding to that observed at 4 and 24 hr postinjection (139 and 79 μg Fe/100 ml, respectively). The results were similar to those found in the above study using *A. hydrophila*. At 266 μg Fe/100 ml the bacteria grew equally well at the afebrile temperatures of 39 and 40°C as at the febrile temperature of 41°C; but at either of the reduced levels of iron, the bacteria grew well only at the afebrile temperatures (21).

A criticism of the growth studies described above is that the growth medium did not closely simulate the rabbit's own plasma. In this artificial medium virtually all of the iron would be in the free state, whereas in normal plasma almost all the iron is bound to protein (9). As a result, we have now grown *P. multocida* in plasma obtained either from normal healthy rabbits or from rabbits 24 hr after injection with live *P. multocida*. The plasma was removed under aseptic conditions and checked for sterility by plating a sample on sheep blood agar, any contaminated plasma being discarded. The plasma was then inoculated with *P. multocida* and the growth rate determined over the next 12 hr. In addition, samples of the plasma were removed and the pH determined to ensure that it remained within the normal physiological range (ca. 7.5 to 7.7), as well as to determine the plasma concentrations of iron, zinc, and copper. The results of these growth studies are shown in Figs. 2 and 3. In normal rabbit plasma the bacteria grew at similar rates at temperatures corresponding to afebrile (39 and 40°C) and febrile (41 and 42°C) temperatures. When the bacteria were grown in plasma obtained from rabbits that had been infected with live bacteria 24 hr earlier, the growth rates were not markedly affected at 39 or 40°C, but were reduced at 41 and 42°C. Clearly, changes had occurred in the plasma of the infected rabbits which decreased the growth rate of *P. multocida* at febrile temperatures. Whether these are entirely related to the observed changes in trace metals is not yet known. We are currently determining whether the addition of iron to the growth medium (plasma) at 41 and 42°C restores the growth rate of these bacteria toward that seen in control plasma. In addition, the possible involvement of copper and zinc in the reduction in growth of pathogenic bacteria at febrile temperatures is also being investigated.

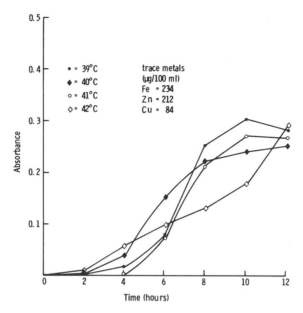

FIG. 2. Growth rate of *P. multocida* in normal rabbit plasma at temperatures corresponding to afebrile (39 and 40°C) and febrile (41 and 42°C) body temperatures of New Zealand rabbits.

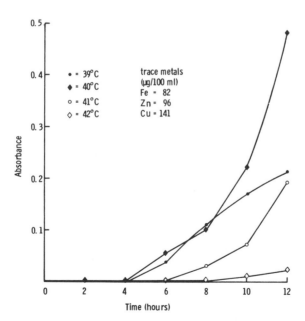

FIG. 3. Growth rate of *P. multocida* in plasma obtained from rabbits 24 hr after infection with pathogenic bacteria at temperatures corresponding to afebrile (39 and 40°C) and febrile (41 and 42°C) body temperatures of New Zealand rabbits.

An additional piece of datum which supports the hypothesis that the changes in trace metals and body temperature which occur during infection are a coordinated host defense response is the evidence that these changes are both mediated by the same substance; that is, the protein responsible for the changes in trace metals (leukocyte endogenous mediator) is probably the same as the protein responsible for inducing a fever (leukocyte endogenous pyrogen) (16,26).

IMPLICATIONS

It is possible that the growth rate of many species of pathogenic microorganisms is reduced at febrile temperatures, particularly in an iron-poor environment. As a result, any form of "therapy" which either lowers body temperature to afebrile levels or raises plasma iron levels to noninfected levels could result in an increased severity of the infection caused by these pathogens.

In addition, Hoffman-Goetz and Kluger (15) have shown that in the protein-deprived rabbit, both the fall in plasma iron concentration and the febrile response are markedly reduced during bacterial infection. For example, at 24 hr after injection with *P. multocida,* plasma iron concentration had fallen an average of 116 μg Fe/100 ml in the protein-deprived rabbits compared to 182 μg Fe/100 ml in the controls ($p < 0.0001$). The average 24-hr fever in the protein-deprived rabbits was 0.26°C versus 1.43°C in the control rabbits ($p < 0.0001$). The failure to lower plasma iron and to raise body temperature to levels found in control animals was the result of a significant reduction in the production of endogenous pyrogens from the white blood cells of the protein-deprived population. If these results can be extrapolated to human beings, then the severe attenuation of the febrile response, coupled with the relative elevation in plasma iron in the protein-deprived individual, could partly account for the increased incidence and severity of many bacterial infections in this group.

ACKNOWLEDGMENTS

This research was supported by NIH Grant AI 13878. I thank Susan Kluger and Alastair J. Turnbull for critically reading this manuscript.

REFERENCES

1. Ashman, R. B., and Nahmias, A. J. (1977): Enhancement of human lymphocyte responses to phytomitogens in vitro by incubation at elevated temperatures. *Clin. Exp. Immunol.,* 29:464–467.
2. Beisel, W. R., Pekarek, R. S., and Wannemacher, R. W., Jr. (1974): The impact of infectious disease on trace-element metabolism of the host. In: *Trace Element Metabolism in Animals,* edited by W. G. Hoekstra, J. W. Suttie, H. E. Ganther, and W. Mertz, pp. 217–240. University Park Press, Baltimore.
3. Bennett, I. L., Jr., and Nicastri, A. (1960): Fever as a mechanism of resistance. *Bacteriol. Rev.,* 24:16–34.
4. Bernheim, H. A., Bodel, P. T., Askenase, P., and Atkins, E. (1978): Effects of fever on host

defense mechanisms after infection in the lizard *Dipsosaurus dorsalis. Br. J. Exp. Pathol.,* 59: 76–84.

5. Bernheim, H. A., and Kluger, M. J. (1976): Fever and antipyresis in the lizard *Dipsosaurus dorsalis. Am. J. Physiol.,* 231:198–203.
6. Bernheim, H. A., and Kluger, M. J. (1976): Fever: Effect of drug-induced antipyresis on survival. *Science,* 193:237–239.
7. Bryant, R. E., DesPrez, R. M., VanWay, M. H., and Rogers, D. E. (1966): Studies on human leukocyte motility. I. Effects of alterations in pH, electrolyte concentration, and phagocytosis on leukocyte migration, adhesiveness, and aggregation. *J. Exp. Med.,* 124:483–499.
8. Bullen, J. J., Rogers, H. J., and Griffiths, E. (1974): Bacterial iron metabolism and immunity. In: *Microbial Iron Metabolism, A Comprehensive Treatise,* edited by J. B. Neilands, pp. 517–551. Academic Press, New York.
9. Bullen, J. J., Rogers, H. J., and Griffiths, E. (1978): Role of iron in bacterial infection. *Curr. Top. Microbiol. Immunol.,* 80:1–35.
10. Carmichael, L. E., Barnes, F. D., and Percy, D.H. (1969): Temperature as a factor in resistance of young puppies. *J. Infect. Dis.,* 120:669–678.
11. Covert, J. B., and Reynolds, W. W. (1977): Survival value of fever in fish. *Nature,* 267: 43–45.
12. Craig, C. P., and Suter, E. (1966): Extracellular factors influencing staphylocidal capacity of human polymorphonuclear leukocytes. *J. Immunol.,* 97:287–296.
13. Garibaldi, J. A. (1972): Influence of temperature on the biosynthesis of iron transport compounds by *Salmonella typhimurium. J. Bacteriol.,* 110:262–265.
14. Grieger, T. A., and Kluger, M. J. (1978): Fever and survival: The role of serum iron. *J. Physiol. (Lond.),* 279:187–196.
15. Hoffman-Goetz, L., and Kluger, M. J. (1979): Protein deprivation: Its effects on fever and plasma iron during bacterial infection in rabbits. *J. Physiol. (Lond.) (in press).*
16. Klempner, M. S., Dinarello, C. A., and Gallin, J. I. (1978): Human leukocyte pyrogen induces release of specific granule contents from human neutrophils. *J. Clin. Invest.,* 61:1130–1336.
17. Kluger, M. J. (1978): The history of bloodletting. *Nautral History,* 87:78–83.
18. Kluger, M. J. (1979): Phylogeny of fever. *Fed. Proc.,* 38:30–34.
19. Kluger, M. J. (1979): *Fever: Its Biology, Evolution, and Function.* Princeton University Press, Princeton, N.J.
20. Kluger, M. J., Ringler, D.H., and Anver, M. R. (1975): Fever and survival. *Science,* 188:166–168.
21. Kluger, M. J., and Rothenburg, B. A. (1979): Fever and reduced iron: Their interaction as a host defense response to bacterial infection. *Science,* 203:374–376.
22. Kluger, M. J., and Vaughn, L. K. (1978): Fever and survival in rabbits infected with *Pasteurella multocida. J. Physiol. (Lond.),* 282:243–251.
23. Kochan, I. (1973): The role of iron in bacterial infections, with special consideration of host-tubercle bacillus interaction. *Cur. Top. Microbiol. Immunol.,* 60:1–30.
24. Kochan, I. (1977): Role of iron in the regulation of nutritional immunity. *Adv. Chem.,* 162: 55–77.
25. Liebermeister, C. (1887): *Vorlesungen über Specielle Pathologie und Therapie.* Verlag von F. C. W. Vogel, Leipzig.
26. Merriman, C. R., Pulliam, L. A., and Kampschmidt, R. F. (1977): Comparison of leukocyte pyrogen and leukocytic endogenous mediator. *Proc. Soc. Exp. Biol. Med.,* 154:224–227.
27. Murray, M. J., Murray, A. B., Murray, M. B., and Murray, C. J. (1978): The adverse effect of iron repletion on the course of certain infections. *Br. Med. J.,* 2:1113–1115.
28. Muschenheim, C., Duerschrer, D. R., Hardy, J. D., and Stoll, A. M. (1943): Hypothermia in experimental infections. III. The effect of hypothermia on resistance to experimental pneumococcus infection. *J. Infect. Dis.,* 72:187–196.
29. Nahas, G. G., Tannieres, M. L., and Lennon, J. F. (1971): Direct measurement of leukocyte motility: Effects of pH and temperature. *Proc. Soc. Exp. Biol. Med.,* 138:350–352.
30. Phelps, P., and Stanislaw, D. (1969): Polymorphonuclear leukocyte mobility in vitro. I. Effect of pH, temperature, ethyl alcohol and caffeine, using a modified Boyden chamber technique. *Arthritis Rheum.,* 12:181–182.
31. Roberts, N. J., Jr., and Steigbigel, R. T. (1977): Hyperthermia and human leukocyte functions: Effects on response of lymphocytes to mitogen and antigen and bactericidal capacity of monocytes and neutrophils. *Infect. Immunol.,* 18:673–679.

32. Sebag, J., Reed, W. P., and Williams, R. C., Jr. (1977): Effect of temperature on bacterial killing by serum and by polymorphonuclear leukocytes. *Infect. Immunol.,* 16:947–954.
33. Teisner, B., and Haahr, S. (1974): Poikilothermia and susceptibility of suckling mice to Coxsackie B₁ virus. *Nature,* 247:568.
34. Toms, G. L., Davies, J. A., Woodward, C. G., Sweet, C., and Smith, H. (1977): The relation of pyrexia and nasal inflammatory response to virus washings of ferrets infected with influenza viruses of differing virulence. *Br. J. Exp. Pathol.,* 58:444–458.
35. Vaughn, L. K., Bernheim, H. A., and Kluger, M. J. (1974): Fever in the lizard *Dispsosaurus dorsalis. Nature,* 252:473–474.
36. Weinberg. E. D. (1974): Iron and susceptibility to infectious disease. *Science,* 184:952–956.
37. Weinberg, E. D. (1978): Iron and infection. *Microbiol. Rev.,* 42:45–66.
38. Yost, R. M., Jr. (1950): Sydenham's philosophy of science. *Osiris,* 9:84–104.

Fever, edited by James M. Lipton.
Raven Press, New York © 1980.

Endogenous Mediators of Fever-Related Metabolic and Hormonal Responses

William R. Beisel and Philip Z. Sobocinski

*U.S. Army Medical Research Institute of Infectious Diseases,
Fort Detrick, Frederick, Maryland 21701*

In 1948 Beeson (3) demonstrated that neutrophilic leukocytes could release an endogenous pyrogenic factor (EP) when engaged in phagocytic activity. EP initiates a febrile response through its effects on CNS temperature-regulating centers (1,10,11). Analogous endogenous substances produced by phagocytic cells have subsequently been found to mediate many of the metabolic and physiologic responses which occur in conjunction with fever (4,8,12–29). Substances that initiate such nonfebrile responses have been termed leukocytic endogenous mediators (LEMs). The relationships between LEM and EP have not been determined with certainty (13,18,19).

ENDOGENOUS PYROGEN AS A MODEL OF OTHER MEDIATORS

Although the molecular mechanisms operative at each step of the fever-producing sequence must still be clarified, an "activation" of pyrogen-releasing cells is the initial event. Under appropriate microenvironmental conditions (10), activated cells then produce and release pyrogenic substances. Although endogenous mediators or pyrogens may be formed through enzymatic conversion of existing precursors, their production via direct *de novo* synthesis is strongly suggested. Studies employing metabolic blocking drugs also indicate that new protein synthesis must take place before EP can be produced (5,10).

Following release from the cell of origin, EP circulates via plasma to the brain. The ensuing febrile response is a neuroregulated event.

In essence, the primary communication mechanism (10) in this fever-producing sequence is quite characteristic of an endocrine regulatory system. Using this concept, EP serves as the hormone, activated phagocytic cells function as multiple individual endocrine glands, and hypothalamic neurons represent the target tissue. The endogenous mediators of other metabolic and physiologic responses appear to follow the EP model (4,8,29), and thus act in the manner of the traditional major hormones.

Note: The view of the authors does not purport to reflect the positions of the Department of the Army or the Department of Defense.

ROLE OF GENERALIZED HOST DEFENSE MECHANISMS

Extreme increases in body temperatures can lead to convulsions, coma, and death. Furthermore, the severity and duration of fever during acute illnesses are roughly proportional to the observed losses of body weight and muscle mass (4). In contrast, a reevaluation of the role of fever in recent years suggests that fever is a defensive response of the body against infections and inflammatory diseases.

If a febrile response is protective, the availability of a hormone-like signal mechanism to initiate a fever would appear to have survival value. Such a system allows either mobile or fixed phagocytic cells at any anatomical site to communicate via a humoral mediator with a distant tissue such as the hypothalamus, liver, or bone marrow. The important fact that a cellular (i.e., inflammatory) defensive response is taking place in some peripheral tissue location is thus made known throughout the body. The number of host defensive cells participating in a peripheral inflammatory response seems to determine the amount of EP or LEM-like endogenous mediating substances released into the circulation. Mediator concentrations in plasma would appear to indicate the magnitude, severity, and duration of the threat (27,28).

Both mobile phagocytic cells and nonmobile macrophages serve as the earliest guardians against microorganisms and other particulate substances. In this capacity, these cells are ideally suited to function as an "early warning" system. In addition to their direct local actions, the phagocytes serve to "spread the alarm" via humoral messages that set generalized mechanisms of host defense into motion. Similar types of cells can also be activated by humoral stimuli which initiate mediator production.

Fever is only one of an extensive series of generalized nonspecific host defensive measures observed during periods of inflammatory or infectious diseases (4). The numerous nonfebrile, nonspecific components of host defense include the mobilization of neutrophilic leukocytes from the bone marrow and the secretion of many hormones. Hepatic cells begin to synthesize a variety of intracellular and extracellular proteins, but at the same time their synthesis of albumin is partially suppressed. Even before the onset of fever, the liver begins to take up free amino acids from plasma. A rapid redistribution of several trace elements also begins within certain body tissues (4,27,28).

Trace elements redistributions are represented by the rapid early movement (flux) of iron and zinc from plasma into the liver. The iron is deposited as ferritin or in hemosiderin granules and the zinc forms a complex with newly synthesized metallothioneine (24). Shortly thereafter, copper begins to move out of the liver and into plasma. The movement of copper from the liver can be explained by the accelerated hepatic synthesis and release of ceruloplasmin, the principal copper-binding protein of plasma. In this regard, accelerated production of ceruloplasmin typifies that of the other acute-phase plasma proteins that are manufactured in increased amounts by hepatocytes during inflammatory and infectious illnesses (4,9,29). The acute-phase reactants are all glycoproteins. In addition to ceruloplasmin, they include fibrinogen, the third component of complement, C-reactive protein, α_1-acid glycoprotein (orosomucoid), α_1-antitrypsin, haptoglobin, and in the rat, α_2-macrofetoprotein. These acute-phase reactants serve to modulate or amplify a variety of host defensive mechanisms.

Along with the nonspecific metabolic and physiologic responses and in coincidence with the onset of a febrile reaction, the body also rearranges its priorities for use of internal cellular metabolic pathways. The new priorities serve to provide additional energy substrates that cells need during periods of fever. To meet the increased cellular demands for energy-yielding substrates, glycogen stores are utilized and the rates of gluconeogenesis are accelerated within the liver. The pancreatic islets release increased amounts of both insulin and glucagon. Adrenal glucocorticoid hormone production increases two- to fivefold in response to stimulation by ACTH, and, in some illnesses, plasma concentrations of growth hormone and the catecholamines are increased as well (4).

The substrates required to permit an increase in hepatic gluconeogenesis are obtained in large part from two free plasma amino acids, alanine and glutamine. These gluconeogenic amino acids are formed *de novo* at an accelerated rate through transamination reactions in skeletal muscle, or they are released directly by the accelerated catabolism of protein in muscle and other somatic tissues. Lactate and pyruvate, emerging from peripheral cellular metabolism are recycled back to the liver to serve as additional substrates for gluconeogenesis; glycerol released from triglycerides is also used.

SPECIFIC VERSUS NONSPECIFIC ASPECTS OF HOST DEFENSE

Many nonspecific host defensive responses begin to occur at about the same time as the onset of fever (4). The weight of evidence (8) suggests that each of these responses contributes in some purposeful manner to the maintenance of host defenses during episodes of infectious or inflammatory diseases. In this regard, the many metabolic and hormonal responses can be considered to represent, along with fever, a combined but essentially nonspecific complex of host defensive mechanisms. Certain conponents of this complex are phylogenetically quite ancient.

These responses are classified as "nonspecific" because of their repeated and consistent participation during each of the many different types of infections or inflammatory diseases that may occur throughout life. The relatively stereotyped patterns of the nonspecific responses contrast with the specialized competence of the immune system. Immune functions deal primarily with recognizing and defending against single foreign, i.e., "specific," antigens (or against groups of specific microbial antigens that might be encountered in simultaneous combinations whenever a microorganism invades the body). The "memory" component of a fully competent host immune system allows lymphocytes and/or immuno-globulins to recognize previously encountered specific foreign antigens. Such specificity is not achieved by the more primitive body defense mechanisms. Rather, any infectious or phlogistic stimulus can trigger the nonspecific compo-nents of host defense via the activation of mediator production by phagocytic cells. Unlike lymphocytic cells, EP/LEM producers are not responsive to the uniqueness of a specific antigen.

CONTROL MECHANISMS FOR THE NONSPECIFIC RESPONSES

The frequent similarity of nonspecific host responses does not imply that all inflammatory or infectious stresses evoke identical response patterns, involv-ing all potential defensive mechanisms to an equal degree (7). A given pattern of clinical fever may characterize certain infections but not others. Some infec-tions stimulate an outpouring of granulocytic white blood cells whereas others do not. Further, the various acute-phase reactants seem to vary independently in their individual concentrations depending on the illness to which they are responding (7). These differences in response patterns, as well as differences in their timing, would be difficult to explain if all responses were initiated and sustained by the effects of a single mediating substance on a single target cell population. Although the various nonspecific responses may have a common purpose, they emerge as individual components of a broad host defensive system. Differences observed during diseases suggest that each defense system component may be regulated by its own mediator. With this concept a single mediator could evoke a varied response by stimulating several kinds of responding cells, or a single cell type could respond differently to stimuli from different mediators.

Since single hepatic cells appear to generate a dozen or more of the identifiable nonspecific host defensive components, a single initiating stimulus could not be expected to regulate all hepatic cell responses. These often show subtle but detectable differences. Rather, differences in hepatic cellular responses would appear to require individual delicately controlled molecular mechanisms such as those that typify other known regulatory systems of the body. A "family" of closely related mediators could conceptually meet this apparent need for a complex network of regulatory controls.

Much has been learned about the different cellular varieties of EPs and their role in initiating fever. It is important to gain equivalent knowledge concerning the nature and variety of signal transmitting mechanisms that initiate other components of nonspecific host defense. Several major organs and tissues contrib-ute to these nonfebrile defenses, including bone marrow, liver, kidneys, pancreas, endocrine glands, hypothalamus, and skeletal muscle. It is pertinent to ask how each of these diverse tissues is stimulated to initiate its portion of the overall defensive response. We also need to learn how these responses are sus-tained and eventually terminated.

ROLE OF ENDOGENOUS MEDIATORS OF NONPYROGENIC RESPONSES

During the past decade, studies conducted in several laboratories (2,4,8,12–29) have shown that phagocytic cells release endogenous mediating substances. These appear to initiate many of the diverse metabolic and physiological defensive responses which are independent of those related directly to the induction of fever. Endogenous pyrogen thus seems to serve as a model of LEM-like signal mechanisms for nonspecific metabolic responses.

Methods virtually identical to those used to obtain EPs are used also for LEMs. Activated neutrophils are collected from the peritoneal cavity of rabbits 16 hr after an earlier injection of shellfish glycogen, an irritant. The cells are washed and incubated for 2 hr in sterile normal saline. Supernatant fluid contains the secreted LEM. Initial findings (13,20,21) suggested that this crude fluid product contained LEM as a heat-labile protein. The active component could be destroyed by pronase and trypsin but not by lipase. Using a bioassay system involving the inoculation of log-based doses of crude LEM or EP/LEM) into the peritoneal cavity of normal rats, the mediator was shown to produce a number of characteristic metabolic responses. These included a rapid dose-related decrease in plasma concentrations of iron, zinc, and amino acids; a rapid flux of iron, zinc, and amino acids into the liver; and a stimulation (at a slower rate) of a protein synthetic response in the liver. This last response included an initial transcription of RNA species, followed closely by accelerated synthesis and release of acute-phase reactant proteins from the liver (9,26,29), and the production of certain intracellular proteins (4,24).

Work in several laboratories (8,14,17,18) showed that crude EP/LEM preparations stimulated a release of white blood cells from the marrow and an increased secretion of both insulin and glucagon from the pancreas (12).

Other bioassay information revealed that LEM, or some substance with similar biological activities, began to circulate in the plasma of human subjects during the early course of an infection-induced fever. The plasma of volunteers exposed to typhoid fever bacilli began to contain heat-labile LEM-like mediators a day or two before the onset of fever (27). These biologically active substances remained in the plasma as long as fever persisted. However, the LEM-like substances could not be detected in plasma obtained from the volunteers either before or after their illness (27). LEM-like activity was demonstrated in serum of patients hospitalized with various generalized bacterial infections or malaria and in some patients with bacterial diarrhea. Similar assays performed in volunteers during experimentally induced sandfly fever also demonstrated the presence of LEM-like substances in plasma during the febrile episode, but in smaller concentrations than those seen in patients with generalized bacterial diseases (28). Most recently, substances with LEM-like activity were demonstrated by bioassay in human plasma during acute febrile exacerbations of regional enteritis

(25), although similar assays of plasma were not positive in patients with quiescent disease. Bioassays also revealed the *de novo* appearance of LEM-like mediators in the plasma of laboratory animals during infections or inflammatory states (20–22). Direct effects of plasma LEM have been demonstrated on cultured hepatic cells as well (23).

SITES OF MEDIATOR ACTIONS

Even though the nature of the mediator substances remains to be clarified, questions must be raised about their possible sites of action in order to explain their multi-organ, multi-locational effects. One could postulate that each endogenous mediator acts in a primary, direct manner on an individual type of responsive cell or tissue. Such a postulation would mean that liver cells, bone marrow cells, hypothalamic neurons, pancreatic islets, and possibly skeletal muscle tissue would each be a primary target for one or more of the LEM-like mediators.

The direct action of an endogenous mediator on the liver has recently been reported by Rupp and Fuller (23) who demonstrated that fibrinogen biosynthesis was induced in cultured fetal rat hepatocytes. Earlier studies (29) demonstrated a direct effect of crude LEM on the liver by showing that it stimulated amino acids uptake during *in vitro* liver perfusions. Adult rat hepatocytes, however, did not show a detectable uptake of amino acids or an increase in protein synthesis when studied in culture (P.G. Canonico, *personal communication*). Kampschmidt and Upchurch (14) also demonstrated a direct action of LEM after partial purification by butanol extraction. This LEM preparation stimulated an increase in colony numbers in rat bone marrow cultures in the presence of rat serum and glass-adherent marrow cells.

Alternatively, one could postulate that the LEM-like mediators would be directly analogous to, or identical with, the endogenous pyrogens in terms of their target tissue. They would thus have a single primary target area in the thermoregulatory hypothalamic neurons, or, alternatively, target areas involving several different types of neurons within adjacent hypothalamic regions. Some experimental evidence suggests that the CNS does participate in the multiple metabolic effects attributable to LEM. An inoculation of minute amounts of crude LEM into a lateral ventricle of the brain in rats (2,12) stimulates the various hepatic, pancreatic, and bone marrow effects attributed to LEM. Such minute amounts of LEM are ineffective in causing these changes if given by any other route. On the other hand, crude LEM contains components that have toxic or irritant qualities (15). The intraventricular inoculation of LEM is followed by an infiltration of inflammatory cells into adjacent brain tissues. It is possible that these newly mobilized inflammatory cells release additional mediators *in vivo* and that these, in turn, initiate peripheral effects by a direct action on target tissues.

If all primary effects of the endogenous mediators were localized within the hypothalamus, some additional mechanisms for signaling distant tissues would need to exist. The effector response as typified by EP could employ direct neurological pathways. Alternatively, an indirect signal might employ neurosecretory hormones as intermediate messengers. These in turn could act on distant target tissues or on the nearby anterior pituitary to stimulate the release of trophic hormones such as ACTH and TSH, or growth hormone, each with its own stimulatory effects on distant cells.

None of the endocrine responses observed during infections or inflammatory illnesses appear to involve nonconventional regulatory mechanisms (4). On the other hand, there is no explanation as to how such endocrine responses are initiated during early prodromal periods of inflammatory illness. Certain LEM-initiated hepatic effects do not require functioning adrenal, pituitary, or thyroid glands (29). However, the permissive presence of adrenal glucocorticoid hormones is required before hepatocytes can produce new RNA and synthesize new acute-phase plasma proteins in response to LEM (26,29). LEM does not act primarily by stimulating the adenylate cyclase-cAMP system in liver (29), although this system may be activated as a secondary response after LEM-stimulated glucagon release (12).

MOLECULAR STRUCTURE OF ENDOGENOUS MEDIATORS

Much uncertainty remains concerning the molecular structure of the endogenous mediators.

LEM and EP may be identical substances (13,19), but some data reveal differences (8,17,18). First, no single substance can be defined as the "only" EP (10). Rather, each cell type known to produce EP appears to produce a subspecies that is characteristic of the cell of origin and distinguishable from EP produced by other cell lines or tissues (1,6,10,11). More than one form of pyrogen may be detected in partially purified preparations (10). It is possible, however, that most endogenous pyrogens share a fundamental protein moiety that could account for their cross-order and cross-class activities (11).

Second, many individual lots of crude LEM prepared in our laboratories from rabbit peritoneal leukocytes did not produce fever when tested by appropriate methods, even though they stimulated all other metabolic effects ascribed to LEM (17,18).

Third, if EP was present in some preparations of crude LEM, it could be removed by adding glass beads to the supernatant fluids (17,18). Endogenous pyrogen adhered to glass, and the bead-treated preparations lost their pyrogenicity when tested in rabbits. In contrast, LEM remained in solution and demonstrated its various metabolic or physiological effects when tested in assay rats.

Fourth, the apparent release of EP from white cells was inhibited by 3 to 5 mM concentrations of K^+ (18), but biological activities attributed to LEM were not. Kampschmidt et al (13), however, reported that release of both EP and LEM was inhibited by 5 mM K^+.

Fifth, endogenous pyrogens are said to be released only by intact cells, whereas

Mapes and Sobocinski (17,18) have shown that some LEM activities can be obtained from broken cell preparations as well.

Few of the most highly purified EP preparations have been tested to determine whether or not they possessed LEM-like actions. Merriman et al. (19) did, however, use an accepted EP purification scheme with slight modifications and showed the EP properties and those of LEM migrated as a single unit during isoelectric focusing in polyacrylamide gels.

Although early studies suggested that LEM was a small, heat-labile protein, recent data of Mapes et al. (16) indicated that biologically active lipid components such as the prostaglandins influenced the production and release of LEM and were also present in crude LEM preparations. Mapes and Sobocinski (17) separated various subspecies of LEM from each other by a combination of procedures which included fractionation with 40% ammonium sulfate, butanol, and treatment with Amberlite CG-50. Each LEM subspecies appeared to initiate a different metabolic or physiologic response when tested in assay rats. Thus preparations of LEM with predominant zinc-fluxing activity could be isolated and differentiated from preparations that stimulated neutrophil release from bone marrow (17). Furthermore, if added to the incubation media of rabbit peritoneal white blood cells, single prostaglandins were each found to stimulate the production of a different individual subspecies of LEM, i.e., 2 μM prostaglandin E led to subspecies that stimulated hepatic amino acid uptake whereas 2 μM of prostaglandin F caused the production of zinc-fluxing LEM (18). In addition, the production of LEM by stimulated cells was prevented by the addition of aspirin or indomethacin to the incubation media (18).

The possibilities that EP or LEM subspecies might each contain a different lipid or prostaglandin component or analog remain as open questions. Protein-lipid complexes may comprise the fully active mediators, since partially purified preparations contain considerably more lipid than protein (16). In fact, the protein content of highly purified EP/LEM preparations may be too low for accurate quantitation, and the localization of EP/LEM within a gel may require identification by biological activity assays instead. Mapes et al. (16) suggest that prostaglandin-like activities may reside within the LEM molecule. Lipids extracted from crude LEM preparations, including hydroxy fatty acids, induce effects in assay rats which physiologically resemble those of LEM (16). It is possible that each subspecies of LEM or EP contains a common amino acid sequence or fundamental protein component (11), to which may be attached an effect-determining active moiety. If the latter were a lipid, its structure might be responsible for producing a discrete effector action (16–18).

The available evidence suggests that activated phagocytic cells could therefore produce a family of closely related mediator substances including pyrogenic and nonpyrogenic varieties. Each subspecies in this mixture could be responsible for triggering at least one of the specific effects attributed to either EP or LEM.

To resolve the unsettled possibilities about the true relationships between EP and LEM, it will be necessary to isolate and purify at least some of the major subspecies of these mediators. The molecular composition, structure, and biological activities of high purified individual subspecies must then be differentiated with careful side-by-side comparisons.

SUMMARY

When appropriately activated, nonlymphocytic cells of bone marrow origin release endogenous mediating substances. These mediators exert hormone-like stimulatory effects on a variety of distant body cells and tissues. Although their molecular nature remains to be defined, these endogenous substances appear to initiate or modulate fever as well as many of the generalized metabolic and physiologic responses of the host that accompany an infectious or inflammatory disease.

REFERENCES

1. Atkins, E., and Bodel, P. (1979): Clinical fever: Its history, manifestations, and pathogenesis. *Fed. Proc.*, 38:57–63.
2. Bailey, P. T., Abeles, F. B., Hauer, E. C., and Mapes, C. A. (1976): Intracerebroventricular administration of leukocytic endogenous mediators (LEM) in the rat. *Proc. Soc. Exp. Biol. Med.*, 153:419–423.
3. Beeson, P. B. (1948): Temperature-elevating effect of a substance obtained from polymorphonuclear leukocytes. *J. Clin. Invest.*, 27:524 (abstr.).
4. Beisel, W. R. (1977): Magnitude of the host nutritional responses to infection. *Am. J. Clin. Nutr.*, 30:1236–1247.
5. Bodel, P. (1970): Studies on the mechanism of endogenous pyrogen production. I. Investigation of new protein synthesis in stimulated human blood leukocytes. *Yale J. Biol. Med.*, 43:145–163.
6. Bodel, P., Wechsler, A., and Atkins, E. (1969): Comparison of endogenous pyrogens from human and rabbit leukocytes utilizing Sephadex filtration. *Yale J. Biol. Med.*, 41:376–387.
7. Bostian, K. A., Blackburn, B. S., Wannemacher, R. W., Jr., McGann, B. G., Beisel, W. R., and DuPont, H. L. (1976): Sequential changes in the concentration of specific serum proteins during typhoid fever infection in man. *J. Lab. Clin. Med.*, 87:577–585.
8. Canonico, P. G., McManus, A. T., and Powanda, M. C. (1979): Biochemistry and function of the neutrophil in infected, burned and traumatized hosts. In: *Lysosomes in Biology and Pathology,* edited by J. T. Dingle and P. Jacques, pp. 289–328. Elsevier, New York.
9. Cockerell, G. L. (1973): Changes in plasma protein-bound carbohydrates and glycoprotein patterns during infection, inflammation and starvation. *Proc. Soc. Exp. Biol. Med.*, 142:1072–1076.
10. Dinarello, C. A. (1979): Production of endogenous pyrogen. *Fed. Proc.*, 38:52–56.
11. Dinarello, C. A., and Wolff, S. M. (1978): Pathogenesis of fever in man. *N. Engl. J. Med.*, 298:607–612.
12. George, D. T., Abeles, F. B., Mapes, C. A., Sobocinski, P. Z., Zenser, T. V., and Powanda, M. C. (1977): Effect of leukocytic endogenous mediators on endocrine pancreas secretory responses. *Am. J. Physiol.* 233:E240–E245.
13. Kampschmidt, R. F., Pulliam, L. A., and Merriman, C. R. (1978): Further similarities of endogenous pyrogen and leukocytic endogenous mediator. *Am J. Physiol.*, 235:C118–C121.
14. Kampschmidt, R. F., and Upchurch, H. F. (1977): Possible involvement of leukocytic endogenous mediator in granulopoiesis. *Proc. Soc. Exp. Biol. Med.*, 155:89–93.
15. Liu, C. T., Sanders, R. P., Hadick, C. L., and Sobocinski, P. Z. (1979): Effects of intravenous infusion of leukocytic endogenous mediator on cardiohepatic functions in rhesus macaques. *Am. J. Vet. Res.*, 40:1035–1039.
16. Mapes, C. A., George, D. T., and Sobocinski, P. Z. (1977): Possible relation of prostaglandins

to PMN-derived mediators of host metabolic responses to inflammation. *Prostaglandins,* 13: 73–85.

17. Mapes, C. A., and Sobocinski, P. Z. (1976): Multiple leukocytic factors that induce reactions characteristic of the inflammatory responses. In: *Army Science Conference Proceedings, Vol. 2,* pp. 405–419. Deputy Chief of Staff for Research, Development, and Acquisition, Department of the Army, Washington, D.C.

18. Mapes, C. A., and Sobocinski, P. Z. (1977): Differentiation between endogenous pyrogen and leukocytic endogenous mediator. *Am. J. Physiol.,* 232:C15–C22.

19. Merriman, C. R., Pulliam, L. A., and Kampschmidt, R. F. (1977): Comparison of leukocytic pyrogen and leukocytic endogenous mediator. *Proc. Soc. Exp. Biol. Med.,* 154:224–227.

20. Pekarek, R. S., and Beisel, W. R. (1971): Characterization of the endogenous mediator(s) of serum zinc and iron depression during infection and other stresses. *Proc. Soc. Exp. Biol. Med.,* 138:728–732.

21. Pekarek, R. S., Wannemacher, R. W., Jr., Chapple, F. E., III, Powanda, M. C., and Beisel, W. R. (1972): Further characterization and species specificity of leukocytic endogenous mediator (LEM). *Proc. Soc. Exp. Biol. Med.,* 141:643–648.

22. Pekarek, R., Wannemacher, R., Powanda, M., Abeles, F., Mosher, D., Dinterman, R., and Beisel, W. (1974): Further evidence that leukocytic endogenous mediator (LEM) is not endotoxin. *Life Sci.,* 14:1765–1776.

23. Rupp, R. G., and Fuller, G. M. (1979): The effects of leukocytic and serum factors on fibrinogen biosynthesis in cultured hepatocytes. *Exp. Cell Res.,* 118:23–30.

24. Sobocinski, P. Z., Canterbury, W. J., Jr., Mapes, C. A., and Dinterman, R. E. (1978): Involvement of hepatic metallothioneins in hypozincemia associated with bacterial infection. *Am. J. Physiol.,* 234:E399–E406.

25. Solomons, N. W., Elson, C. O., Pekarek, R. S., Jacob, R. A., Sandstead, H. H., and Rosenberg, I. H. (1978): Leukocytic endogenous mediator in Crohn's disease. *Infect. Immun.,* 22:637–639.

26. Thompson, W. L., Abeles, F. B., Beall, F. A., Dinterman, R. E., and Wannemacher, R. W., Jr. (1976): Influence of the adrenal glucocorticoids on the stimulation of synthesis of hepatic ribonucleic acid and plasma acute-phase globulins by leucocytic endogenous mediator. *Biochem. J.,* 156:25–32.

27. Wannemacher, R. W., Jr., DuPont, H. L., Pekarek, R. S., Powanda, M. C., Schwartz, A., Hornick, R. B., and Beisel, W. R. (1972): An endogenous mediator of depression of amino acids and trace metals in serum during typhoid fever. *J. Infect. Dis.,* 126:77–86.

28. Wannemacher, R. W., Jr., Pekarek, R. S., Klainer, A. S., Bartelloni, P. J., DuPont, H. L., Hornick, R. B., and Beisel, W. R. (1975): Detection of a leukocytic endogenous mediator-like mediator of serum amino acid and zinc depression during various infectious illnesses. *Infect. Immun.,* 11:873–875.

29. Wannemacher, R. W., Jr., Pekarek, R. S., Thompson, W. L., Curnow, R. T., Beall, F. A., Zenser, T. V., DeRubertis, F. R., and Beisel, W. R. (1975): A protein from polymorphonuclear leukocytes (LEM) which affects the rate of hepatic amino acid transport and synthesis of acute-phase globulins. *Endocrinology,* 96:651–661.

Fever, edited by James M. Lipton.
Raven Press, New York © 1980.

Metabolic Alterations Elicited by Endogenous Pyrogens

Ralph F. Kampschmidt

Biomedical Division, The Samuel Roberts Noble Foundation, Inc., Ardmore, Oklahoma 73401

A number of early studies indicated that material occurring in pus or inflammatory exudates would cause fever and other host alterations (23,47). It now seems likely that much of the activity in these early experiments could have been due to endotoxin contamination. The first demonstration of an endogenous product with pyrogenic activity clearly distinct from endotoxin was by Beeson (6). There also were early indications that crude endogenous pyrogen (EP) preparations from peritoneal exudates caused granulocytosis (42,59), lowering of plasma iron (33), and delayed inflammatory responses (52). Most methods for the preparation of EP involved the induction of peritoneal granulocytes in rabbits by injecting large volumes of saline and a small amount of irritant. The granulocytes were then washed and incubated for 2 to 4 hr in saline at 37°C to cause the release of EP into the supernatant. It is now known that such crude EP preparations are relatively free of endotoxin contamination (4,10,40,58). When injected into rats or rabbits these crude preparations lowered plasma iron (35) and plasma zinc (37,55) and increased plasma copper (56). These injections caused the release of bone marrow neutrophils (27), promoted granulopoiesis (39), and stimulated the synthesis of fibrinogen (38), haptoglobin (38), α_1-macrofetoprotein, α_2-macrofetoprotein (19), ceruloplasmin (56), hemopexin (50), and c-reactive protein (48). A crude mediator preparation from rat peritoneal leukocytes also caused a flux of amino acids from muscle to liver (67). Owing to its source and the multiplicity of host alterations produced (Fig. 1), the active material(s) has been called leukocytic endogenous mediator (LEM) and its properties have been reviewed recently (25).

HOW MANY DIFFERENT FACTORS ARE INVOLVED?

Among many unanswered questions, a prominent one is whether the protein known as EP is responsible for a variety of host alterations in addition to fever (31,45). The activities of EP and LEM seem to be associated with proteins (1,25), since both are destroyed by pronase, trypsin (15,57,60), or heat (10,15,57). Reviews frequently state that EP can be destroyed by heating at 56°C for 1

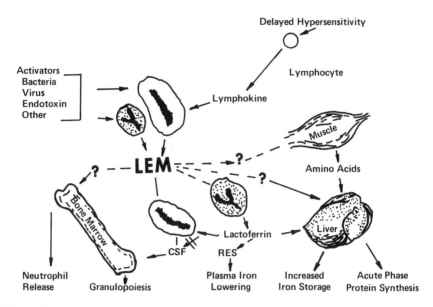

FIG. 1. Diagrammatic representation of some of the activators and cells which synthesize leukocytic endogenous mediator. Also shown are some of the alterations produced when LEM is injected into rabbits, rats, or mice along with some postulated pathways that might explain how these changes occur.

hr (1) and that LEM is not inactivated at this temperature (12). However, there are few data to support either statement. Both LEM and EP activities can be destroyed at 90°C (25), but no direct comparisons of heat inactivation have been made at lower temperatures. Both LEM and EP require free sulfhydryl groups for activity (40,44). The activity is therefore lost in an oxidative environment, but it can be restored by sulfhydryl-reducing agents (40,44).

Most of the studies on LEM have used either rabbit or rat peritoneal granulocytes (25), but a limited amount of data indicates that rat Kupffer cells and peritoneal macrophages, after appropriate activation, will produce LEM (32). Peripheral blood leukocytes from rabbits, rats, and humans when activated *in vitro* by endotoxin or heat-killed staphylococci produced LEM (30,32). Neither EP nor LEM is produced spontaneously from blood leukocytes, and activators which promote the synthesis of EP and LEM appear to be similar (1,25).

Endotoxin, bacteria, virus, and the injection of certain colloidal materials cause fever and LEM activities in intact animals (14,34). Delayed hypersensitivity reactions cause fever, and there is evidence that this fever results from the production of EP brought about by the activation of monocytes with a lymphokine (2,3). Elicitation of a delayed hypersensitivity reaction in either rats or rabbits results in all the changes normally seen after an injection of LEM (28).

Blood monocytes from humans or rabbits produce more EP than an equal number of neutrophils (9,15). Recently it was shown that monocytes from these species yield about 10-fold more LEM activity than neutrophils, and that both a high and low molecular weight pyrogen produced by these monocytes had LEM activity (30).

The process by which cells become activated to produce and release EP has been the subject of numerous studies (8,24,54,61,64); however, comparable studies have not been conducted for LEM. There is some evidence that LEM and EP release from PMN cells of rabbit peritoneal exudates are inhibited to about the same extent when K^+ or Ca^{2+} ions are added to the incubation medium (7,13,21,31).

All of the biological activities of LEM can be produced in endotoxin-tolerant rats or rabbits (32,35,37,58). Repeated injections of LEM or EP do not lead to tolerance for the alterations they produce (1,26,39).

Although EP and LEM thus appear biologically closely related, chemical proof that they are the same protein has not been obtained. Both activities have been shown to elute in the same fractions after column chromatography on Sephadex (10,36,49). They also migrate at the same rates during acrylamide gel electrophoresis (40,49). The most highly purified preparations of EP were obtained by Murphy et al. (52) in a five-step procedure. When a slightly modified version of this procedure was used, both LEM and EP activities were closely associated at each purification step and in the final product (49). To obtain a truly homogenous product will probably require a more abundant source than the granulocytes of rabbit peritoneal exudates. Loss of activity due to the absorption of protein onto glass surfaces and the difficulty in keeping the sulfhydryl groups reduced make improvement of the yields difficult (49,53). With the methods currently available, it would therefore be necessary to use exudates from several hundred rabbits to obtain sufficient material to test for homogeneity.

Recently Dinarello et al. (16) have prepared rabbit antibodies to EP from human monocytes by continuing the booster injections for 7 to 13 months. This antibody was then used to help purify the pyrogen; after the EP was labeled with ^{125}I, a radioimmunoassay was used to detect small amounts of the pyrogen (17). Since crude human monocyte pyrogen has both EP and LEM activities in rabbits (15,30) and rats (30), it should be possible to check for LEM activity in these species with the purified preparation (17).

There have been some results which indicate that LEM and EP are different proteins. Mapes and Sobocinski (45) found that EP adhered more readily to glass surfaces than did LEM. They also observed that during the summer months their preparations lost pyrogenic but not LEM activities and that EP release was more sensitive to inhibition by potassium ions than LEM release (45). Other investigators have not observed the marked seasonal variation (10,31) or differential loss of EP and LEM onto glass during purification (49), and inhibition of release by potassium ions was found to be about equal for EP and LEM (31). Mapes and Sobocinski also found, unlike most investigators who work with EP (8,9,20,21,51,54), that homogenates of rabbit peritoneal granulocytes produced LEM-like activity (45). These discrepancies could be due to differences in the methods used by Mapes and Sobocinski and those used by most other investigators in mediator preparation. Although most of the studies with EP have used low-speed centrifugation for short periods of time (10,31, 42,52), Mapes and Sobocinski removed cells by centrifugation at 62,000 × g for 30 min (45). It therefore seems possible that high-speed centrifugation may be releasing a contaminant that also causes numerous host alterations when injected. It would be interesting to know whether this factor is truly endogenous (i.e., no tolerance after repeated injections), is released under *in vivo* conditions, and is released from the more durable peripheral blood leukocytes.

The multiple effects produced by LEM suggest that it must act at a variety of target sites such as the bone marrow, liver, and the hypothalamus. This has led some investigators to suggest the formation of an apoLEM which then binds to other effector molecules (12), but evidence in support of this suggestion is lacking. Perhaps LEM does not act directly on the target tissue, but instead induces production of other mediators (25).

LEM AS A CENTRAL MEDIATOR

In a liver perfusion system the addition of LEM and cortisol stimulated both the incorporation of orotate into ribosomes and the intracellular accumulation of α-aminoisobutyric acid (65,68). These studies suggest that LEM acts directly on liver to stimulate the hepatic uptake of free amino acids and synthesis of acute-phase proteins. Primary cultures of fetal rat liver cells also indicated that LEM acted directly on hepatocytes to increase the synthesis of fibrinogen (62). On the other hand, studies using liver slices showed no direct effect of LEM, but plasma from LEM-injected rats stimulated fibrinogen synthesis (38), suggesting the possibility that the effect of LEM on acute phase protein occurred indirectly through another mediator.

Mechanisms whereby plasma iron is lowered during infections and inflammation have not been clearly established. Although it has been shown that LEM injections will lower plasma iron (26,33,35,55), there are also indications that lactoferrin may be involved (46,66). Quite recently Klempner et al. (43) have shown that a highly purified human EP induced neutrophils to selectively release lactoferrin. It seems possible, therefore, that both LEM and lactoferrin are involved in plasma iron lowering. Infection may promote the synthesis of LEM, which then causes neutrophils to release the more proximate iron lowering compound lactoferrin.

The number of neutrophils in the blood was markedly increased after giving a rat 10 or more daily injections of LEM (39). Some of this increase was caused by the release of neutrophils from the bone marrow (27), but there was also an increased granulopoiesis which could be related to the increased colony-stimulating factor found in the plasma when more LEM injections were given (39). When added to bone marrow cultures, LEM will stimulate colony formation if the population of adherent cells is present (39). LEM seems to be acting on mature macrophages, causing them to release colony-stimulating factor which stimulates the bone marrow cultures to form colonies. Recently it has been shown that lactoferrin may be a granulocyte-derived inhibitor of colony-stimulating activity production (11). Thus LEM, by inducing the release of colony-stimulating factor from macrophages and lactoferrin from neutrophils, has a potential to stimulate or inhibit granulopoiesis. Figure 1 indicates some of the possible interrelationships between LEM and other mediators.

During the acute stages of infection or inflammation, a number of metabolic alterations can be observed which seem to involve numerous biochemical pathways in the body. The similarity of these changes during a variety of stresses led early investigators to refer to these collective alterations as "autonomic shift" or "emergency reactions" (22). Some investigators believed that these changes were initiated by the central nervous system, since bleeding into certain areas of the brain or traumatic lesions caused most of these nonspecific reactions (22). When LEM was injected intracisternally it was no more effective than when it was administered intravenously (41). Bailey et al. (5), however, found that doses of LEM that were inactive by i.v. injection had activity when injected into the lateral cerebral ventricle of rats. These results were obtained with a crude preparation and need to be confirmed with a partially purified LEM preparation. It is at present difficult to understand how LEM can act directly on some tissues (62,65) and also through the central nervous system.

Many of the changes occurring during infection, inflammation, or other stresses have been attributed to hormones from the adrenals or pituitary (63). If the primary mechanism of action of LEM was through these hormones, LEM would be expected to have little effect in animals where the glands producing these hormones had been removed. However, changes that typically occur in normal animals after an injection of LEM occur in adrenalectomized or hypophysectomized rats (41,65,68).

The search for a better understanding of the metabolic changes that occur during the acute stages of infection or inflammation has spanned several decades. The investigations have persisted because the alterations seem to be important in early defense of the host following infection, trauma, or inflammation. Recent evidence would seem to confirm the role of these alterations in host defense, since injections of LEM will protect the rat against a usually fatal dose of *Salmonella typhimurium* (29) or *Streptococcus pneumoniae* (12). Unfortunately, even those host changes that have been studied most thoroughly, such as fever, still elude us as we attempt to understand the finer details of how it occurs and its possible role in defense.

The synthesis and release of EP and/or LEM probably constitute just one of several early mediators during infection or inflammation, and some of them may be acting through other more proximate mediators. Thus EP may be a central mediator for only a small, but apparently important, portion of the early nonspecific defense mechanisms. If all of us persist in our investigations, perhaps the time for an eventual understanding of at least this portion of the host's alterations during infection or inflammation might be measured in years rather than decades.

REFERENCES

1. Atkins, E., and Bodel, P. (1974): Fever. In: *The Inflammatory Process, 2nd Ed.*, edited by B. W. Zweifach, L. Grant, and R. T. McCluskey, pp. 467–513. Academic Press, New York.
2. Atkins, E., Feldman, J. P., Francis, L., and Hursh, E. (1972): Studies on the mechanism of fever accompanying delayed hypersensitivity. The role of the sensitized lymphocyte. *J. Exp. Med.*, 135:1113–1132.
3. Atkins, E., Francis, L., and Bernheim, H. A. (1978): Pathogenesis of fever in delayed hypersensitivity: Role of monocytes. *Infect. Immun.*, 21:813–820.
4. Atkins, E., and Snell, E. S. (1965): Fever. In: *The Inflammatory Process, 1st Ed.*, edited by B. W. Zweifach, L. Grant, and R. T. McCluskey, pp. 495–534. Academic Press, New York.
5. Bailey, P. T., Abeles, F. B., Hauer, E. C., and Mapes, C. A. (1976): Intracerebroventricular administration of leukocytic endogenous mediators (LEM) in the rat. *Proc. Soc. Exp. Biol. Med.*, 153:419–423.
6. Beeson, P. B. (1948): Temperature-elevating effect of a substance obtained from polymorphonuclear leucocytes. *J. Clin. Invest.*, 27:524.
7. Berlin, R. D., and Wood, W. B., Jr. (1964): Studies on the pathogenesis of fever. XII. Electrolytic factors influencing the release of endogenous pyrogen from polymorphonuclear leukocytes. *J. Exp. Med.*, 119:697–714.
8. Bodel, P. (1970): Studies on the mechanism of endogenous pyrogen production. I. Investigation of new protein synthesis in stimulated human blood leukocytes. *Yale J. Biol. Med.*, 43:145–163.
9. Bodel, P. (1974): Studies on the mechanism of endogenous pyrogen production. III. Human blood monocytes. *J. Exp. Med.*, 140:954–965.
10. Bornstein, D. L., and Walsh, E. C. (1978): Endogenous mediators of the acute-phase reaction. I. Rabbit granulocytic pyrogen and its chromatographic subfractions. *J. Lab. Clin. Med.*, 91:236–245.
11. Broxmeyer, H. E., Smithyman, A., Eger, R. R., Meyers, P. A., and DeSousa, M. (1978): Identification of lactoferrin as the granulocyte-derived inhibitor of colony-stimulating activity production. *J. Exp. Med.*, 148:1052–1067.
12. Canonico, P. G., McManus, A. T., and Powanda, M. C. (1979): Biochemistry and function of the neutrophil in infected, burned, and traumatized hosts. In: *Lysosomes in Biology and Pathology, Vol. 6*, edited by J. T. Dingle and P. Jacques. Academic Press, New York *(in press)*.
13. Cheuk, S. F., Hahn, H. H., Moore, D. M., Krause, D. N., Tomasulo, P. A., and Wood, W. B., Jr. (1970): Studies on the pathogenesis of fever. XX. Suppression and regeneration of pyrogen-producing capacity of exudate granulocytes. *J. Exp. Med.*, 132:127–133.
14. Dinarello, C. A. (1979): Production of endogenous pyrogen. *Fed. Proc.*, 38:52–56.
15. Dinarello, C. A., Goldin, N. P., and Wolff, S. M. (1974): Demonstration and characterization of two distinct human leukocytic pyrogens. *J. Exp. Med.*, 139:1369–1381.
16. Dinarello, C. A., Renfer, L., and Wolff, S. M. (1977): The production of antibody against human leukocytic pyrogen. *J. Clin. Invest.*, 60:465–472.
17. Dinarello, C. A., Renfer, L., and Wolff, S. M. (1977): Human leukocytic pyrogen: Purification and development of a radioimmunoassay. *Proc. Natl. Acad. Sci. U.S.A.*, 74:4624–4627.
18. Eddington, C. L., Upchurch, H. F., and Kampschmidt, R. F. (1971): Effect of extracts from rabbit leukocytes on levels of acute phase globulins in rat serum. *Proc. Soc. Exp. Biol. Med.*, 136:159–164.
19. Eddington, C. L., Upchurch, H. F., and Kampschmidt, R. F. (1972): Quantitation of plasma alpha-2-AP globulin before and after stimulation with leukocytic extracts. *Proc. Soc. Exp. Biol. Med.*, 139:565–569.
20. Fessler, J. H., Cooper, K. E., Cranston, W. I., and Vollum, R. L. (1961): Observations on the production of pyrogenic substances by rabbit and human leucocytes. *J. Exp. Med.*, 113:1127–1137.
21. Hahn, H. H., Cheuk, S. F., Moore, D. M., and Wood, W. B., Jr. (1970): Studies on the

pathogenesis of fever. XVII. The cationic control of pyrogen release from exudate granulocytes *in vitro. J. Exp. Med.,* 131:165–178.

22. Hoff, F. (1959): Nonspecific resistance and nonspecific therapy. *Stanford Med. Bull.,* 17:133–141.
23. Homburger, F. (1945): A plasma fibrinogen-increasing factor obtained from sterile abscesses in dogs. *J. Clin. Invest.,* 24:43–45.
24. Kaiser, H. K., and Wood, B. W., Jr. (1962): Studies on the pathogenesis of fever. X. The effect of certain enzyme inhibitors on the production and activity of leucocytic pyrogen. *J. Exp. Med.,* 115:37–47.
25. Kampschmidt, R. F. (1978): Leukocytic endogenous mediator. *J. Reticuloendothel. Soc.,* 23:287–297.
26. Kampschmidt, R. F. (1979): Role of RES and leukocytic endogenous mediator in iron, zinc, and copper metabolism. In: *Macrophages and Lymphocytes: Nature, Functions and Interaction,* edited by M. R. Escobar and H. Friedman, pp. 403–411. Plenum Press, New York.
27. Kampschmidt, R. F., Long, R. D., and Upchurch, H. F. (1972): Neutrophil releasing activity in rats injected with endogenous pyrogen. *Proc. Soc. Exp. Biol. Med.,* 139:1224–1226.
28. Kampschmidt, R. F., and Pulliam, L. A. (1974): Effect of delayed hypersensitivity on plasma iron and zinc concentration and blood leukocytes. *Proc. Soc. Exp. Biol. Med.,* 147:242–244.
29. Kampschmidt, R. F., and Pulliam, L. A. (1975): Stimulation of antimicrobial activity in the rat with leukocytic endogenous mediator. *J. Reticuloendothel. Soc.,* 17:162–169.
30. Kampschmidt, R. F., and Pulliam, L. A. (1978): Effect of human monocyte pyrogen on plasma iron, plasma zinc, and blood neutrophils in rabbits and rats. *Proc. Soc. Exp. Biol. Med.,* 158:32–35.
31. Kampschmidt, R. F., Pulliam, L. A., and Merriman, C. R. (1978): Further similarities of endogenous pyrogen and leukocytic endogenous mediator. *Am. J. Physiol.,* 235:C118–C121.
32. Kampschmidt, R. F., Pulliam, L. A., and Upchurch, H. F. (1973): Sources of leukocytic endogenous mediator in the rat. *Proc., Soc. Exp. Biol. Med.,* 144:882–886.
33. Kampschmidt, R. F., and Upchurch, H. F. (1962): Effects of bacterial endotoxin on plasma iron. *Proc. Soc. Exp. Biol. Med.,* 110:191–193.
34. Kampschmidt, R. F., and Upchurch, H. (1968): Toxohormone. *Proc. Soc. Exp. Biol. Med.,* 127:632–635.
35. Kampschmidt, R. F., and Upchurch, H. F. (1969): Lowering of plasma iron concentration in the rat with leukocytic extracts. *Am. J. Physiol.,* 216:1287–1291.
36. Kampschmidt, R. F., and Upchurch, H. F. (1970): A comparison of the effects of rabbit endogenous pyrogen on the body temperature of the rabbit and lowering of plasma iron in the rat. *Proc. Soc, Exp. Biol. Med.,* 133:128–130.
37. Kampschmidt, R. F., and Upchurch, H. F. (1970): The effect of endogenous pyrogen on the plasma zinc concentration of the rat. *Proc. Soc. Exp. Biol. Med.,* 134:1150–1152.
38. Kampschmidt, R. F., and Upchurch, H. F. (1974): Effect of leukocytic endogenous mediator on plasma fibrinogen and haptoglobin. *Proc, Soc. Exp. Biol. Med.,* 146:904–907.
39. Kampschmidt, R. F., and Upchurch, H. F. (1977): Possible involvement of leukocytic endogenous mediator in granulopoiesis. *Proc. Soc. Exp. Biol. Med.,* 155:89–93.
40. Kampschmidt, R. F., Upchurch, H. F., Eddington, C. L., and Pulliam, L. A. (1973): Multiple biological activities of a partially purified leukocytic endogenous mediator. *Am. J. Physiol.,* 224:530–533.
41. Kampschmidt, R. F., Upchurch, H. F., and Pulliam, L. A. (1973): Investigations on the mode of action of endogenous mediator. *Proc. Soc. Exp. Biol. Med.,* 143:279–283.
42. King, M. K. (1960): Pathogenesis of fever: Effects of various endogenous pyrogens upon the level of circulating granulocytes in normal rabbits. *J. Exp. Med.,* 112:809–819.
43. Klempner, M. S., Dinarello, C. A., and Gallin, J. I. (1978): Human leukocytic pyrogen induces release of specific granule contents from human neutrophils. *J. Clin. Invest.,* 61:1330–1336.
44. Kozak, M. D., Hahn, H. H., Lennarz, W. J., and Wood, W. B., Jr. (1968): Studies on the pathogenesis of fever. XVI. Purification and further chemical characterization of granulocytic pyrogen. *J. Exp. Med.,* 127:341–357.
45. Mapes, C. A., and Sobocinski, P. Z. (1977): Differentiation between endogenous pyrogen and leukocytic endogenous mediator. *Am. J. Physiol.,* 232:C15–C22.
46. Masson, P. L., Heremans, J. F., and Schonne, E. (1969): Lactoferrin, an iron-binding protein in neutrophilic leukocytes. *J. Exp. Med.,* 130:643–656.

47. Menkin, V. (1956): *Biochemical Mechanisms in Inflammation.* Charles C Thomas, Springfield, Ill.
48. Merriman, C. R., Pulliam, L. A., and Kampschmidt, R. F. (1975): Effect of leukocytic endogenous mediator on C-reactive protein in rabbits. *Proc. Soc. Exp. Biol. Med.,* 149:782–784.
49. Merriman, C. R., Pulliam, L. A., and Kampschmidt, R. F. (1977): Comparison of leukocytic pyrogen and leukocytic endogenous mediator. *Proc. Soc. Exp. Biol. Med.,* 154:224–227.
50. Merriman, C. R., Upchurch, H. F., and Kampschmidt, R. F. (1978): Effects of leukocytic endogenous mediator on hemopexin, transferrin, and liver catalase. *Proc. Soc. Exp. Biol. Med.,* 157:669–671.
51. Moore, D. M., Cheuk, S. F., Morton, D., Berlin, R. D., and Wood, W. B., Jr. (1970): Studies on the pathogenesis of fever. XVIII. Activation of leukocytes for pyrogen production. *J. Exp. Med.,* 131:179–188.
52. Moses, J. M., Ebert, R. H., Graham, R. C., and Brine, K. L. (1964): Pathogenesis of inflammation. I. The production of an inflammatory substance from rabbit granulocytes *in vitro* and its relationship to leucocyte pyrogen. *J. Exp. Med.,* 120:57–81.
53. Murphy, P. A. Chesney, P. J., and Wood, W. B., Jr. (1974): Further purification of rabbit leukocyte pyrogen. *J. Lab. Clin. Med.,* 83:310–322.
54. Nordlund, J. J., Root, R. K., and Wolff, S. M. (1970): Studies on the origin of human leukocytic pyrogen. *J. Exp. Med.,* 131:727–743.
55. Pekarek, R. S., and Beisel, W. R. (1971): Characterization of the endogenous mediator(s) of serum zinc and iron depression during infection and other stresses. *Proc. Soc. Exp. Biol. Med.,* 138:728–732.
56. Pekarek, R. S., Powanda, M. C., and Wannemacher, R. W., Jr. (1972): The effect of leukocytic endogenous mediator (LEM) on serum copper and ceruloplasmin concentration in the rat. *Proc. Soc. Exp. Biol. Med.,* 141:1029–1031.
57. Pekarek, R. S., Wannemacher, R. W., Jr., Chapple, F. W., III, Powanda, M. C., and Beisel, W. R. (1972): Further characterization and species specificity of leukocytic endogenous mediator (LEM). *Proc. Soc. Exp. Biol. Med.,* 141:643–648.
58. Pekarek, R., Wannemacher, R. W., Jr., Powanda, M., Abeles, F., Mosher, D., Dinterman, R., and Beisel, W. (1974): Further evidence that leukocytic endogenous mediator (LEM) is not endotoxin. *Life Sci.,* 14:1765–1776.
59. Petersdorf, R. G., Keene, W. R., and Bennett, I. L. (1957): Studies on the pathogenesis of fever. IX. Characteristics of endogenous serum pyrogen and mechanisms governing its release. *J. Exp. Med.,* 106:787–809.
60. Rafter, G. W., Cheuk, S. F., Krause, D. W., and Wood, W. B., Jr. (1966): Studies on the pathogenesis of fever. XIV. Further observations on the chemistry of leukocytic pyrogen. *J. Exp. Med.,* 123:433–444.
61. Root, R. K., Nordlund, J. J., and Wolff, S. M. (1970): Factors affecting the quantitative production and assay of human leukocytic pyrogen. *J. Lab. Clin. Med.,* 75:679–693.
62. Rupp, R. G., and Fuller, G. M. (1979): The effects of leucocytic and serum factors on fibrinogen biosynthesis in cultured hepatocytes. *Exp. Cell Res.,* 118:23–30.
63. Selye, H. (1950): *Stress.* Acta Inc., Montreal, Canada.
64. Siegert, R., Philipp-Dormston, W. K., Radsak, K., and Menzel, H. (1976): Mechanism of fever induction in rabbits. *Infect. Immun.,* 14:1130–1137.
65. Thompson, W. L., Abeles, F. B., Beall, F. A., Dinterman, R. E., and Wannemacher, R. W., Jr. (1976): Influence of the adrenal glucocorticoids on the stimulation of synthesis of hepatic ribonucleic acid and plasma acute-phase globulins by leucocytic endogenous mediator. *Biochem. J.,* 156:25–32.
66. Van Snick, J. L., Masson, P. L., and Heremans, J. F. (1974): The involvement of lactoferrin in the hyposideremia of acute inflammation. *J. Exp. Med.,* 140:1068–1084.
67. Wannemacher, R. W., Jr., Pekarek, R. S., and Beisel, W. R. (1972): Mediator of hepatic amino acid flux in infected rats. *Proc. Soc. Exp. Biol. Med.,* 139:128–132.
68. Wannemacher, R. W., Jr., Pekarek, R. S., Thompson, W. L., Curnow, R. T., Beall, F. A., Zenser, T. V., DeRubertis, F. R., and Beisel, W. R. (1975): A protein from polymorphonuclear leukocytes (LEM) which affects the rate of hepatic amino acid transport and synthesis of acute-phase globulins. *Endocrinology,* 96:651–661.

Fever, edited by James M. Lipton.
Raven Press, New York © 1980.

Fever and Gastric Function

Adelbert S. J. P. A. M. van Miert

Institute of Veterinary Pharmacology and Toxicology, Faculty of Veterinary Medicine, The State University, 3572 BP Utrecht, The Netherlands

It would be a pity to start my chapter without referring to the early studies done by Dr. Carlson and his colleagues from the Hull Physiology Laboratory of the University of Chicago. The results of their studies were reported in 1917 and 1918. However, this work received little attention. Carlson observed that dogs with distemper or pneumonia refused food and showed complete atony of the stomach with absence of hunger contractions, especially during fever episodes. In addition, they performed some experiments in which fever was evoked by pyrogens, such as sodium nucleinate and a killed culture of *Serratia marcescens.* They concluded that gastric secretion and hunger contractions were absent in marked fever and that these effects were associated with anorexia as long as fever was present. *In vitro* experiments showed that these pyrogens did not have any direct effect on the stomach smooth muscle. The splanchnic nerves did not appear to be involved either. However, after transection of the vagus nerve, gastric hunger contractions persisted during pyrexia (30,31).

Since that time, other investigators have confirmed the inhibition of gastric secretion by pyrogens, although little has been done to elucidate the mechanisms underlying this inhibitory effect (2,3,7,8,54,65). Furthermore, little is known about the effect of pyrogens on the gastric emptying rate (52). In veterinary medicine it is well known that acute febrile diseases cause gastrointestinal dysfunction in most animal species. Especially in ruminants, inhibition of forestomach motility is a frequent complication in febrile diseases (9,10,13,17,18.)

The inhibition of gastric motility may have serious consequences in some patients. For example, diminished forestomach contractions during clinical fever inhibit the microbial degradation of ingested feed and the elimination of fermentation gases in ruminants. Moreover, the diminished gastric emptying rate in febrile diseases poses potential therapeutic problems by altering the absorption of drugs administered orally to treat these conditions (21,22).

Normal forestomach contractions consist of (a) weak, localized intrinsic movements occurring six to nine times per minute: and (b) characteristic, powerful extrinsic contraction sequences, which occur approximately once per minute and which are wholly dependent on reflex mechanisms involving afferent and efferent pathways in vagal nerves and bilateral "gastric centers" in the medulla oblongata (26). The forestomach compartments (reticulum, rumen, and omasum) are separated from the true acid-secreting stomach (abomasum). We have studied the extent to which motility of the reticulorumen was inhibited during hyperthermia and in various forms of experimentally induced fever. In parallel studies we examined the inhibitory effect of endotoxin on gastric secretion and motility in rats.

Goats were trained to stand quietly during actual recording sessions by repeatedly placing them in the experimental cage for several hours at a time passing nasal catheters into the rumen. Recordings of intragastric pressure changes were made by means of an open-ended water-filled polyethylene tube passed into the rumen and connected to a pressure transducer. The frequency (RF) and the amplitude (RA) of the rumen contractions were measured every 15 min and expressed as percentages of the initial value. Rectal temperatures were measured with an electrothermometer. A fever index, the area under the curves, was calculated. A frequency and amplitude index for rumen contractions was calculated in a similar way. Heartbeat frequency was taken from electrocardiograph recordings (37,38,42,43,48).

EFFECTS OF EXOGENOUS PYROGENS

Intravenous injection of exogenous pyrogens such as endotoxins (from *Escherichia coli* or *Salmonella typhimurium*), Newcastle disease virus, Poly 1:Poly C, sodium nucleinate from yeast, or johnin challenge after vaccination with *Mycobacterium johnei* induced fever, changes in heart rate, and inhibition of extrinsic ruminal contractions, although there were differences in latency time and the shape of the temperature curves (40,42). From these experiments we concluded that in conditions associated with fever, there is an inhibition of forestomach contractions. This is in agreement with observations made in patients during febrile episodes.

The reactions of adult goats to the intravenous administration of *E. coli* endotoxin were studied in more detail. The main symptoms observed were depression, anorexia, increased respiration rate, occasional coughing fits, micturition, increased defecation rate, and salivation. Other clinical symptoms were shivering, a rise in body temperature, simultaneous inhibition of the reticuloruminal contractions (Fig. 1) changes in heart rate, leukopenia, and hyperglycemia followed by hypoglycemia.[1] Latency to response, duration of shivering, the shape of the temperature curves, and the magnitude of the inhibition of the ruminal contractions were all dose dependent (36). If the inhibition of rumen motility (amplitude and frequency index) and the change in body temperature (fever index) are plotted against the dose of *E. coli* endotoxin injected (the latter in

---

[1] Moreover, Cakala (12) observed a diminution of abomasal secretion during endotoxin-induced fever.

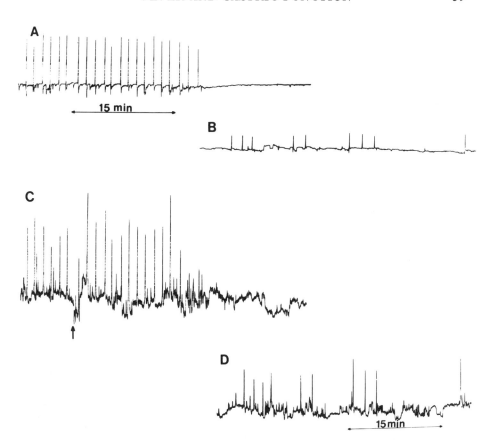

FIG. 1. The effect of pyrogen on extrinsic contractions of the reticulum **(A,B)** and rumen **(C,D)** in a conscious goat. After i.v. injection (↑) of *E. coli* LPS 0.2 µg/kg body weight, there was a latent period during which 15 reticulorumen contraction sequences of normal form and amplitude occurred. Thereafter a complete stasis developed. **B** and **D**: Spontaneous reappearance of the contractions 280 min after the injection. (From van Miert et al., ref. 48a, with permission.)

a logarithmic scale), the relationship between the dose and these effects can be seen (Fig. 2). It is concluded from this experiment that inhibition of rumen motility is not secondary to rise in body temperature.

It has been suggested that there is a good correlation between increase in heart rate and rise in body temperature during fever. Such a correlation, for instance, exists in human patients with viral pneumonia (15). However, in our experiments we did not find such correlation (40,42). Moreover, no such correlation was observed in goats infected with *Trypanosoma vivax (62)* or cattle infected with *E. coli* mastitis (63).

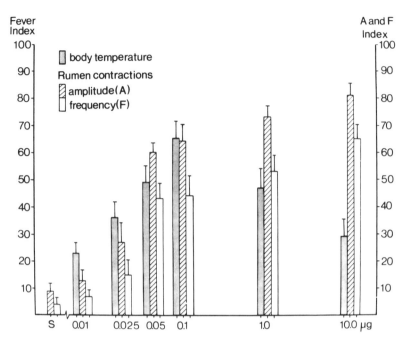

FIG. 2. Pyrogenicity and changes in rumen motility after *E. coli* LPS (batch 481424). Fever index, rumen amplitude (A) index, and rumen frequency (F) index were calculated for a 5-hr period after i.v. injection of the pyrogen for a group of 5 goats given varying doses as indicated. These doses (per kg body weight) were given at intervals of 3 weeks to avoid the development of tolerance. S = saline 0.1 ml/kg body weight i.v. Mean value ± SE are shown. (Modified from van Miert, ref. 36).

EFFECT OF ENDOGENOUS PYROGEN AND HYPERTHERMIA

The temperature responses induced with exogenous pyrogens were biphasic (40,42). The basis for the biphasic response is a matter of speculation. Some investigators believe that the first temperature peak observed after endotoxin administration is produced by direct action of this pyrogen on thermoregulatory centers and the second peak is due to released endogenous pyrogen (4,51). We have demonstrated the presence of endogenous pyrogen in the blood of goats during endotoxin-induced fever (37,38,40). Heat-labile endogenous pyrogen evoked febrile responses characterized by monophasic temperature curves and by a shorter latency time, a more rapid rise to peak fever, and a quicker return to the initial temperature level than produced by the relatively heat-stable exogenous pyrogens. However, a marked inhibitory effect on the extrinsic ruminal contractions was not observed (40). Moreover, an inhibition of rumen motility was not seen during fever evoked by intramammary administered endotoxin (an example is shown in Fig. 3).

It is known that a physically induced rise of body temperature affects gastric

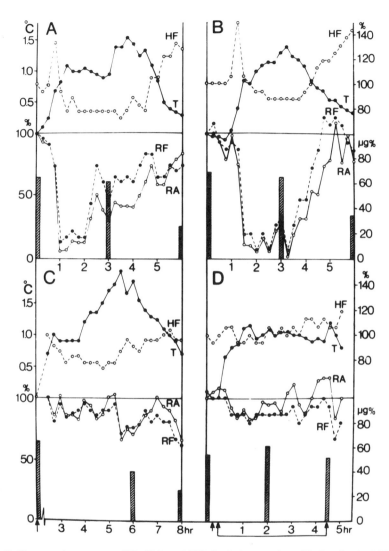

FIG. 3. Changes in rumen motility (RA and RF), body temperature (T), heart rate (HF), and plasma zinc level *(bars)* after pyrogen administration in a conscious goat. *E. coli* LPS (batch 614378) was given: **A,** intravenously 0.1 μg/kg; **B,** intramuscularly 1 μg/kg; **C,** intramammary 1 mg. These experiments were done at intervals of 3 weeks to avoid the development of tolerance. Thereafter tolerance was induced by 10 daily injections of *E. coli* LPS 0.1 μg/kg body weight. Next, leukocytic pyrogen was administered **(D)**. A priming injection of 5 ml/kg was given followed by a continuous infusion at the rate of 2 ml/min (total dose 665 ml ∼ 9.10[9] leukocytes). RF, frequency of rumen contractions per 15 min expressed in percentages of the initial value; RA, summation derived from 15-min intervals of amplitude expressed in percentages of the initial value. (From Verheÿen, ref. 63.)

secretion (2,8). It therefore seemed of interest to investigate the effect of hyper-thermia on the motility of forestomachs (32). The evidence obtained in this experiment suggests that body temperature elevation itself is a factor in the depression of gastric motility. This is in agreement with the observations made in monogastric species during hyperthermia (30,49). Still, it is difficult to compare the effects during hyperthermia and fever as such. For instance, respiratory alkaloses due to overventilation can be observed during severe hyperthermia (5), whereas a decrease in blood pH is a consistent finding during fever (20,50).

ROLE OF CATECHOLAMINES

It is known that during hyperthermia (1,58) and also during endotoxin-induced fever (55,59), a marked increase of catecholamines occurs. Moreover, in rumi-nants, hyperglycemia can be observed during endotoxin-induced fever (11,36,50). On the basis of *in vitro* observations, we concluded that in the ruminal smooth muscle both α-stimulatory and β-inhibitory adrenergic receptors are present (46). In the intact animal, α- and β-adrenergic drugs both interfere with extrinsic reticuloruminal contractions, probably by reflex inhibition (33,34).

However, an intravenous infusion with α- and β-adrenergic receptor-blocking agents did not oppose the action of endotoxin on heart rate and rumen motility. Moreover, adrenalectomy or transection of the splanchnic nerves did not an-tagonize the inhibition of rumen contractions to endotoxin either (35). Pretreat-ment with α-methyldopa caused a significant dose-related decrease in fever re-sponse to endotoxin. The temperature response to endogenous pyrogen was also reduced or abolished (39). Pretreatment with α-methyldopa had only a partial antagonistic influence on endotoxin-induced ruminal stasis (35). Since the inhibition of ruminal contractions also occurred under conditions in which there was no rise in body temperature, it was concluded that the inhibition is not primarily due to the temperature response.

In our experiments with rats, *E. coli* endotoxin did not induce fever (45). Nevertheless, inhibition of gastric secretion (29) and gastric emptying rate (47) was observed. Pretreatment with α-methyldopa did not reduce the inhibitory effect of endotoxin on gastric emptying rate in the rat (47). In other words, the effects of endotoxin on thermoregulation and on the stomach seem to be due to different mechanisms. In the rat, too, adrenalectomy or adrenergic recep-tor blocking agents did not oppose the inhibitory effects of endotoxin on gastric function (29,47).

EFFECT OF NONSTEROIDAL ANTI-INFLAMMATORY AGENTS

The intravenous injection of PGE or PGF$_{2\alpha}$ caused inhibition of extrinsic ruminal contractions in conscious goats (61). In rabbit plasma both PGE and PGF concentrations increased considerably during fever evoked by *E. coli* endo-

TABLE 1. Fever and inhibition of rumen motility by endotoxins and modification of these effects by flurbiprofen[a]

Test agents	Dose per kg i.v. (μg)	Fever index ± SEM			Rumen amplitude index ± SEM			Rumen frequency index ± SEM			N[b]
		0–1.5	1.5–3	3–5 hr	0–1.5	1.5–3	3–5 hr	0–1.5	1.5–3	3–5 hr	
LPS E. coli	0.01	4.1 ± 0.8	12.9 ± 1.7	14.8 ± 2.6	5.8 ± 1.2	11.9 ± 2.8	15.3 ± 4.5	3.9 ± 0.8	8.2 ± 2.9	13.1 ± 4.5	7
LPS + drug	0.01	−2.9 ± 0.9c	−3.1 ± 1.0c	−2.5 ± 1.9c	3.6 ± 0.9	11.9 ± 4.0	17.8 ± 4.6	3.9 ± 1.2	6.4 ± 1.4	13.8 ± 4.5	
LPS E. coli	0.1	6.3 ± 1.7	16.0 ± 3.7	27.6 ± 3.1	14.0 ± 1.6	24.1 ± 0.6	30.9 ± 3.2	11.4 ± 2.2	20.3 ± 2.1	23.1 ± 2.3	4
LPS + drug	0.1	−2.7 ± 1.0c	−1.7 ± 1.2c	0.1 ± 1.6c	2.2 ± 1.0c	12.2 ± 2.1c	24.3 ± 2.9	2.3 ± 1.1c	8.8 ± 1.3c	18.6 ± 2.7	
LPS S. typhimurium	0.3	7.0 ± 1.1	17.2 ± 2.6	31.0 ± 4.2	11.1 ± 1.9	22.7 ± 1.1	29.4 ± 2.1	8.4 ± 1.9	16.4 ± 1.6	27.4 ± 1.8	7
LPS + drug	0.3	−1.3 ± 0.4c	−3.2 ± 0.9c	−3.4 ± 2.5c	4.5 ± 1.0c	18.2 ± 1.7	30.3 ± 2.1	3.3 ± 0.8c	13.5 ± 2.2	24.7 ± 3.2	

[a] Sodium flurbiprofen, dissolved in saline, was given i.v. 2 mg/kg body weight, immediately followed by i.v. administration of the pyrogen.
[b] Number of goats.
[c] Significantly different, $p < 0.05$.

toxin (57). Philipp-Dormston and Siegert (57) suggested that the enhanced PG concentrations in the plasma might be responsible for the various pathological effects observed during fever, such as diarrhea and abortion. Nonsteroidal anti-inflammatory agents such as flurbiprofen inhibited the prostaglandin synthetase system (6,14,16). In our experiments, the febrile responses to pyrogens were completely abolished by the prior intravenous administration of flurbiprofen (41,42,48). Nevertheless, endotoxin-induced inhibition of forestomach motility occurred (42,48). The drug had no significant effect on ruminal stasis induced by a small dose of *E. coli* endotoxin (0.01 µg/kg). However, the same dose of flurbiprofen had a significant partial antagonistic influence if higher doses of endotoxin were used (Table 1). Pretreatment with other antipyretic agents such as sodium meclofenamate, acetaminophen, and phenylbutazone also had a partial antagonistic influence on endotoxin-induced ruminal stasis if higher doses of the pyrogen were used (48). Therefore, it is likely that the change in forestomach motility after i.v. injection of exogenous pyrogens is the combined result of two different mechanisms: a temperature-dependent and a temperature-independent inhibitory mechanism. This could also explain the effect of α-methyldopa on endotoxin-induced ruminal stasis.

RESULTS OF ELECTROPHYSIOLOGICAL STUDIES

Reticuloruminal responses to endotoxin similar to those of conscious sheep and goats were also obtained in halothane-anesthetized sheep, allowing a closer analysis of the mechanisms underlying the action of the pyrogen. Endotoxin-induced inhibition of extrinsic reticulum contractions was present even after (a) transection of the brainstem at the level of the pons so that the gastric centers were no longer under the influence of higher centers, including the thermoregulatory regions of the hypothalamus; and (b) removal of the abomasum. Abomasal acidity is a potent excitatory stimulus for the extrinsic forestomach contractions. Endotoxin-induced stasis, however, was not secondary to a reduction in gastric acid secretion and hence reduced excitatory input to the gastric centers.

During stasis, electrical stimulation of the efferent gastric vagal fibers evoked extrinsic contractions similar to those obtained before endotoxin administration. In other words, endotoxin did not induce a neuromuscular blockade. Conversely, electrical stimulation of the afferent gastric vagal fibers did not evoke reflex contractions except during an initial period lasting about 5 to 10 min after the onset of stasis and until the spontaneous reappearance of extrinsic contractions. This observation may mean that gastric center depression is a major cause of all except the initial part of the period of stasis. During this initial episode, no electrical activity was observed in the afferent gastric vagal fibers, perhaps as a result of smooth muscle relaxation. During the later part of stasis, supranormal bursts of electrical activity occurred. These were interpreted as being due to more forceful intrinsic contractions. These discharges, however, did not induce reflex extrinsic contractions, because of the gastric center depression described above.

The overall conclusions (27,28,34) were that endotoxin-induced stasis could be explained on the basis that (a) there is a latent period, after which the pyrogen may induce the release of intermediates which cause changes in smooth muscle tone; (b) the initial part of the stasis is due to smooth muscle relaxation in the gastric wall, which causes reflex inhibition by reduced excitatory input to the gastric centers; and (c) the later part of the stasis is due to the depression of the gastric centers.

ROLE OF HUMORAL SUBSTANCES IN RELATION TO THE PERIPHERAL EFFECTS INDUCED BY INTRAVENOUS ENDOTOXIN ADMINISTRATION

Several pharmacologically active substances including histamine, serotonin, plasma kinins, and prostaglandins have been implicated in the mechanism of endotoxin shock (19,23–25,56,64). Little is known about the influence of small

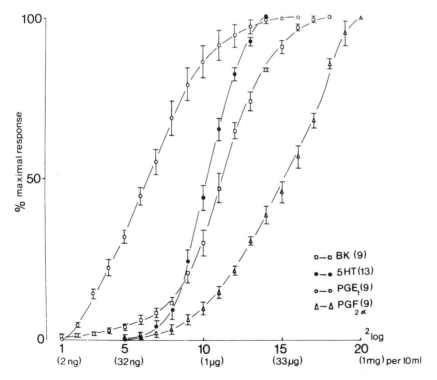

FIG. 4. Log dose-response curves for contraction of goat ruminal smooth muscle strips by bradykinin (BK), serotonin (5HT), prostaglandin E_1 (PGE$_1$), and prostaglandin $F_{2\alpha}$ (PGF$_{2\alpha}$). Mean values $\pm$ SE are given. Number of experiments in parentheses. (From Veenendaal, ref. 60.)

pyrogenic doses of endotoxin on the synthesis and/or release of these substances. The question as to which humoral substance is primarily responsible for mediating the forestomach responses induced by small pyrogenic doses of endotoxin cannot be answered conclusively from our experiments. Certain conclusions can, however, be drawn. *In vitro* experiments showed that neither endotoxin nor endogenous pyrogen had any effect on the ruminal smooth muscle (34). However, bradykinin, serotonin, PGE_1, and $PGF_{2\alpha}$ induced a dose-dependent increase in smooth muscle tonus (Fig. 4). Histamine caused different types of responses: contraction (H1 receptors), relaxation (H2 receptors), or contraction followed by relaxation (53). Intravenous injection of these substances evoked inhibition of extrinsic ruminal contractions in conscious goats, probably by reflex mechanisms (44,60,61). No change of whole blood serotonin level was found during endotoxin-induced fever, and only a small increase of the whole blood bradykinin-like activity could be detected (62). Attempts to detect changes in plasma prostaglandin concentrations during endotoxin-induced fever were unsuccessful (60). Moreover, intravenous infusion or injection with H1, H2, or serotonin receptor blocking agents did not oppose the action of endotoxin on rumen motility (44,60).

From experiments with antipyretic agents such as flurbiprofen, it seems unlikely that the inhibition of forestomach motility by endotoxin is primarily due to a release of prostaglandins (42,48). Although it seems unlikely that inhibition of reticuloruminal motility by exogenous pyrogens is simply due to a peripheral release of the humoral substances mentioned before, it still may be considered that a combination of these factors or other unknown mediators might be responsible for mediating the changes in gastric smooth muscle tonus during fever.

EFFECTS OF INTRACEREBRAL INJECTION OF ENDOTOXIN

The administration of a small dose of endotoxin (0.01 μg *E. coli* LPS) into the third ventricle of conscious goats induced shivering, a biphasic rise in body temperature, and inhibition of extrinsic ruminal contractions (43). A similar dose of this pyrogen given i.v. was much less effective (Fig. 5). The changes in arterial blood pressure and reticulum motility that resulted from an endotoxin injection near the left and right dorsal vagal nuclei in an anesthetized ewe were similar to those produced by intravenous injection of this pyrogen (34,43). The equivalent effects on blood pressure and rumen motility required an i.v. dose of *E. coli* endotoxin about 100 times larger than that required on injection into the medulla oblongata. This demonstrates that the effects were not due to a leakage of the pyrogen into the systemic circulation. These findings indicate that biphasic temperature response and inhibition of reticulorumen motility can be reproduced by an action of endotoxin within the central nervous system. However, the clinical symptoms were preceded by a certain time lag, which suggests that the action of endotoxin within the CNS is an indirect one. A

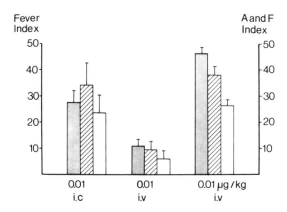

FIG. 5. Fever index, rumen amplitude (A) index, and rumen frequency (F) index calculated for a 4-hr period after injection of *E. coli* LPS (batch 487989) into the third ventricle of the brain (i.c.) or given by the intravenous route (i.v.). The effects of 0.01 μg/kg body weight are shown on the right-hand side. Mean values ± SE are given (*N* = 4). (See also Fig. 2.)

detailed study of the processes within the CNS responsible for pyrogen-induced gastric dysfunction is still required.

REFERENCES

1. Andersson, B., Gale, C. C., Hökfelt, B., and Ohga, A. (1963): Relation of preoptic temperature to the function of the sympathico-adrenomedullary system and the adrenal cortex. *Acta Physiol. Scand.,* 61:182–191.
2. Bandes, J., Hollander, F., and Bierman, W. (1948): The effect of physically induced pyrexia on gastric acidity. *Gastroenterology,* 10:697–707.
3. Baume, P. E., Nicholls, A., and Baxter, C. H. (1967): Inhibition of gastric acid secretion by a purified bacterial lipopolysaccharide. *Nature,* 215:59–60.
4. Bennett, I. L., and Cluff, L. E. (1957): Bacterial pyrogens. *Pharmacol. Rev.,* 9:429–475.
5. Bianca, W., and Findlay, J. D. (1962): The effect of thermally induced hyperpnoea on the acid-base status of the blood of calves. *Res. Vet. Sci.,* 3:38–49.
6. Blackham, A., and Owen, R. T. (1975): Prostaglandin synthetase inhibitors and leucocytic emigration. *J. Pharm. Pharmacol.,* 27:201–202.
7. Blickenstaff, D. and Grossman, M. I. (1950): A quantitative study of the reduction of gastric acid secretion associated with pyrexia. *Am. J. Physiol.,* 160:567–571.
8. Brodie, D. A., and Kundrats, S. K. (1964): The effect of pyrexia on rat gastric secretion. *Gastroenterology,* 47:171–178.
9. Brunaud, M. (1954): Données actuelles sur la physiologie et la pharmacodynamie des estomacs des ruminants. *Rev. Med. Vet.,* 105:535–580.
10. Burgess, G. W., and Spradbrow, P. B. (1977): Studies on the pathogenesis of bovine ephemeral fever. *Aust. Vet. J.,* 53:363–368.
11. Cakala, S. (1965): Studies on the fever in sheep. II. Influence of fever on certain physiological indices in blood of sheep. *Bull. Vet. Inst. Pulawy,* 9:111–127.
12. Cakala, S. (1968): Influence of bacterial pyrogens and of insulin on the rumen motility and the abomasal secretion in goats. *Pol. Arch. Weter.,* 11:95–109.
13. Clark, R. (1956): Refresher courses in physiology. The mechanics of the ruminant stomach. *J. S. Afr. Vet. Assoc.,* 27:75–104.
14. Cook, C., and Collins, A. J. (1975): Prostaglandin synthetase activity from human rheumatoid

synovial tissue and its inhibition by nonsteroidal anti-inflammatory drugs. *Prostaglandins,* 9:857–868.

15. Cooper, K. E. (1971): Some physiological and clinical aspects of pyrogens. In: *Pyrogens and Fever,* edited by G. E. W. Wolstenhome and J. Birch, pp. 5–21. Churchill-Livingstone, Edinburgh.

16. Crook, D., Collins, A. J., and Rose, A. J. (1976): A comparison of the effect of flurbiprofen on prostaglandin synthetase from human rheumatoid synovium and enzymatically active animal tissue. *J. Pharm. Pharmacol.,* 28:535.

17. Diernhofer, K. (1953): Diagnose und Behandlung der Indigestionen des Rindes. *Wien. Tieraerztl. Wochenschr.,* 40:531–547.

18. Diernhofer, K. (1959): Vormagenerkrankungen des Rindes, Probleme und Erfahrungen. *Dtsch. Tieraerztl. Wochenschr.,* 66:141–149.

19. Erdös, E. G., and Miwa, I. (1968): Effect of endotoxin on the kallikrein kinin system of the rabbit. *Fed. Proc.,* 27:92–95.

20. Going, H., and Kaiser, P. (1966): Aufbau und Wirkungsweise bakterieller Endotoxine. In: *Ergebnisse der Mikrobiologie, Immunitätsforschung und experimentellen Therapie,* Vol. 39, edited by W. Henle, W. Kikuth, R. F. Meyer, E. G., Nauck, and J. Tomcsik, pp. 243–326. Springer-Verlag, Berlin.

21. Groothuis, D. G. (1980): The pharmacokinetic behaviour of antimicrobial drugs in veal calves and their antibacterial activity in relation to salmonellosis *(S. dublin).* Ph.D. thesis, University of Utrecht, The Netherlands.

22. Groothuis, D. G., van Miert, A. S. J. P. A. M., Ziv, G., and Nouws, J. F. M. (1978): Effects of experimental *E. coli* endotoxaemia on ampicillin-amoxycillin blood levels after oral and parenteral administration in calves. *J. Vet. Pharmacol. Ther.,* 1:81–84.

23. Herman, A. G., and Vane, J. R. (1974): On the mechanism of the release of prostaglandins E_2 and $F_{2\alpha}$ in renal venous blood during endotoxin-hypotension. *Arch. Int. Pharmacodyn. Ther.,* 208:365–366.

24. Herman, A. G, and Vane, J. R. (1976): Release of renal prostaglandins during endotoxin-induced hypotension. *Eur. J. Pharmacol.,* 39:79–90.

25. Hinshaw, L. B. (1964): The release of vasoactive agents by endotoxin. In: *Bacterial Endotoxins,* edited by M. Landy and W. Braun, pp. 118–125. Rutgers University Press, New Brunswick, N.J.

26. Leek, B. F. (1969): Reticulo-ruminal function and dysfunction. *Vet. Rec.,* 84:238–243.

27. Leek, B. F., and van Miert, A. S. J. P. A. M. (1971): An analysis of the pyrogen-induced inhibition of gastric motility in sheep. *J. Physiol. (Lond.),* 215:28P-29P.

28. Leek, B. F., and van Miert, A. S. J. P. A. M. (1971): An analysis of the gastric stasis induced by pyrogen: The effects on intrinsic and extrinsic movements of the ruminant forestomach. *Rendic. Rom. Gastroenterol.,* 3:163–167.

29. Leenen, F. H. H., and van Miert, A. S. J. P. A. M. (1969): Inhibition of gastric secretion by bacterial lipopolysaccharide in the rat. *Eur. J. Pharmacol.,* 8:228–231.

30. Meyer, J., and Carlson, A. J. (1917): Contributions to the physiology of the stomach. XLIII. Hunger and appetite in fever. *Am. J. Physiol.,* 44:222–233.

31. Meyer, J., Cohen, S. J., and Carlson, A. J. (1918): Contribution to the physiology of the stomach. XLVI. Gastric secretion during fever. *Arch. Intern. Med.,* 21:354–365.

32. Miert, A. S. J. P. A. M. van (1969): The effect of bacterial pyrogen and hyperthermia on rumen motility in the goat. *Acta Physiol. Pharmacol. Neerl.,* 15:57–58.

33. Miert, A. S. J. P. A. M van (1969): The effect of α- and β-sympathicomimetics on rumen motility and heart rate frequency in conscious goats. *J. Pharm. Pharmacol.,* 21:697–699.

34. Miert, A. S. J. P. A. M. van (1970): Inhibition of reticulo-rumen motility during fever induced by bacterial pyrogen—lipopolysaccharides from Gram-negative bacteria—in sheep and goats. Ph. D. thesis, University of Utrecht, Utrecht, The Netherlands.

35. Miert, A. S. J. P. A. M. van (1971): Inhibition of gastric motility by endotoxin (bacterial lipopolysaccharide) in conscious goats and modification of this response by splanchnectomy, adrenalectomy or adrenergic blocking agents. *Arch. Int. Pharmacodyn. Ther.,* 193:404–415.

36. Miert, A. S. J. P. A. M. van (1973): Clinical symptoms induced by *E. coli* endotoxin in goats. *Zentralbl. Veterinaermed. [A],* 20:614–623.

37. Miert, A. S. J. P. A. M. van, and Atmakusuma, A. (1970): Comparative observations on the production of fever by bacterial pyrogens and leucocytic pyrogen in goats and rabbits. *Zentralbl. Veterinaermed. [A],* 17:174–184.

38. Miert, A. S. J. P. A. M. van, and Atmakusuma, A. (1971): Fever induced with leucocytic or bacterial pyrogen in young and adult goats. *J. Comp. Pathol.*, 81:119–127.
39. Miert, A. S. J. P. A. M. van, and van Duin, C. T. M. (1972): The antipyretic effect of α-methyldopa in experimental fever. *J. Pharm. Pharmacol.*, 24:988–990.
40. Miert, A. S. J. P. A. M. van, and van Duin, C. T. M. (1974): The effects of bacterial pyrogens and leucocytic pyrogen upon gastric motility and heart rate frequency in conscious goats. *Zentralbl. Veterinaermed. [A]*, 21:692–702.
41. Miert, A. S. J. P. A. M. van, and van Duin, C. T. M. (1977): The antipyretic effect of flurbiprofen. *Eur. J. Pharmacol.*, 44:197–204.
42. Miert, A. S. J. P. A. M. van, and van Duin, C. T. M. (1979): The effect of flurbiprofen upon fever and ruminal stasis induced by *E. coli* endotoxin, Poly I:Poly C and sodium nucleinate from yeast in conscious goats. *J. Vet. Pharmacol. Ther.*, 2:69–79.
43. Miert, A. S. J. P. A. M. van, van Duin, C. T. M., and Leek, B. F. (1978): Effects on reticulo-rumen motility and body temperature of *E. coli* endotoxin on injection into the medulla oblongata and third ventricle of small ruminants. *Zentralbl. Veterinaermed. [A]*, 25:718–726.
44. Miert, A. S. J. P. A. M. van, van Duin, C. T. M., and Veenendaal, G. H. (1976): Role of histamine in the genesis of pyrogen (endotoxin)-induced reticulo-ruminal stasis in goats. *Zentralbl. Veterinaermed. [A]*, 23:819–826.
45. Miert, A. S. J. P. A. M. van, and Frens, J. (1968): The reaction of different animal species to bacterial pyrogens. *Zentralbl. Veterinaermed. [A]*, 15:532–543.
46. Miert, A. S. J. P. A. M. van, and Huisman, E. A. (1968): Adrenergic receptors in the ruminal wall of sheep. *J. Pharm. Pharmacol.*, 20:495–496.
47. Miert, A. S. J. P. A. M. van, and de la Parra, D. A. (1970): Inhibition of gastric emptying by endotoxin (bacterial lipopolysaccharide) in conscious rats and modification of this response by drugs affecting the autonomic nervous system. *Arch. Int. Pharmacodyn. Ther.*, 184:27–33.
48. Miert, A. S. J. P. A. M. van, van der Wal-Komproe, L. E., and van Duin, C. T. M. (1977): Effects of antipyretic agents on fever and ruminal stasis induced by endotoxins in conscious goats. *Arch. Int. Pharmacodyn. Ther.*, 225:39–50.
48a. Miert, A. S. J. P. A. M. van, Veenendaal, G. H., and van Genderen, H. (1976): Pharmakologische Untersuchungen über die Hemmung der Magenmotilität bei experimentellem Fieber. *Dtsch. Tieraertzl. Wochenschr.*, 83:188–192.
49. Misiewicz, J. J., Waller, S. L., Fox, R. H., Goldsmith, R., and Hunt, T. J. (1968): The effect of elevated body temperature and of stress on the motility of stomach and colon in man. *Clin. Sci.*, 34:149–159.
50. Mullenax, C. H., Keller, R. F., and Allison, M. J. (1966): Physiologic responses of ruminants to toxic factors extracted from rumen bacteria and rumen fluid. *Am. J. Vet. Res.*, 27:857–868.
51. Myers, R. D., Rudy, T. A., and Yaksh, T. L. (1973): Evocation of a biphasic febrile response in the rhesus monkey by intracerebral injection of bacterial endotoxins. *Neuropharmacology*, 12:1195–1198.
52. Necheles, H., Dommers, P., Weiner, M., Olson, W. H., and Rychel, W. (1942): Depression of gastric motility without elevation of body temperature following the injections of pyrogens. *Am. J. Physiol.*, 137:22–29.
53. Ohga, A., and Taneike, T. (1978): H_1- and H_2-receptors in the smooth muscle of the ruminant stomach. *Br. J. Pharmacol.*, 62:333–337.
54. Olson, W. H., Walker, L., and Necheles, H. (1954): Depression of gastric secretion without elevation of temperature following injection of pyrogens. *Am. J. Physiol.*, 176:393–395.
55. Ouellette, J. J., Chosy, J. J., and Reed, C. H. (1967): Catecholamine excretion and bronchial response to methacholine after *Salmonella enteriditis* endotoxin in a normal and an "asthmatic subject." *J. Allergy*, 39:234–237.
56. Parratt, J. R., and Sturgess, R. M. (1977): The possible roles of histamine, 5-hydroxytryptamine and prostaglandin $F_{2\alpha}$ as mediators of the acute pulmonary effects of endotoxin. *Br. J. Pharmacol.*, 60:209–219.
57. Philipp-Dormston, W. K., and Siegert, R. (1974): Plasma prostaglandins of the E and F series in rabbits during fever induced by Newcastle disease virus, *E. coli* endotoxin, or endogenous pyrogen. *Z. Naturforsch.*, 29c:773–776.
58. Robertshaw, D., and Whittow, G. C. (1966): The effect of hyperthermia and localized heating of the anterior hypothalamus on the sympathoadrenal system of the ox *(Bos taurus)*. *J. Physiol. (Lond.)*, 187:351–360.

59. Serafimov, N. (1962): Urinary excretion of catecholamines in endotoxin-induced fever in rabbits. *Acta Physiol. Scand.,* 54:354–358.
60. Veenendaal, G. H. (1979): Role of circulating inflammatory substances in the genesis of pyrogen (endotoxin)-induced ruminal stasis in goats. Ph.D. thesis, University of Utrecht, Utrecht, The Netherlands.
61. Veenendaal, G. H., and van Miert, A. S. J. P. A. M. (1979): Responses of ruminal smooth muscle to serotoin, bradykinin and prostaglandins in vitro and in vivo. *Res. Vet. Sci. (in press).*
62. Veenendaal, G. H., van Miert, A. S. J. P. A. M., van de Ingh, T. S. G. A. M., Schotman, A. J. H., and Zwart, D. (1976): A comparison of the role of kinins and serotonin in endotoxin induced fever and *Trypanosoma vivax* infections in the goat. *Res. Vet. Sci.,* 21:271–279.
63. Verheijden, J. H. M. (1979): Acute coliform mastitis in cattle. Ph.D. thesis, University of Utrecht, Utrecht, The Netherlands.
64. Vick, J. A., Mehlman, B., and Heiffer, M. H. (1971): Early histamine release and death due to endotoxin. *Proc. Soc. Exp. Biol. Med.,* 137:902–906.
65. Wyllie, J. H., Limbosch, J. M., and Nyhuis, L. M. (1967): Inhibition of gastric acid secretion by bacterial lipopolysaccharide. *Nature,* 215:879.

Fever, edited by James M. Lipton.
Raven Press, New York © 1980.

Central Inactivation of Endogenous Pyrogens

James M. Lipton

Physiology and Neurology Departments, Southwestern Medical School, University of Texas Health Science Center at Dallas, Dallas, Texas 75235

Despite the importance of defervescence in clinical medicine, little attempt has been made to explain the events responsible for termination of fever. The presumption has been that defervescence occurs when pathological processes responsible for endogenous pyrogen release abate and the level of circulating pyrogen diminishes as a result of both (a) reduced pyrogen formation and (b) its continued catabolism. As a result of reduction in circulating pyrogen, fever is not maintained, and body temperature returns to normal. This presumption is plausible, but it offers no specific hypothesis about the fate of endogenous pyrogen that reaches the brain. Because pyrogen produces fever only by acting on CNS temperature controls, the process of central inactivation of pyrogen is of crucial importance to defervescence. Much as for central neurotransmitters, the action of which must be terminated through some local process, so it must be for endogenous pyrogen within the brain. If there were no means of terminating the central action of pyrogen, fevers caused by infection and injury, once initiated, would persist indefinitely. Since this does not occur, it follows that the brain handles pyrogen such that it becomes ineffective in producing fever.

Study of the central events responsible for defervescence is complicated by lack of knowledge of the precise physical characteristics of the endogenous pyrogen that reaches the brain and by the possibility that additional substances are involved in central mediation of fever. Leukocytic pyrogen (LP) is believed to be composed of acidic protein, and two distinct LPs derived from human leukocytes have been described (4), one with a molecular weight of 15,000 and the other of about 40,000 daltons. These molecules are larger than one might expect for a substance presumed to readily enter the brain, and it may be that fragments of the proteins act centrally to produce fever. Prostaglandins (PG) of the E series (5,11) have also been proposed to be essential to fever. If these autacoids are involved in fever, then defervescence might depend on their central inactivation.

PROLONGATION OF FEVER BY CENTRAL ADMINISTRATION OF TAURINE

Endogenous pyrogen may be inactivated in the brain by transport from receptor sites. This possibility was suggested by the observation that taurine (2-aminoethanesulfonic acid), a sulfonated amino acid which is highly concentrated in the brain, prolonged fever when infused into the cerebral ventricles of rabbits (6). Fever produced by intravenous administration of *Salmonella typhosa* endotoxin was inhibited by giving a priming dose and an infusion of taurine (Fig. 1). After the infusion was stopped, hyperthermia recurred and lasted 8.75 to 17.5 hr, much longer than the usual 6-hr fever produced by endotoxin in control experiments. Infusion of a similar amount of taurine into the cerebral ventricles of the same animals when they were afebrile did not cause hypothermia, and no fever developed when infusion was stopped. These results indicate that there is an essential relation between pyrogen that reaches the brain and taurine treatment in production of prolonged fevers. The effect of central taurine on fever appears to be specific for endogenous pyrogen since the amino acid did not prolong hyperthermia induced by intracerebroventricular (i.c.v.) injection of PGE_1 or by i.v. amphetamine, a drug which acts both peripherally and centrally to raise body temperature. Because the endotoxin-induced taurine-prolonged fevers resembled long-term fevers caused by central injection of LP, it was concluded that taurine infusion inhibits central inactivation of endogenous pyrogen, resulting in accumulation of the pyrogen in the brain and, therefore, a prolongation of its action on central temperature controls. This conclusion was supported by a necessity to increase the rate of taurine infusion after endotoxin in order to hold rectal temperature at baseline levels.

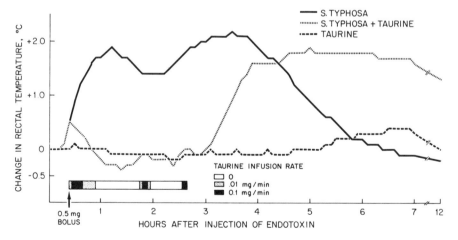

FIG. 1. Taurine infused into the lateral cerebral ventricle inhibited the development of fever in response to peripheral endotoxin and caused prolonged fever when infusion was stopped. Examples from a single rabbit showing normal febrile response to i.v. *Salmonella typhosa* endotoxin, initial inhibition of the febrile response by a bolus and controlled infusion of taurine followed by prolonged fever when infusion was stopped in another experiment, and the lack of effect of taurine control injections and infusion made in the same animal when it was afebrile. (From Harris and Lipton, ref. 6, with permission.)

PROLONGATION OF FEVER BY CENTRAL
ADMINISTRATION OF PROBENECID

The increase in fever duration after central infusion of taurine suggests that increased levels of the amino acid reduce the rate of inactivation of endogenous pyrogen within the brain. Taurine and other small neutral nonessential amino acids are constantly produced within the CNS, and it is likely that their concentration in the brain extracellular space is regulated not so much by restriction of entry but by outwardly directed capillary transport mechanisms (3). Taurine is one of the more prevalent amino acids within the brain, and it is transported by a structurally specific, saturable, high-affinity transport system that is both temperature and energy dependent (10). Because catabolism of this amino acid is very slow in brain tissue, removal through facilitated transport may be the primary route of its central inactivation. The idea that taurine inhibits inactivation of LP and that this amino acid is actively transported raised the hypothesis that LP may also be inactivated by removal from receptor sites via such a transport process. To test this idea, we gave probenecid (PBCD), an inhibitor of facilitated transport, i.c.v. to rabbits made febrile by i.v. LP.

When this drug was injected centrally, it caused dose-related augmentation of LP-induced fevers whether the rabbits were in thermoneutral, hot, or cold environments (Fig. 2) (2). When 0.5 mg PBCD was given at the peak of LP fever, 70 to 80 min later, and again 1 hr after the second injection, the normal fever duration of 2 to 3 hr was extended to over 12 hr. Initial i.c.v. injection plus infusion of PBCD for 1 hr beginning 10 min after LP was administered increased the area under the fever curve nearly twofold (Fig. 3). The higher fevers were associated with prolonged vasoconstriction in the ears during the

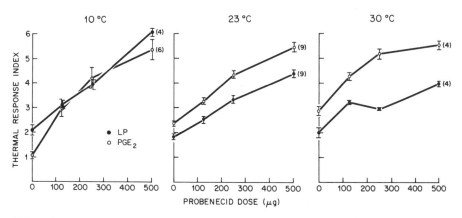

FIG. 2. Augmentation of hyperthermic responses to i.v. LP (0.10 ml) and i.c.v. PGE$_2$ (0.5 μg) by 10 min prior i.c.v. injection of probenecid in animals tested in three ambient temperatures. Scores represent mean ($\pm$ SE) 5-hr thermal response indexes. Numbers of animals are given in parentheses. (From Crawford et al., ref. 2, with permission.)

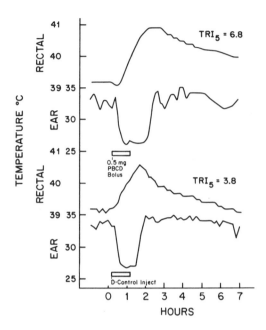

FIG. 3. A single i.c.v. PBCD injection plus infusion (50 μg/min) 10 min after i.v. LP enhanced and prolonged fever *(upper). Lower panel* shows fever after control injection and infusion of diluent. LP given at zero. Examples from a single rabbit. (From Crawford et al., ref. 2, with permission.)

chill phase. Defervescence was slow and also marked by reductions in ear temperature indicative of periods of vasoconstriction. PBCD given peripherally (100 mg/kg, intraperitoneally) 1 hr after *S. typhosa* endotoxin (1 μg/kg i.v.) caused rectal temperature to remain at high levels for over 12 hr whereas the control fever duration averaged 6 hr. This indicates that PBCD given systemically can prolong fever evoked by endogenously released LP.

PBCD also prolonged hyperthermia caused by central administration of PGE_2 provided that the transport inhibitor was given before PGE_2 administration (Fig. 2). Hyperthermia associated with the combined treatment sometimes reached lethal levels, and antipyretics were ineffective in lowering body temperature. The PGE concentration of CSF samples also increased during PBCD-prolonged LP-induced fever. The parallel augmentation of LP and PGE_2 hyperthermias by PBCD and the finding that PGE concentrations of CSF increased during fever prolonged by PBCD suggested that the transport inhibitor might prolong fever by influencing PGE concentration, rather than LP concentration, in the brain. However, control infusions of PBCD diluent increased PGE concentrations of CSF on some occasions even though there was no change or a decrease in rectal temperature. Even stronger evidence against the idea that PBCD prolongs fever by delaying inactivation of centrally released PGE was the finding that when the usual response to LP would have ended, acetaminophen and indomethacin both lowered LP-induced fever prolonged by PBCD. If the fever at the time of antipyretic administration was solely due to accumulation of prostaglandin, the antipyretics should have been ineffective since they do not inhibit hyperthermia caused by i.c.v. and intracerebral injections of PGE. It is therefore more likely that probenecid inhibited inactivation of LP itself, or of some related central mediator other than PGE. Probenecid inhibits the transport of centrally released prostaglandins, the main avenue of inactivation of these autacoids (1). However, the relation between this effect of PBCD and the central mediation of fever is uncertain.

PROLONGATION OF FEVER BY CENTRAL ADMINISTRATION OF TAURINE ANALOGS

With the hypothesis that taurine prevents termination of the effect of central LP by interfering with its transport, amino acids which compete with taurine for transport in CNS tissue (7) were given to see if they also prolong fever (8). Intracerebroventricular injection and infusion of taurine and of its sulfinic and carboxyl analogs hypotaurine and β-alanine were initiated when rectal temperature of rabbits given homologous LP i.v. had risen 0.3°C. In all animals taurine inhibited the normal increase in body temperature and caused fever to be prolonged when infusion was stopped (Fig. 4), much as it did in earlier experiments when endotoxin was given. Acetaminophen reduced the prolonged

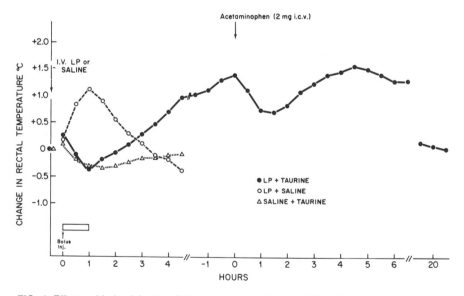

FIG. 4. Effects of bolus injection (0.5 mg) plus 1 hr infusion (0.01–0.2 mg/min) of taurine on LP fever. Scores are means of observations on 5 animals. At a time when the febrile response is generally ending, rectal temperature after taurine rose and remained elevated. Acetaminophen (2 mg) divided into 3 equal doses given 10 min apart around the time indicated by the arrow reduced the prolonged fever for 2–3 hr, but did not prevent a return of body temperature to elevated levels. The time between taurine infusion and acetaminophen injections was not the same in all animals (note break in line). (From Lipton and Ticknor, ref. 8, with permission.)

fevers, again suggesting that taurine does not extend fever by inhibiting termination of the effects of PGE. Similar taurine treatments only inhibited hyperthermia caused by i.c.v. injections of PGE_2. Hypotaurine injected (Fig. 5) or infused i.c.v. during the chill phase of LP fever inhibited the development of fever, increased the peak fever, and prolonged the febrile response. The initial rise in temperature was also consistently inhibited when β-alanine was given. Maximum fever was increased by this taurine analog in 60% of the experiments, and fever duration was increased in 80%.

These results support the hypothesis that taurine interferes with termination of the effect of endogenous pyrogen within the brain, but that it does not do so by interfering with central inactivation of PGE. Inhibition of fever develop-

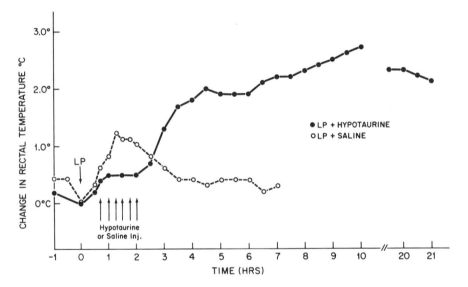

FIG. 5. Effects of repeated i.c.v. injections of hypotaurine (1 mg) on fever produced by i.v. LP in a single rabbit. (From Lipton and Ticknor, ref. 8, with permission.)

ment and production of hypothermia by taurine was observed again and is presumed to result from inhibitory effects on central pathways which control vasomotor tone, heat production, and arousal. The finding that all three amino acids prolong fever suggests that taurine and its analogs are transported via carriers that are also involved in termination of the effects of LP or related central mediators. Infusion of these amino acids into the brain can occupy the carrier system and delay termination of the pyrogen action. Endogenous pyrogen then accumulates in the brain so that when the amino acid infusion is stopped, fever develops and persists for prolonged periods, much as when LP is injected i.c.v. or into the preoptic/anterior hypothalamic region.

EFFECTS ON FEVER OF CENTRAL ADMINISTRATION OF OTHER TRANSPORT INHIBITORS

Three anion transport systems are known: the iodide system, inhibited by perchloric acid; the hippurate or H system, inhibited by *p*-aminohippuric acid (PAH); and the L or liver-like system, inhibited by iodipamide. Probenecid, shown to prolong fever in experiments described above, is a transport inhibitor of low specificity and is known to influence both the H and L systems. To determine whether the transport processes essential to central inactivation of endogenous pyrogen could be assigned to one or more of the anion transport systems, the inhibitors of the three systems were given to rabbits made febrile by i.v. LP (9). Intracerebroventricular injection of iodipamide 10 min before LP augmented the ensuing fevers in a dose-related fashion (Fig. 6). With 0.25, 0.5, and 1.0 mg iodipamide, the area under the fever curve was increased above control levels 21, 38, and 42%, respectively. These doses did not increase body temperature when given to the same animals in the absence of LP. Central administration of PAH and perchloric acid did not augment fever produced by LP or cause hyperthermia when given alone. Iodipamide administered 10 min before 0.5 μg PGE$_2$ i.c.v. also augmented the resulting hyperthermia, but PAH and perchloric acid did not (Fig. 6). Because iodipamide augmented both LP fever and PGE$_2$ hyperthermia, the question again arose as to whether the inhibitor augmented LP-induced fever by promoting accumulation of central PGE released by the endogenous pyrogen. Transport of PGE out of the brain

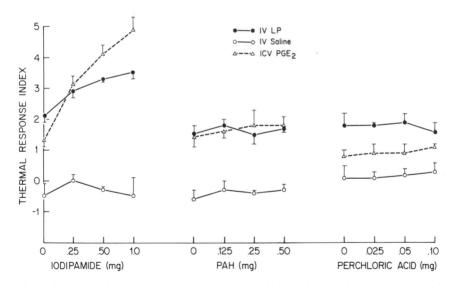

FIG. 6. Effects on the temperature response to i.v. LP, i.v. saline, or i.c.v. PGE$_2$ of 10 min prior i.c.v. injection of iodipamide, PAH, or perchloric acid. Scores are mean ($\pm$ SE) temperature response of 5 rabbits. (From Lipton et al., ref. 9, with permission.)

has been shown to be inhibited by iodipamide (1). However, acetaminophen injected i.c.v. when rectal temperature was near the peak in animals given iodipamide and LP abolished the prolongation of fever by iodipamide, which suggests that this transport inhibitor reduced central inactivation of LP *per se*.

Since iodipamide also appears to reduce inactivation of PGE_2 injected into the cerebral ventricles, it may be that central LP and PGE share an inactivation pathway through transport by the L system. The inactivation pathways of LP and PGE may not be exactly the same since the L system is thought to be a composite system. That transport systems other than the L system may be involved in the central inactivation of LP is suggested by the finding that the augmentation of LP fever by iodipamide is much less than that caused by PBCD, the "catch-all" transport inhibitor.

ROLE OF TRANSPORT PROCESSES IN ANTIPYRESIS

From the preceding results, the question arose as to the role of transport processes in the central action of antipyretics. Rabbits were given 50 μl of rabbit LP i.c.v. followed 4 and 8 hr later by acetaminophen (1.0 mg), PBCD (0.5 mg) plus acetaminophen (1.0 mg), or saline control injections (Fig. 7). Acetaminophen reduced fever caused by the pyrogen after both the 4- and 8-hr injections. This antipyretic effect was decreased when acetaminophen injection was preceded by PBCD administration, indicating an antagonism between the two agents. Since there is no previous indication that these substances compete for receptor sites in brain tissue, it seems reasonable to assume that PBCD antagonizes the antipyretic effect of acetaminophen by inhibiting transport processes. It may be that PBCD prevents acetaminophen from reaching receptor

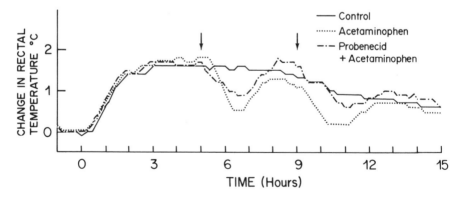

FIG. 7. Mean changes in fever caused by acetaminophen and probenecid plus acetaminophen in 10 rabbits. LP (50 μl) injected i.c.v. at zero time. Acetaminophen (1 mg), probenecid (0.5 mg) plus acetaminophen (1 mg), or saline injected i.c.v. at 5 and 9 hr *(arrow)* after LP.

sites by inhibiting its transport across neuronal membranes. This would imply that the antipyretic normally exerts its action within the neuron. On the other hand, if acetaminophen acts in part by enhancing transport of endogenous pyrogen, PBCD may simply reduce this action. It is not clear from the present data and from other data on sodium salicylate (J. M. Lipton, *unpublished observations*) which of the possibilities is correct. However, the findings are consistent in indicating that transport processes are essential to the normal effects of antipyretics.

SUMMARY

Although it is generally agreed that fever depends on an action of endogenous pyrogen on CNS temperature controls, the local processes within the brain which underlie defervescence have not been described. Recent data suggest that transport processes are involved in the central inactivation of LP that reaches the brain. Taurine, an amino acid that is actively extruded from the brain, and its analogs may prolong fever by competing with LP for transport. It is speculated that taurine and similar amino acids preferentially occupy the carrier required for central inactivation of LP. It is clear that taurine does not interfere with central inactivation of PGE, a presumed central mediator of fever. Probenecid, a well-known inhibitor of transport, also prolongs fever, which supports the idea that facilitated transport processes are required for central inactivation of both LP and central PGE_2. Finally, there is evidence that inhibition of transport processes reduces the effects of antipyretics. The broad conclusions from the results are that defervescence requires central inactivation of endogenous pyrogen through a facilitated transport process and that normal transport processes are essential to antipyretic action.

ACKNOWLEDGMENT

This research was supported by Grant NS 10046 from the National Institute of Neurological and Communications Disorders and Stroke.

REFERENCES

1. Bito, L. Z., Davson, H., and Hollingsworth, J. R. (1976): Facilitated transport of prostaglandins across the blood-cerebrospinal fluid and blood-brain barriers. *J. Physiol. (Lond.)*, 256:273–285.
2. Crawford, I. L., Kennedy, J. I., Lipton, J. M., and Ojeda, S. R. (1979): Effects of central administration of probenecid on fevers produced by leukocytic pyrogen and PGE_2 in the rabbit. *J. Physiol. (Lond.)*, 287:519–533.
3. Cutler, R. W. P., and Coull, B. M. (1978): Amino acid transport in the brain. In: *Taurine and Neurological Disorders*, edited by A. Barbeau and R. J. Huxtable, pp. 95–107. Raven Press, New York.
4. Dinarello, C. A., Goldin, N. P., and Wolff, S. M. (1974): Demonstration and characterization of two distinct human leukocytic pyrogens. *J. Exp. Med.*, 139:1369–1381.
5. Feldberg, W., and Saxena, P. N. (1971): Fever produced by prostaglandin E_1. *J. Physiol. (Lond.)*, 217:547–556.

6. Harris, W. S., and Lipton, J. M. (1977): Intracerebroventricular taurine in rabbits: Effects on normal body temperature, endotoxin fever and hyperthermia produced by PGE_1 and amphetamine. *J. Physiol. (Lond.)*, 266:397–410.

7. Kaczmarek, L. K., and Davison, A. N. (1972): Uptake and release of taurine from rat brain slices. *J. Neurochem.*, 19:2355–2362.

8. Lipton, J. M., and Ticknor, C. B. (1979): Central effect of taurine and its analogues on fever caused by intravenous leukocytic pyrogen in the rabbit. *J. Physiol. (Lond.)*, 287:535–543.

9. Lipton, J. M., Whisenant, J. D., Gean, J. T., and Ticknor, C. B. (1979): Effects on fever of central administration of transport inhibitors. *Brain Res. Bull.*, 4:297–300.

10. Lombardini, J. B. (1978): High affinity transport of taurine in the mammalian central nervous system. In: *Taurine and Neurological Disorders,* edited by A. Barbeau and R. J. Huxtable, pp. 119–135, Raven Press, New York.

11. Milton, A. S., and Wendlandt, S. (1971): Effects on body temperature of prostaglandins of the A, E and F series on injection into the third ventricle of unanesthetized cats and rabbits. *J. Physiol. (Lond.)*, 218:325–336.

Fever, edited by James M. Lipton.
Raven Press, New York © 1980.

Central Neurology of Homeothermy and Fever

John Bligh

Institute of Arctic Biology, University of Alaska, Fairbanks, Alaska 99701

The effect of a pyrogen is to readjust the thermoregulatory set-point mechanism in an upward direction. Undoubtedly, this is a valid description: homeothermy implies the existence of some kind of set-point process, and the normality of thermoregulatory responses to thermal disturbance during the plateau phase of a fever (23) is clear evidence of an upward shift in the set-point. But what is the nature of the set-point mechanism, and how do pyrogens act on it to cause its upward readjustment? There are several tentative answers to these questions, but none is regarded as firmly established.

At the neurophysiological level, the set-point has been considered more in biochemical terms with little regard to control theory: a balanced release of two neurotransmitter substances, or a balance in the concentrations of calcium and sodium ions in the environment of particular neurons. Neither of these concepts involves the definition of an actual set-point determinant, since something else must be determining the release of the transmitters, or the balance of specific ions in the environment of neurons. Such theories deal only with possible components of systems and not with the fundamental principles of systems.

A theoretical concept of the biological thermostat is based on physical systems in which a disturbance signal is compared with one derived from a reference signal generator (Fig. 1A). A neuronal thermoregulatory set-point could operate on this principle (5) if a temperature-insensitive spontaneously active neuron

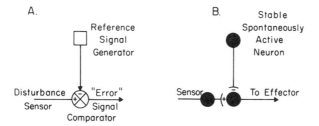

FIG. 1. A: Principle of the comparison of a disturbance signal with a stable reference signal in the creation of a set-point. **B:** Neuronal equivalent of this function in which a synapse acts as the comparator in an excitatory signal from a sensor and an inhibitory signal from a stable spontaneously active neuron in the brain.

supplied the reference signal (Fig. 1B). A pyrogen-induced rise in the set-point could result from a change in the reference signal or in the disturbance signal relative to temperature.

The neuronal signal generator is not, however, an imperative hypothesis. Two populations of sensors reacting in opposing ways to temperature changes is an equally well-established physical principle, and it has also been suggested that the known existence of two populations of thermosensors could be the basis of homeothermy (5,25,31). In such a system, a change in the activity/temperature characteristics of the sensors or otherwise induced changes in the signal passing to thermoregulatory effectors could account for a pyrogen-induced elevation in the set-point temperature.

FORMULATION OF A NEURONAL MODEL
OF THERMOREGULATION

From established relationships between thermal disturbances and thermoregulatory responses, it can be argued that there need be only quite simple neuronal connections between thermosensors and thermoregulatory effectors (5). The null- or set-point between the activities of heat production and heat loss effectors well-demonstrated in man (3,13) could be the consequence of signal generating neurons in the CNS (Fig. 2A) or simple crossing inhibition between two opposing effector pathways (Fig. 2B).

The thermoregulatory effects of intracerebroventricular (i.c.v.) injections of the putative transmitter substances norepinephrine (NE) and 5-hydroxytryptamine (5-HT) and the cholinomimetic substance carbamylcholine (CCh) into

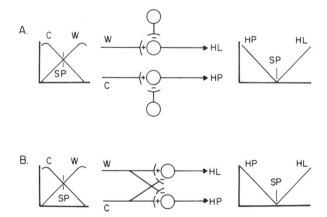

FIG. 2. A: Creation of the demonstrated central null-point between heat production and heat loss effector functions could be due to converging inhibitory influences, creating synaptic gates. **B:** The null-point could also be created simply by opposing inhibitory influences between two direct pathways from the opposing thermosensors to the opposing thermoregulatory effectors. C, cold sensor; W, warm sensor; HL, heat loss; HP, heat production; SP, set-point.

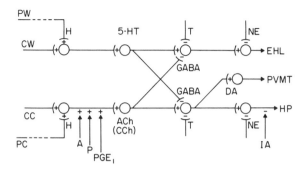

FIG. 3. Modification of a model used by Bligh (6) to describe the apparent points of actions of the many putative transmitter substances which have been found to affect thermoregulation when introduced into a lateral cerebral ventricle of the sheep. PW, peripheral warm sensor; CW, central warm sensor; PC, peripheral cold sensor; CC, central cold sensor; EHL, evaporative heat loss (respiratory frequency); PVMT, peripheral vasomotor tone (of the ears); HP, heat production (EMG or $\dot{V}O_2$); A, aspartate; ACh, acetylcholine; CCh, carbamylcholine; DA, dopamine; GABA, γ-aminobutyric acid; H, histamine; 5-HT, 5-hydroxytryptamine; IA, indoleamine; NE, norepinephrine; P, pyrogenic end activator of a TAB vaccine-induced fever; PGE_1, prostaglandin E_1; T, taurine.

sheep, goats, and rabbits have been described in terms of a simple neuronal format (7) which is essentially the same as that derived from disturbance/response analyses. Subsequent studies have since been done on sheep to test this basic hypothesis and to determine the effects of other putative transmitter substances (see ref. 6). The results are summarized in Fig. 3.

FEVER IN RELATION TO THE NEURONAL MODEL

If Fig. 3 is a valid description of the neuronal connections between thermosensors and thermoregulatory effectors, the action of pyrogens should also be expressible within this format. Fever is a state of raised heat storage due to an increase in heat production (HP) and/or peripheral vasomotor tone (PVMT), and an inhibition of evaporative heat loss (EHL). The simplest way by which a pyrogen could operate to cause these effects would be for it to act at one point only, so as to increase heat production and decrease heat loss. In terms of the neuronal model (Fig. 3), this one point of action would have to be between the cold sensors and the point of origin of the crossing inhibitory influence on evaporative heat loss, and perhaps before a cholinergic synapse on the pathway from cold sensors. The results of experiments done to test this proposition are summarized below:

1. The thermoregulatory responses to an i.v. injection of typhoid A and B (TAB) vaccine (8) or an i.c.v. injection of prostaglandin E_1 (PGE_1) (9) in the sheep caused thermoregulatory effects which were essentially the same as those resulting from an i.c.v. injection of CCh—an increase in HP and/or an increase in PVMT and/or a reduction in EHL.

2. A prior i.c.v. injection of atropine sulfate attenuated the thermoregulatory responses to (a) a low ambient temperature, (b) an i.v. injection of TAB vaccine, and (c) an i.c.v. injection of PGE_1 (10).

3. An i.c.v. injection of NE during the rising phase of a TAB vaccine-induced fever caused the cessation of shivering and a halt in the rise in body temperature. The i.c.v. NE was, however, without effect on the already depressed EHL (4,8).

4. An i.c.v. injection of 5-HT during the rising phase of a fever caused by an i.v. TAB vaccine caused a reduction in HP, a reduction in PVMT, and an increase in EHL. Because of this complete reversal of the activities of the thermoregulatory effector processes, not only was the rise in body temperature halted, but the direction of change was reversed (4,8).

This evidence is in accord with the neuronal format (Fig. 3), and indicates that the direct or indirect actions of a bacterial endotoxin or a prostaglandin E are on the cold sensors or on the pathway from the cold sensors, before a cholinergic synapse, and before the point of origin of an inhibitory influence on heat loss processes.

FURTHER STUDIES WITH OTHER PUTATIVE TRANSMITTERS AND FEVER

The thermoregulatory effects of the other putative transmitters which have subsequently been found to have thermoregulatory effects when injected into the cerebral ventricles of sheep can all be expressed in terms of the neuronal model without any basic change in its configuration. The relative positions of the actions of these substances have been deduced from the effect of specific receptor blocking agents. Figure 3 includes a recent finding that γ-aminobutyric acid (GABA) may be the terminal transmitter of the crossing inhibitory influences (11).

With these further details of the apparent configuration of the synapses at which several transmitter substances are involved in the regulation of body temperature, many further experiments can now be designed to determine the point of action of a pyrogen.

The evidence of the points of action of i.c.v. histamine and aspartic acid somewhere between peripheral cold sensors and the cholinergic synapse on the pathway to heat production effectors has afforded an opportunity to consider whether the pyrogen acts on the cold sensors or somewhere along the pathway from them. The histamine receptor blocker mepyramine blocks the input from peripheral cold sensors somewhere before the cholinergic synapse, since it does not block the thermoregulatory effects of i.c.v. CCh (1). We have now found that mepyramine does not interfere with the course of a fever induced by i.v. TAB vaccine (J. Bligh and C. A. Smith, *unpublished observations*). It is also known that an i.c.v. injection of the aspartate receptor blocker pimelic acid in a quantity that blocks the signals from cold sensors also does not alter the course of a TAB vaccine fever (A. Silver, *unpublished observations*). These results clearly indicate that the point of action of the pyrogen is efferent to the point or points at which histamine and aspartate act, and afferent to the point of action of ACh. This finding fits with an observation that the activity/temperature profiles of a cold sensor on the tongue of the rabbit is unaffected by a pyrogen-induced fever (20). There is, however, no evidence that hypothalamic thermosensors are unaffected by pyrogen and some evidence that they are.

PERTINENT COMPARATIVE STUDIES BY OTHERS ON RABBITS

All our studies with putative synaptic transmitters and of the interactions of pyrogens and synaptically active substances can be expressed in terms of the neuronal model, but they have been done mostly on the one species, the sheep, and there is much evidence of differences between species in the effects of i.c.v. or intrahypothalamically administered putative transmitter substances. Thus the evidence may be considered too specific to be the basis for a general hypothesis. However, the original study of Bligh et al. (7) with 5-HT, CCh, and NE was done on sheep, goats, and rabbits, with similar results for all three species; and several studies on fever in relation to the roles of endogenous hypothalamic 5-HT, ACh, and NE have been done in other laboratories on the rabbit. Thus we can inquire whether the results from these independent experiments accord with the neuronal concept.

From the neuronal model it would be expected that depletion of the endogenous stores of 5-HT or NE in the preoptic/anterior hypothalamic (PO/AH) area of the brain would not greatly modify the course of an induced fever, since neither substance appears to be a transmitter substance acting "on-line" between the supposed point of action of the pyrogen and the thermoregulatory effectors. These predictions, however, need qualification. The effect of the removal of NE might depend on the extent of the NE-transmitted inhibitory tone normally acting on the pathways from thermosensors to thermoregulatory effectors. The removal of such tone could change the magnitude of effector activities in response to a pyrogen, but the influence on the displacement of body temperature would probably not be great. The anticipated effect of endogenous 5-HT depletion must also be qualified. The resultant blockade of the influence of warm sensors could result in an exaggerated fever response, and such exaggeration would also occur if the drug used to empty the 5-HT reservoir also blocked the suspected inhibitory action of an endogenous non-5-HT indoleamine on heat production (see Fig. 3).

In contrast, the depletion or blockade of ACh which does appear to act "on-line" between the supposed point of action of the pyrogen and the effectors of a fever would be expected to markedly attenuate or even to block the febrile response to a pyrogen.

An induced fever in the rabbit is attenuated by an i.c.v. injection of 5-HT (26). This tallies with the observed interaction of pyrogen and i.c.v. 5-HT in the sheep. Some reports of the effect of the depletion of 5-HT stores with para-chlorophenylalanine (PCPA) on fever are that this treatment is without effect (12,15,19,29); others are of an increase in the height of a pyrogen-induced fever (21,26). This evidence is essentially consistent with the thermoregulatory role of endogenous PO/AH 5-HT and its involvement in the genesis of fever proposed in Fig. 3.

There is one contrary result: heptadine was used to interfere with the natural role of 5-HT, and was found to attenuate the febrile response to a pyrogen (14). This study is also singular in the agent used to interfere with the availability of endogenous 5-HT; there could be something particular about the effects of this substance which accounts for the observed effect on fever.

The reduction in the endogenous NE in the PO/AH of the rabbit induced by pretreatment with α-methyl-p-tyrosine was found to cause no change in the course of an induced fever (18), or to cause some attenuation of an induced fever (24).

In other experiments on rabbits, pretreatment with reserpine was used to deplete the endogenous monomines, which include both 5-HT and NE. This was found to depress the febrile response to a pyrogen (18), although the depletion of NE alone (18) or the depletion of 5-HT alone (19) was found to have no effect on fever. It was thus suspected that reserpine has some other action unrelated to NE or 5-HT depletion. However, Veale and Cooper (30) were unable to confirm that reserpine pretreatment modified the course of an induced fever in the rabbit.

Again, the general pattern of these results agrees with those predictable from the neuronal model. Evidently endogenous NE and 5-HT do not play essential roles in the genesis of fever. However, 5-HT does seem to play an essential ("on-line") role in normal thermoregulation whereas NE apparently plays a modulatory ("off-line") role, and consequently their additions to or removal from the PO/AH does exert modulatory effects on the course of a fever.

As with sheep, pretreatment of a rabbit with an i.c.v. injection of atropine sulfate attenuates fever (17). Tangri et al. (28) also found that an acetylcholine (ACh) blocking agent caused the attenuation of an induced fever, but obtained this effect with the nicotinic ACh receptor blocker hemicholinium, whereas the muscarinic receptor blocker atropine was without effect. Cooper et al. (16) were unable to confirm this finding of Tangri et al., and found fever to be attenuated only by atropine.

Despite the doubt about the classification of the central ACh receptor, this independent evidence from the rabbit is in accord with that from the sheep in indicating an "on-line" cholinergic synapse between the point of action of a pyrogen and the final pathways to the thermoregulatory effectors by which heat storage of the body is increased.

Generally speaking, these studies on rabbits have involved the measurement only of body temperature, and not of changes in the activities of thermoregulatory effectors, and generally, they were done at only one ambient temperature. More information is necessary for a complete analysis of the effects, and therefore of the possible points of action, of substances which interfere with thermoregulation (2). Thus a full assessment of the extent to which these results on rabbits are truly consistent with the proposed neuronal model is not possible. The independent studies noted above do, however, substantiate the original findings that the effects on thermoregulation of i.c.v. 5-HT, ACh (or CCh), and NE are basically the same in the sheep and the rabbit (7) and indicate that pyrogens, too, act in essentially the same way in the two species.

GENERAL DISCUSSION OF THE MODEL IN RELATION TO SPECIES DIFFERENCES

This concurrence of evidence with sheep and rabbit still leaves the problem of the apparent species differences in the roles of central transmitters in the regulation of body temperature.

In the rat, for example, in which the thermoregulatory effects of i.c.v. or intrahypothalamic injections of carbachol have generally been found to be different from those in the sheep and rabbit, i.c.v. injections of neither a muscarinic (atropine) or nicotinic (mecamyline) receptor blocker attenuated a fever induced by PGE_1 injected directly into the PO/AH (27). It was concluded, therefore, that in this species there is no cholinergic synapse between the point of action of PGE_1 and the heat production effector.

Unlike the rabbit and sheep, cats have been found to respond to i.c.v. 5-HT with vasoconstriction, shivering, and a rise in body temperature; yet, as with rabbits and sheep, pretreatment with PCPA to lower brain 5-HT did not attenuate the fever induced by i.c.v. PGE_1 (22).

These inconsistent results might relate to the current debates on whether normal fever involves prostaglandins, and on the alleged species differences in the roles of synaptic transmitter substances in the central regulation of body temperature, but they do not necessarily run counter to the thesis presented here. There is no *a priori* reason why the same transmitter substances should not occur at more than one location on a multisynaptic pathway, nor why the same transmitter should not have a function on each of two pathways which are concerned with the operation of opposing effector functions in a control system (6). For reasons relating to species differences in the sizes of brains and in brain structures, in the ease of diffusion of injected substances, or in gross (supracellular) anatomy, such as the nearness of pathways to the cerebral ventricles, injected substances could have different consequences in different species without there being any true species differences at the level of cellular organization, or in the roles played by transmitters.

Furthermore, even if there are true species differences in the roles of transmitter substances, these would not necessarily nullify the validity of the proposition presented here, since the basic thesis of two thermosensor pathways with crossing inhibitory influences between them is equally well derived from thermal disturbance/thermoregulatory response analyses as it is from synaptic interference studies.

Fever may involve more than one terminal pyrogenic agent acting at more than one location in the CNS, since (a) the biphasic pattern of the febrile response to a bacterial endotoxin has two time courses which are separable pharmacologically, and (b) we have never succeeded in totally preventing the febrile response to a bacterial endotoxin by means of i.c.v. atropine sulfate. The residual fever pattern after atropine could be interpreted as evidence of the blockade of the agent responsible for the first fever peak, but not of the second. Perhaps here we have been considering the point of action only of one component of fever. This possibility indicates a need for further studies in which the changes in the pattern of the fever, as well as in the magnitude of the fever, are investigated in relation to synaptic interferences, and the neuronal model discussed here.

ACKNOWLEDGMENT

This work was supported by NIH Biomedical Research Support Grant 5S07RR07001–11.

REFERENCES

1. Bacon, M. J., Bligh, J., Silver, A., and Smith, C. A. (1980): The use of histamine receptor blockers to investigate the role of histamine in thermoregulation in the sheep. *J. Thermal Biol. (in press).*
2. Baumann, I. R., and Bligh, J. (1975): The influence of ambient temperature on drug-induced disturbances of body temperature. In: *Temperature Regulation and Drug Action,* edited by P. Lomax, E. Schonbaum, and J. Jacob, pp. 241–251. S. Karger, Basel.
3. Benzinger, T. H., Kitzinger, C., and Pratt, A. W. (1963): The human thermostat. In: *Temperature—Its Measurement and Control in Science and Industry, Vol. 3, Pt. 3,* edited by J. D. Hardy, pp. 637–665. Reinhold, New York.
4. Bligh, J. (1974): Neuronal models of hypothalamic temperature regulation. In: *Recent Studies of Hypothalamic Function,* edited by K. Lederis and K. E. Cooper, pp. 315–327. S. Karger, Basel.
5. Bligh, J. (1978): Thermal regulation: What is regulated and how? In: *New Trends in Thermal Physiology,* edited by Y. Houdas and J. D. Guieu, pp. 1–10. Masson, Paris.
6. Bligh, J. (1979): The central neurology of mammalian thermoregulation. *Neuroscience,* 4:1213–1236.
7. Bligh, J., Cottle, W. H., and Maskrey, M. (1971): Influence of ambient temperature on the thermoregulatory responses to 5-hydroxytryptamine, noradrenaline and acetylcholine injected into the lateral cerebral ventricles of sheep, goats and rabbits. *J. Physiol. (Lond.),* 212:377–392.
8. Bligh, J., and Maskrey, M. (1971): The interactions between the effects of thermoregulation of TAB vaccine injected intravenously and monoamines injected into a lateral cerebral ventricle of a Welsh mountain sheep. *J. Physiol. (Lond.),* 213:60–62P.
9. Bligh, J., and Milton, A. S. (1973): The thermoregulatory effects of prostaglandin E_1 when infused into a lateral cerebral ventricle of the Welsh mountain sheep at different ambient temperatures. *J. Physiol. (Lond.),* 229:30–31P.
10. Bligh, J., Silver, A., Bacon, M., and Smith, C. A. (1978): The central role of a cholinergic synapse in thermoregulation in the sheep. *J. Thermal Biol.,* 3:147–151.

11. Bligh, J., and Smith, C. A. (1980): Central GABA and thermoregulation in sheep. In: *Thermoregulatory Mechanisms and Their Therapeutic Implications,* edited by P. Lomax, A. S. Milton, and E. Schönbaum. S. Karger, Basel *(in press).*

12. Borsook, D., Laburn, H. P., Rosendorff, C., Willies, G. H., and Woolf, C. J. (1977): A dissociation between temperature regulation and fever in the rabbit. *J. Physiol. (Lond.),* 266:423–433.

13. Cabanac, M., and Massonnet, B. (1977): Thermoregulatory responses as a function of core temperature in humans. *J. Physiol. (Lond.),* 265:587–596.

14. Canal, N., and Ornesi, A. (1961): La serotiniana quale agente ipertermizzante. *Atti Accad. Med. Lomb.,* 16:64–69.

15. Carruba, M. O., and Bächtold, H. P. (1976): Pyrogen fever in rabbits pretreated with *p*-chlorophenylalanine or 5,6-dihydroxytryptamine. *Experientia,* 32:729–730.

16. Cooper, K. E., Preston, E., and Veale, W. L. (1976): Effects of atropine, injected into a lateral cerebral ventricle of the rabbit, on fevers due to intravenous leucocyte pyrogen and hypothalamic and intraventricular injections of prostaglandin E_1. *J. Physiol. (Lond.),* 254:729–741.

17. Cooper, K. E., and Veale, W. L. (1974): An abnormal drive to the heat conserving and producing mechanisms. In: *Recent Studies of Hypothalamic Function,* edited by K. Lederis and K. E. Cooper, pp. 315–322. S. Karger, Basel.

18. Des Prez, R., Helman, R., and Oates, J. A. (1966): Inhibition of endotoxin fever by reserpine. *Proc. Soc. Exp. Biol. Med.,* 122:746–749.

19. Des Prez, R. M., and Oates, J. A. (1968): Lack of relationship of febrile response to endotoxin and brain stem 5-hydroxytryptamine. *Proc. Soc. Exp. Biol. Med.,* 127:793–794.

20. Evans, M. H., Frens, J., and Bligh, J. (1972): Unaltered activity of tongue temperature sensors after administration of pyrogen to rabbit. *Eur. J. Pharmacol.,* 18:333–337.

21. Giarman, N. J., Tanaka, C., Mooney, J., and Atkins, E. (1968): Serotonin, norepinephrine and fever. *Adv. Pharmacol.,* 6:307–317.

22. Harvey, C. A., and Milton, A. S. (1973): The effect of parachlorophenylalanine on the response of the conscious cat to intravenous and intraventricular prostaglandin E_1. *J. Physiol. (Lond.),* 234:12–13P.

23. MacPherson, R. K. (1959): The effect of fever on temperature regulation in man. *Clin. Sci.,* 18:281–287.

24. Metcalf, G., and Thompson, J. W. (1975): The effect of various amine-depleting drugs on the fever response exhibited by rabbits to bacterial or leucocyte pyrogen. *Br. J. Pharmacol.,* 53:21–27.

25. Mitchell, D., Snellen, J. W., and Atkins, A. R. (1970): Thermoregulation during fever: Change in set-point or change in gain. *Pflüegers Arch.,* 321:293–302.

26. Peindaries, R., and Jacob, J. (1971): Interactions between 5-hydroxytryptamine and a purified bacterial pyrogen when injected into the lateral cerebral ventricle of the wake rabbit. *Eur. J. Pharmacol.,* 13:347–355.

27. Rudy, T. A., and Viswanathan, C. T. (1975): Effect of central cholinergic blockade on the hyperthermia evoked by prostaglandin E_1 injected in the rostral hypothalamus of the rat. *Can. J. Physiol. Pharmacol.,* 53:321–324.

28. Tangri, K. K., Bhargava, A. K., and Bhargava, K. P. (1975): Significance of central cholinergic mechanism in pyrexia induced by bacterial pyrogen in rabbits. In: *Temperature Regulation and Drug Action,* edited by P. Lomax, E. Schonbaum, and J. Jacob, pp. 65–74. S. Karger, Basel.

29. Teddy, P. J. (1969): The effects of alterations in hypothalamic monoamine content on fever in the rabbit. *J. Physiol. (Lond.),* 204:140P.

30. Veale, W. L., and Cooper, K. E. (1974): Evidence for the involvement of prostaglandins in fever. In: *Recent Studies of Hypothalamic Function,* edited by K. Lederis and K. E. Cooper, pp. 289–300. S. Karger, Basel.

31. Vendrik, A. J. H. (1959): The regulation of body temperature in man. *Ned. Tijdschr. Geneeskd.,* 103:240–244.

Fever, edited by James M. Lipton.
Raven Press, New York © 1980.

Activity of Thermoresponsive Neurons in Fever

Eugene P. Schoener

*Department of Pharmacology, Wayne State University School of Medicine,
Detroit, Michigan 48201*

The term "fever" is now generally applied to the sustained elevation of body temperature that occurs in homeotherms as a reaction to a pyrogenic substance. Mechanistically, we regard fever as a regulated upward adjustment of the thermoregulatory set-point in the temperature control system. That is, fever reflects a disturbance of control elements which determine the "desired output" of the system, or the core temperature.

Although a precise understanding of the anatomical components which subserve temperature control functions has thus far eluded us, attention has long been focused on the preoptic/anterior hypothalamic (PO/AH) region of the brain as the primary seat of such activity. Definitive evidence for the importance of this brain region was first provided by Ranson (24) and his colleagues using localized ablation techniques as well as electrical and thermal stimulation. Thermoregulatory responses were elicited by local stimulation and could be selectively dissociated by lesions in different parts of the hypothalamus. With the advent of technology for neuronal recording some 20 years later, activity of thermosensitive neurons in the PO/AH was identified by varying local hypothalamic temperature (8,11,12,16,22). Both warm and cold receptor activities were characterized. In addition to these primary thermodetector cells, the presence of units responsive to thermal stimulation elsewhere in the body was soon appreciated (13,14,18,35). Thus a picture developed of the extensive neuronal "hardware" for thermoregulation in the PO/AH, and a rather complex model of the apparatus was constructed by Hardy and Guieu (10). In essence, all of the various neuronal components presumably related to PO/AH temperature controlling functions can be distilled down to three elemental categories: (a) units directly excited by increase of local temperature in the physiological range; (b) units directly inhibited by increase of local temperature in the physiological range; and (c) units excited or inhibited by increase of temperature at peripheral and/or central thermodetectors. This last classification pertains to neurons we regard as interneurons, i.e., they may or may not possess primary thermosensitivity, but receive and integrate information from thermodetectors in the PO/AH, at the body surface, and perhaps elsewhere. This particular unit, with its convergence of thermal information, possesses the qualities of a "summing junction" in the temperature control system, and this type of cell most consistently reflects an alteration of the set-point, although it may not bear ultimate responsibility for generation of the set-point.

CNS, PYROGENS, AND FEVER

The location of possible central nervous system sites of pyrogen action drew increased attention in the early 1960s, at the same time that interest in the specific neuronal activities concerned with thermoregulatory function was growing. Villablanca and Myers (33) first presented evidence that *Salmonella typhosa* provokes fever in cats when injected into or near the hypothalamus and, particularly, into the anterior hypothalamus. Shortly thereafter, other endotoxins (*Shigella dysenteriae* and *Escherichia coli*) were also found to cause fever when injected into the anterior hypothalamus (21). These observations have since been confirmed in several species including the rabbit (3), monkey (21), and rat (29).

Inquiries next turned to putative endogenous mediators of endotoxin-induced fever, for it was aptly reasoned that the large size of the endotoxin molecule would preclude its entry into the CNS. In 1967 three laboratories independently reported that a pyrogenic substance produced by leukocytes would elicit fever with greater potency and/or shorter latency than endotoxin when injected into the same PO/AH sites in rabbits and cats (3,15,25). We now generally agree that production and release of endogenous pyrogen is the obligatory first step in the pathogenesis of fever caused by exogenous pyrogens (6).

PYROGENS AND PO/AH NEURONAL ACTIVITY

The influence of pyrogens on neuron function in the PO/AH area has been explored in several laboratories. There are four reports of pyrogen effects on single-unit activity in the literature. These studies were all performed on urethane-anesthetized animals, thus obviating the demonstration of concurrent change in "thermoregulatory" neuronal discharge and body temperature. Therefore, the functional roles of PO/AH units in the febrile reaction have been inferred from their thermoresponsive characteristics.

Cabanac and co-workers (1) examined the response of PO/AH neurons in the rabbit to intravenous typhoid vaccine. The units were identified as thermosensitive (warm and cold) and insensitive by their responses to tissue warming and cooling with locally implanted thermodes. No attempt was made to distinguish between thermodetectors and interneurons, but warm-sensitive neurons could be separated into two groups on the basis of their pyrogen response. Half of these units displayed complete inhibition of spontaneous discharge, whereas the others were only partially depressed. The latter group exhibited decreased thermosensitivity during subsequent thermal challenge. Some of the neurons found to be cold sensitive were excited after the pyrogen and, although most of those identified as insensitive to local temperature change did not show any significant change in discharge rate after pyrogen, one was completely depressed. The latency observed with these various neuronal effects of systemic pyrogen was very much in accord with the usual time to onset of fever in the animal, a point of support in the absence of actual hyperthermia. No recovery to control activity was reported.

Although they also administered endotoxin systemically, Wit and Wang (36) approached the study of PO/AH neurons in the cat from a different perspective. In their experimental protocol, neurons were identified by warming of the body surface and were classified as responsive to peripheral and/or central thermal stimulation. The effect of pyrogen was tested on thermoresponsive neurons whose discharge rate was enhanced by elevation of PO/AH temperature. Carotid arterial infusion of the endotoxin pyrogen (Piromen®) during maintained hyperthermia was followed by significant depression of neuronal discharge and of the induced thermal polypnea. Further elevation of PO/AH temperature revealed that neuronal thermosensitivity was greatly reduced after pyrogen depression. Temperature-insensitive neurons were also unresponsive to pyrogen as well.

Eisenman (7) sought to distinguish between thermodetector cells and thermoregulatory interneurons in the cat PO/AH area before studying their response to endotoxin (pyromen). By local warming and cooling of the PO/AH area, he identified two unique thermoresponsive profiles: one was a smooth, continuous change in discharge rate with heating or cooling; the second—interrupted by a discontinuity in responsiveness—a plateau where further change in temperature did not alter neuronal firing rate. The former units were presumed to be primary thermodetectors, and the latter, thermoregulatory interneurons. They were both influenced by endotoxin, but in apparently different ways. At a constant PO/AH temperature, the firing rate of warm-sensitive thermodetector units was unchanged by intravenous pyrogen, whereas the basal discharge of warm-sensitive interneurons was reduced. However, comparison of pre- and postpyrogen thermosensitivities disclosed depression of this variable for both types of cells. Recovery of neuronal activity to pretreatment control levels was observed in some experiments with interneurons at 75 to 90 min after administration of pyrogen.

In an effort to determine whether leukocyte pyrogen, the proposed endogenous mediator of endotoxin fever, influenced thermoregulatory neurons directly, I employed the microinjection technique together with PO/AH neuron recording (26). Thermoresponsive neurons were identified by body surface warming, as in the studies of Wit and Wang (35), while skin, rectal, and hypothalamic temperatures were monitored. The inherent delay in elevation of central temperature permitted independent assessment of peripheral and central thermoresponsiveness. The effect of locally applied pyrogen was investigated on both warm and cold responsive interneurons, i.e., cells whose discharge increased or decreased, respectively, with elevation of skin temperature alone or of both skin and PO/AH temperature. The predominant response of warm-sensitive units to the pyrogen was a decrease of firing rate which began within the 3-

to 5-min injection period, reached nadir about 5 min after the administration was completed, and persisted for a time which varied directly with the dose administered. Recovery to the control discharge rate was observed in all cases and, in several experiments, the pyrogen test was repeated after recovery with a resulting depression of activity that equaled or surpassed the initial inhibition. Interneurons with negative thermoresponsive characteristics were excited after pyrogen was administered, with essentially the same kinetics as the inhibition of warm-sensitive units. Repeated pyrogen tests on these neurons produced equi-effective excitation.

This series of investigations clearly demonstrated that the activity of thermoresponsive neurons located in the classic thermoregulatory center of the CNS is selectively modulated by endotoxin and endogenous pyrogen. The consistency of observations from laboratories using different techniques serves to corroborate the conclusion that pyrogens are capable of influencing "thermoregulatory" neuronal activity in accordance with the set-point hypothesis. However, the explicit site of pyrogen action cannot be attributed to any given type of thermoregulatory neuron on the basis of the foregoing studies.

SALICYLATE AND PO/AH NEURONS

It has been appreciated for many years that salicylates lower body temperature of febrile but not normothermic subjects. The presumption has been that the "classic" hypothalamic thermoregulatory apparatus was the site of salicylate action. The first definitive evidence supporting this thesis, however, was that provided by Wit and Wang (36) in their examination of acetylsalicylate effects on PO/AH neurons. In the urethane-anesthetized hyperthermic cat preparation, they administered sodium acetylsalicylate systemically after a pyrogen reaction had been established and found that recovery to the pre-pyrogen control rate of firing was greatly accelerated. Because the effective dose of salicylate by the intravenous route was two to three times greater than that by the intracarotid route, Wit and Wang concluded that the site of salicylate action was in the central nervous system, most probably in the hypothalamus.

Following these initial recording studies, several reports appeared which further delineated the putative central site of salicylate antipyresis. Cranston and co-workers (4) narrowed consideration to brain regions accessible to the ventricular space by demonstrating in febrile rabbits that less than 1% of the intravenous salicylate dose was required for antipyresis when infused directly into the cerebral ventricles. Shortly thereafter, Chai et al. (2) corroborated these findings with similar studies in monkeys. Both groups of investigators subsequently localized the primary site of salicylate action in the central nervous system to the PO/AH area by discrete microinjection studies (5,19).

Once I had determined that leukocyte pyrogen directly modulates "thermoregulatory" neuronal activity, I inquired if salicylate would counter the pyrogen effects at this same level (26). When the drug was microinjected in the vicinity of a neuron pretreated with endogenous pyrogen, the pyrogen-displaced discharge rate immediately returned toward control level. This was the case for both warm- and cold-sensitive units; the former were inhibited by the pyrogen and disinhibited by the acetylsalicylate, whereas the latter exhibited opposite behavior. Direct application of sodium acetylsalicylate to the PO/AH area without pretreatment with pyrogen elicited no consistent neuronal response. Thus it appeared that salicylate had the capacity to "reset" the discharge rate of pyrogen-offset neurons in the PO/AH, prompting the suggestion that drug and pyrogen might interact directly.

I undertook consideration of this proposal, employing a slightly different experimental protocol for its study (27). Having noted that discrete microinjection of pyrogen in the PO/AH on one side of the brain could alter the discharge of identified thermoresponsive neurons in the contralateral PO/AH (with latency similar to ipsilateral injection), I administered sodium acetylsalicylate at this unpretreated site. In all cases, administration of the antipyretic agent was followed by a change in neuronal discharge consistent with its thermoresponsive behavior, i.e., the firing rate of warm units increased while that of cold units decreased. Administration of pyrogen ipsilateral to the neuron and acetylsalicylate contralateral to it resulted in qualitatively similar observations. It was concluded, therefore, that the antagonism between endogenous pyrogen and salicylate at the neuronal level is not one of simple receptor competition and that it most likely involves an additional substrate of interaction.

PYROGENIC ACTION OF PROSTAGLANDINS

In 1970 Milton and Wendlandt (20) reported that PGE_1 would evoke a fever in unanesthetized cats when injected into the cerebroventricular space. This observation was confirmed in rabbits and rats in the following year (9) and extended to PGE_2 (23). Concurrently, Vane (32) presented evidence that salicylate had the capacity to inhibit the synthesis of prostaglandins. Because synthesis and release of prostaglandins are virtually equitable, Vane reasoned that inhibition of prostaglandin synthesis represented a major mechanism of action for salicylates. Since that time, it has also been demonstrated that endogenous pyrogen significantly accelerates the cerebral prostaglandin synthetase system *in vitro* and that this action can be inhibited by antipyretic agents (37).

Thus the stage was set for a closer examination of the neuronal mechanisms involved with fever and defervescence. Utilizing a discrete injection technique, Stitt (30) found that the primary locus of PGE_1 sensitivity was the PO/AH region, the same region that is sensitive to endogenous pyrogen. Dose-dependent fever could be generated by infusion of 20 ng to 1 μg PGE_1 into this area. Recent attempts to map PGE_1-sensitive sites more extensively in the rat brain have reconfirmed the PO/AH as the most reactive region in the brain for mediation of prostaglandin fever (34).

My studies then turned to the question of whether PGE might mediate the effects of leukocyte pyrogen on PO/AH neurons (28). A necessary condition for this would be the production of similar neuronal changes with both pyrogen and PGE. In urethane-anesthetized cats, the activity of single PO/AH units was isolated, identified as thermoresponsive (with interneuron-like characteristics), and tested with locally applied PGE_1. The neuronal reaction was not exactly the same as that with pyrogen under all conditions; depending on the PGE_1 dose employed, uni- or bidirectional responses were obtained. When 50 ng of PGE_1 was injected, warm-responsive units were depressed and cold-responsive units were excited, much as with leukocyte pyrogen. However, when 100 ng was administered, half of the cells tested exhibited a secondary reversal phenomenon, e.g., warm units that had been inhibited spontaneously and rapidly increased their rate of firing to a level above control. In experiments with repeated administration of PGE_1, the secondary component was found to decrease progressively whereas the primary one did not. I concluded that the complexity of neuronal responses to PGE_1 may reflect a multiplicity of pharmacologic effects, including modulation of local blood flow as well as direct membrane action. Under certain conditions, it was possible to mimic the actions of leukocyte pyrogen with PGE_1.

Other workers have attempted to elucidate the actions of PGE on PO/AH neurons with microiontophoresis of the agent at the recording site. This technique greatly restricts drug distribution, presumably to the immediate vicinity of the micropipette tip ($\sim 5 \mu$m) from which it is expelled, and thus it represents a more discrete mode of administration than microinjection. Unfortunately, these efforts have not yielded consistent data. Iontophoresis of PGE_1 in PO/AH areas of both the rabbit (31) and cat (17) were found to alter the neuronal activity of only 10% of the units studied. A review of the data indicates that there was no correlation between neuronal excitation or depression by PGE_1 and thermoresponsive behavior. Indeed, Stitt and Hardy noted that thermally insensitive units were indistinguishable from thermoresponsive ones in PGE_1 reactivity. Furthermore, neither study demonstrated a specific interaction of PGE_1 with biogenic amines that would be consistent with a modulatory role of the agent on fundamental neurotransmitter processes. Further work is necessary to explain the differences between the results of studies with microinjection and those with microiontophoresis.

REFERENCES

1. Cabanac, M., Stolwijk, J. A. J., and Hardy, J. D. (1968): Effect of temperature and pyrogens on single-unit activity in the rabbit's brain stem. *J. Appl. Physiol.*, 24:645–652.
2. Chai, C. Y., Lin, M. T., Chen, H. I., and Wang, S. C. (1971): The site of action of leukocytic pyrogen and antipyresis of sodium acetylsalicylate in monkeys. *Neuropharmacology*, 10:715–723.
3. Cooper, K. E., Cranston, W. I., and Honour, A. J. (1967): Observations on the site and mode of action of pyrogens in the rabbit brain. *J. Physiol.*, 191:325–337.
4. Cranston, W. I., Luff, R. H., Rawlins, M. D., and Rosendorff, C. (1970): The effects of salicylate on temperature regulation in the rabbit. *J. Physiol.*, 208:251–259.

5. Cranston, W. I., and Rawlins, M. D. (1972): Effects of intracerebral micro-injection of sodium salicylate on temperature regulation in the rabbit. *J. Physiol.*, 222:257–266.
6. Dinarello, C. A. (1979): Production of endogenous pyrogen. *Fed. Proc.*, 38:52–56.
7. Eisenman, J. S. (1969): Pyrogen-induced changes in the thermosensitivity of septal and preoptic neurons. *Am. J. Physiol.*, 216:330–334.
8. Eisenman, J. S., and Jackson, D. C. (1967): Thermal response patterns of septal and preoptic neurons in cats. *Exp. Neurol.*, 19:33–45.
9. Feldberg, W., and Saxena, P. N. (1971): Fever produced by prostaglandin E_1. *J. Physiol.*, 217:547–556.
10. Hardy, J. D., and Guieu, J. D. (1971): Integrative activity or preoptic units. II. Hypothetical network. *J. Physiol. (Paris)*, 63:264–267.
11. Hardy, J. D., Hellon, R. F., and Sutherland, K. (1964): Temperature sensitive neurones in the dog's hypothalamus. *J. Physiol.*, 175:242–253.
12. Hellon, R. F. (1967): Thermal stimulation of hypothalamic neurones in unanesthetized rabbits. *J. Physiol.*, 193:318–395.
13. Hellon, R. F. (1970): The stimulation of hypothalamic neurones by changes in ambient temperature. *Pfluegers Arch.*, 321:56–66.
14. Hellon, R. F. (1972): Temperature-sensitive neurons in the brain stem: Their responses to brain temperature at different ambient temperatures. *Pfluegers Arch.*, 335:323–334.
15. Jackson, D. L. (1967): A hypothalamic region responsive to localized injection of pyrogens. *J. Neurophysiol.*, 30:586–602.
16. Jell, R. M., and Gloor, P. (1971): Distribution of thermosensitive and nonthermosensitive preoptic and anterior hypothalamic neurons in unanesthetized cats and effects of some anesthetics. *Can. J. Physiol. Pharmacol.*, 50:890–901.
17. Jell, R. M., and Sweatman, P. (1977): Prostaglandin-sensitive neurones in cat hypothalamus: Relation to thermoregulation and to biogenic amines. *Can. J. Physiol. Pharmacol.*, 55:560–567.
18. Knox, G. V., Campbell, C., and Lomax, P. (1973): Cutaneous temperature and unit activity in the hypothalamic thermoregulatory centers. *Exp. Neurol.*, 40:717–730.
19. Lin, M. T., and Chai, C. Y. (1972): The antipyretic effect of sodium acetylsalicylate on pyrogen-induced fever in rabbits. *J. Pharmacol. Exp. Ther.*, 180:603–609.
20. Milton, A. S., and Wendlandt, S. (1970): A possible role of prostaglandin E_1 as a modulator for temperature regulation in the central nervous system of the cat. *J. Physiol.*, 207:76–77P.
21. Myers, R. D. (1971): Hypothalamic mechanisms of pyrogen action in the cat and monkey. In: *Ciba Foundation Symposium on Pyrogens and Fever*, edited by G. E. W. Wolstenholme and J. Birch, pp. 131–153. Churchill, London.
22. Nakayama, T., Hammel, H. T., Hardy, J. D., and Eisenman, J. S. (1963): Thermal stimulation of electrical activity of single units of the preoptic region. *Am. J. Physiol.*, 204:1122–1126.
23. Potts, W. J., and East, P. F. (1972): Effects of prostaglandin E_2 on body temperature of conscious rats and cats. *Arch. Int. Pharmacodyn. Ther.*, 197:31–36.
24. Ranson, S. W. (1940): Regulation of body temperature. *Res. Publ. Assoc. Nerv. Ment. Dis.*, 20:342–399.
25. Repin, I. S., and Kratskin, I. L. (1967): Hypothalamic mechanisms of fever. *Fiziol. Zh. SSSR*, 53:1206–1211.
26. Schoener, E. P., and Wang, S. C. (1975): Leucocytic pyrogen and sodium acetylsalicylate on hypothalamic neurons in the cat. *Am. J. Physiol.*, 229:185–190.
27. Schoener, E. P., and Wang, S. C. (1975): Observations on the central mechanism of acetylsalicylate antipyresis. *Life Sci.*, 17:1063–1068.
28. Schoener, E. P., and Wang, S. C. (1976): Effects of locally administered prostaglandin E_1 on anterior hypothalamic neurons. *Brain Res.*, 117:157–162.
29. Splawinski, J. A., Gorka, Z., Zacny, E., and Kaluza, J. (1977): Fever produced in the rat by intracerebral *E. coli* endotoxin. *Pfluegers Arch.*, 368:117–123.
30. Stitt, J. T. (1973): Prostaglandin E_1 fever induced in rabbits. *J. Physiol.*, 232:163–179.
31. Stitt, J. T., and Hardy, J. D. (1975): Microelectrophoresis of PGE_1 onto single units in the rabbit hypothalamus. *Am. J. Physiol.*, 229:240–245.
32. Vane, J. R. (1971): Inhibition of prostaglandin synthesis as a mechanism of action for aspirin-like drugs. *Nature [New Biol.]*, 231:232–235.
33. Villablanca, J., and Myers, R. D. (1965): Fever produced by microinjection of typhoid vaccine into hypothalamus of cats. *Am. J. Physiol.*, 208:703–707.

34. Williams, J. W., Rudy, T. A., Yaksh, T. L., and Viswanathan, C. T. (1977): An extensive exploration of the rat brain for sites mediating prostaglandin-induced hyperthermia. *Brain Res.*, 120:251–262.
35. Wit, A., and Wang, S. C. (1968): Temperature-sensitive neurons in preoptic/anterior hypothalamic region: Effects of increasing ambient temperature. *Am. J. Physiol.*, 215:1151–1159.
36. Wit, A., and Wang, S. C. (1968): Temperature-sensitive neurons in preoptic/anterior hypothalamic region: Actions of pyrogen and acetylsalicylate. *Am. J. Physiol.*, 215:1160–1169.
37. Ziel, R., and Krupp, P. (1976): Influence of endogenous pyrogen on cerebral prostaglandin-synthetase system. *Experientia*, 32:1451–1452.

Fever, edited by James M. Lipton.
Raven Press, New York © 1980.

Fever: Intermediary Neurohumoral Factors Serving the Hypothalamic Mechanism Underlying Hyperthermia

R. D. Myers and W. D. Ruwe

Departments of Psychiatry and Pharmacology, University of North Carolina School of Medicine, Chapel Hill, North Carolina 27514

When it was first observed that an endotoxin applied directly to the thermosensitive region of the hypothalamus causes an intense fever (28), one inexplicable fact stood out. A latency of up to 20 min for the beginning of the pyrexic response was noted repeatedly. This suggested at once that some kind of endogenous neurohumoral factor must function as a chemical intermediary between the pyrogen, its local action on the neuronal tissue, and the final efferent responses subserving thermogenesis (29).

Today the idea still persists, perhaps more strongly, that one or more endogenous substances act as mediators of the febrile response (16). Historically, the candidate suspected initially was serotonin (5-HT). Following the intrahypothalamic injection of 5-HT (8), the shivering, vasoconstriction, and sharp rise in temperature, seen almost immediately, provided the clue that this endogenous indoleamine could be a neuronal mediator of a bacterial pyrogen. Further evidence over and above the physiological responses to 5-HT include the findings (8) that 5-HT nerve endings terminate in the thermosensitive zone of the anterior hypothalamus, which is reactive to endotoxin as well as to leukocyte pyrogen; an enhanced release of 5-HT occurs during the intense thermogenesis of a febrile episode; the attenuation of 5-HT hyperthermia can be brought about by an antipyretic; and the increased synthesis of 5-HT within the hypothalamus occurs during fever. On the obverse side, Borsook et al. (2) claim that heat production induced in the rabbit by 5-HT and the febrile response produced by bacterial pyrogen are able to be dissociated pharmacologically.

With the passage of the "amine era" of the 1960s, it is now clear that 5-HT cannot be the sole hypothalamic mediator of a pyrexic response. In fact, a variety of chemical substances which are present in the hypothalamus have been implicated as intermediary factors. A host of experiments show that a specific substance can evoke a substantial rise in core temperature when it is injected into the hypothalamus or infused into the cerebral ventricle of the unanesthetized animal. Selected findings based on these investigations are presented as follows.

PROSTAGLANDINS

Prostaglandin of the E series (PGE) has been proposed as another CNS mediator for the febrile reaction. This is based on two main avenues of evidence: (a) the extreme thermogenic potency of PGE, in the nanogram range, when injected into either the cerebral ventricle or anterior hypothalamus, and (b) the release of PGE into the ventricular fluid during the course of an endotoxin fever (7). Strong evidence has also accumulated recently which coutermands the theory that PGE serves as an intermediary for fever. As reviewed by Veale et al. (27), many experiments fail to reveal any concordance between pyrogen- and PGE-induced fever: (a) PGE is not released from the anterior hypothalamus during endotoxin fever, even from sites sensitive to PGE; (b) an anterior hypothalamic lesion abolished PGE but not pyrogen fever; (c) the newborn lamb develops fever in response to bacterial or leukocyte pyrogen, but exhibits no thermogenic response to PGE; (d) following pyrogen administration, salicylate infusion in a low dose prevents PGE release but not the febrile response; and (e) pharmacological antagonists of PGE block PGE hyperthermia, but fail to prevent pyrogen fever.

In connection with the theory, compounds related to PGE, including lipid A (7) and other fatty acids (1), do cause a marked hyperthermia when they are applied centrally. Again, however, whether or not any of these lipids play a functional role in the genesis of a bacterial fever is uncertain. For example, we know that PGE hyperthermia is not mediated by a change in the presynaptic release of 5-HT or norepinephrine from the rostral hypothalamus (17). Although the activity of cyclic AMP in the cerebrospinal fluid may indeed correlate with the rise in temperature induced by PGE, the specific function of ubiquitous cyclic nucleotides in a given temperature change is controversial (16).

PEPTIDES AND OTHER SUBSTANCES

That the so-called peptidergic neurons, which are located in the hypothalamus and contain putative peptide neurotransmitters (23), may mediate fever is also a possibility. One of the peptides first to be implicated in the central mechanism for the control of body temperature was thyrotropin-releasing hormone (TRH) (14). Although this tripeptide given intracerebrally can evoke a hypo- or hyperthermic response (13), its possible function is clouded by the fact that it exerts no action either on the anterior preoptic thermosensitive region or on the cells of the posterior hypothalamus when microinjected directly into these areas (19).

The gut hormone which is found throughout the entire gastrointestinal tract, vasoactive intestinal polypeptide (VIP), is for no known reason present in the hypothalamus. When infused into the cerebral ventricle of the cat, VIP evokes a dose-dependent rise in temperature (4) which is not only slight (about 0.5°C), but also of a short duration (less than 1 hr). Thus, like TRH, this peptide does not seem to be a candidate likely to serve as a fever mediator.

In both the cat and rat the endogenous opioid enkephalin evokes hyperthermia when injected into the cerebral ventricle in a dose of from 100 to 250 μg (3,9). Although it is unlikely that the pentapeptide could have any role in thermoregulation (3), it is nevertheless of interest to know the site of thermogenic action of an enkephalin, particularly in light of the unusual finding with TRH (19).

Therefore, we implanted guide tubes to rest just above the thermosensitive zone in the cat's anterior preoptic area within coronal plane AP 15.0. At a depth at which 5-HT (3.5 μg), *Salmonella typhosa* (1:10 dilution), or PGE$_1$ (100 ng) all evoked an intense and prolonged rise in body temperature, leu-enkephalin dissolved in artificial CSF was microinjected bilaterally in a volume of 1.0 μl.

As shown in Fig. 1 *(top)* 1.0 μg enkephalin had no effect on the temperature

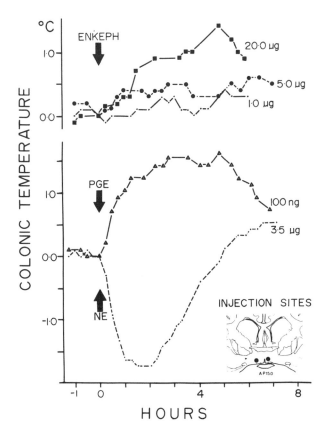

FIG. 1. Body temperature of the unanesthetized cat after microinjections of compounds in a 1.0 μl volume at the two sites shown in the histological inset. (AP 15.0). At the *arrow* **(top)** leu-enkephalin was injected in the doses as indicated at 48-hr intervals. At the *arrows* **(bottom)**, either 100 ng PGE$_1$ or 3.5 μg norepinephrine was microinjected bilaterally. Time is in hours.

of the cat. However, a dose of 5.0 μg caused a modest elevation of 0.5°C over a 1-hr interval. When 20 μg of enkephalin was infused, a gradual increase in the cat's temperature occurred which was quite dissimilar to the sharp rise in core temperature evoked by endotoxin, 5-HT, or PGE. To illustrate, at the same bilateral microinjection sites (Fig. 1, *bottom*), 100 ng PGE_1 induced its typical hyperthermic response characterized by a short latency and rapid rise. Interestingly, the area was also monoamine sensitive as evidenced by the deep fall in the cat's temperature brought about by 3.5 μg norepinephrine (NE) infused again at the same hypothalamic sites.

Thus whether or not an endogenous enkephalin plays any part in the thermoregulatory process within the hypothalamus remains to be seen, particularly in view of its low potency.

CALCIUM IONS

There are now many independent lines of experimental evidence which support the theory that the inherent stability of specific ions within the posterior hypothalamus establishes a "set-point" or reference around which the temperature of the animal is defended (16). Given the validity of the notion that a fever represents an upward displacement of the set-point temperature (5), then a pyrogen ought to disturb the ionic balance in the posterior hypothalamus. However, a serious anatomical incongruency is immediately apparent. How can caudal hypothalamic neurons underpin the perturbation of a temperature set-point value when the site of action of a pyrogen is the rostral hypothalamus?

Recently, a resolution to this morphological dilemma has emerged. It appears that the proposed posterior hypothalamic set-point mechanism, which depends on the ratio of Na^+ to Ca^{2+} ions, receives powerful and direct neuronal input from the anterior hypothalamic thermosensitive zone (21). That is, when the rostral preoptic region is warmed locally, the activity of Ca^{2+} ions in the posterior hypothalamus, as reflected in their local efflux, is sharply reduced. Conversely, when the same anterior region is cooled locally, the efflux of Ca^{2+} ions again within the posterior area is substantially enhanced. Peripheral warming or cooling has precisely the same mutually antagonistic effects on the kinetics of Ca^{2+} ions in the caudal hypothalamus. But in both instances, the warm or cold stress must be intense so as to subject the set-point itself to a severe challenge, i.e., as if one were plunged into an ice-cold bath (21).

Ca^{2+} ions would now appear also to serve as an intermediary along the anatomical pathway involved in the genesis of a fever. In one set of experiments, we found that an endotoxin infused into a lateral cerebral ventricle releases $^{45}Ca^{2+}$ ions into the third ventricle; conversely, an antipyretic given systemically reversed the ventricular efflux of $^{45}Ca^{2+}$ ions as the febrile cat's temperature declined toward its normal base line (15).

A rather striking demonstration of the involvement of Ca^{2+} ions as a thermogenic intermediary is seen in the results of experiments in which the posterior hypothalamus was labeled with $^{45}Ca^{2+}$ ions 18 hr prior to its push–pull perfusion.

As shown in Fig. 2, when the cat's ambient temperature is raised to 40°C for a brief interval, $^{45}Ca^{2+}$ ions are retained in the posterior hypothalamus; but when the ambient temperature is transiently lowered to 0°C, an immediate efflux of Ca^{2+} occurs from the same perfusion site.

Most important, a pyrogen infused directly into a morphologically reactive

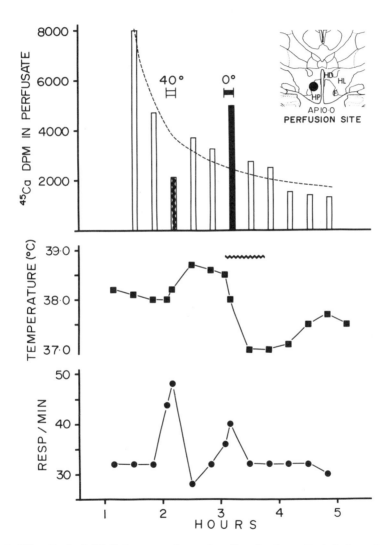

FIG. 2. Efflux **(top)** of $^{45}Ca^{2+}$ in successive push–pull perfusates collected at a rate of 50 μl/min from the perfusion site denoted by the dot in the histological inset. The site had been labeled with 1.0 μCi $^{45}Ca^{2+}$ 18 hr earlier. The chamber temperature of the cat was raised to 40°C or lowered to 0°C just preceding and during the third and sixth perfusions, respectively, as denoted by the *bars*. Colonic temperature **(middle)** and respiratory rate **(bottom)** were recorded continuously. Shivering is designated by the *zig-zag line* **(middle)**. (From Myers et al., ref. 21, with permission.)

site in the anterior hypothalamus evokes an identical ionic shift. Figure 3 presents the same kind of paradigm except that 1:10 dilution of *S. typhosa* was microinjected bilaterally into the cat's anterior hypothalamus as denoted by the arrow. Just before the onset of shivering and the subsequent rise in colonic temperature, a sharp peak in $^{45}Ca^{2+}$ efflux occurred (Fig. 3, *top*). Instead of a "washout"

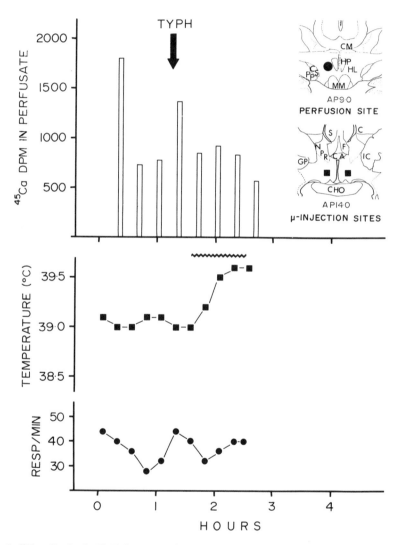

FIG. 3. Efflux **(top)** of $^{45}Ca^{2+}$ in successive push–pull perfusates collected at a rate of 50 μl/min from the perfusion site denoted by the dot in the histological inset. The site had been labeled with 1.0 μCi $^{45}Ca^{2+}$ 18 hr earlier. A $\frac{1}{10}$ dilution of *Salmonella typhosa* (TYPH) was microinjected in a volume of 1.0 μl, before the fourth perfusion, as indicated by the *arrow*, at the injection sites designated by the *squares* in the histological inset. Shivering indicated by the *zig-zag line;* colonic temperature **(middle)** and respiratory rate **(bottom)** are as shown in previous figure. (From Myers et al., ref. 21, with permission.)

of Ca^{2+} ions, typically noted in the control condition, $^{45}Ca^{2+}$ efflux continued to be elevated as the fever developed. A parallel finding is most interesting. When 5-HT was microinjected at homologous loci in the cat's anterior hypothalamus, the calcium response was identical. Figure 4 depicts the same pronounced and sustained efflux of $^{45}Ca^{2+}$ ions from the perfusion site in the cat's posterior hypothalamus after 5-HT was microinjected in a dose of 5.0 μg into the animal's

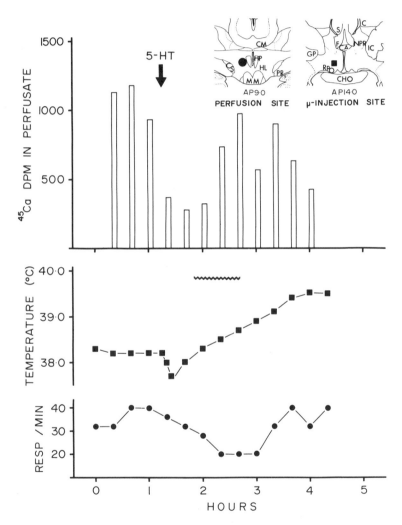

FIG. 4. Efflux **(top)** of $^{45}Ca^{2+}$ in successive push–pull perfusates collected at a rate of 50 μl/min from the perfusion site denoted by the *dot* in the histological inset. The site had been labeled with 1.0 μCi $^{45}Ca^{2+}$ 18 hr earlier. 5.0 μl serotonin (5-HT) was microinjected in a volume of 1.0 μl before the fourth perfusion, as indicated by the *arrow,* at the injection site designated by the *square* in the histological inset. Shivering indicated by the *zig-zag line;* colonic temperature **(middle)** and respiratory rate **(bottom)** are the same as in previous figures. (From Myers et al., ref. 21, with permission.)

anterior hypothalamic preoptic area. It is notable that the most substantial shift in cation output occurs during the interval of shivering and at a level of temperature which was approaching 0.2 to 0.4°C above this individual cat's set-point level of 38.2°C.

Two other points are pertinent. First, PGE_1 exerts virtually the same enhancing effect on the release of $^{45}Ca^{2+}$ from the caudal hypothalamus, whereas NE applied to the same anterior hypothalamic locus attenuates the efflux of the cation. Second, the local anesthetic procaine, when infused into the endotoxin-, PGE-, or amine-sensitive site, totally blocks any change in either direction of $^{45}Ca^{2+}$ activity in the posterior hypothalamus during a severe cold or heat challenge (21).

Overall, these results strongly suggest that a pyrogen, whether acting through 5-HT, PGE, a peptide, or other intermediary factor, affects the thermoregulatory neurons located within the anterior hypothalamus. In turn, these cells transmit impulses to the neurons within a circumscribed portion of the posterior hypothalamic area; and these signals are coded in such a way as to activate a shift in the set-point temperature. The unbinding of Ca^{2+} ions from the membrane or their loss from intracellular mitochondrial stores could constitute the mechanism whereby the intrinsic stability of the posterior hypothalamic neurons is temporarily disrupted. The change in Ca^{2+} stability presumably results in an increased firing rate of efferent cells that activate the pathway for thermogenesis (22).

UNKNOWN PROTEIN FACTOR

The "missing link" in fever, as it were, has made itself further known in a somewhat round about fashion. Among the initial observations made by Takagi and colleagues was that the endotoxin-induced release of 5-HT from blood platelets in the periphery not only is Ca^{2+} dependent, but also requires an additional unknown protein factor (18). Later, it was found that a metabolic inhibitor alters the production of leukocyte pyrogen (10), whereas the inhibition of protein synthesis retards the hyperthermic response to tryptaminergic or pyrogenic substances (12,25). In view of these results, we tested the possibility further that a brain protein substrate may constitute an important neurochemical intermediary in pyrogen fever.

In the first series of experiments, we used the potent inhibitor of protein synthesis cycloheximide; however, because of the nonspecific and highly toxic side effects of cycloheximide (26), we turned to a structurally dissimilar inhibitor, anisomycin, whose effects on protein synthesis are transient, completely reversible, and mainly on ribosomal translocation (24). Flood et al. (11) showed that anisomycin injected peripherally in a comparable concentration inhibits brain protein synthesis up to 90%. When given subcutaneously in a dose of 30 mg/kg, anisomycin completely inhibits a pyrogen fever. In fact, as shown in Fig. 5, the drug given 30 min prior to intravenous typhoid (1.0 ml of 1:10 dilution of 10^8 organisms/ml) causes a gradual but long-acting decline in the cat's colonic temperature. Surprisingly, 10 hr later, the animal is still afebrile.

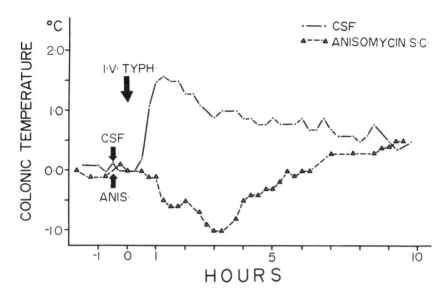

FIG. 5. Body temperature of the unanesthetized cat in two separate experiments in which either 10 ml CSF was given subcutaneously or the same volume of anisomycin (ANIS) was given in a dose of 30 mg/kg. In both cases, 1.0 ml of 1:10 dilution of typhoid vaccine was injected intravenously 30 min later. Time is in hours.

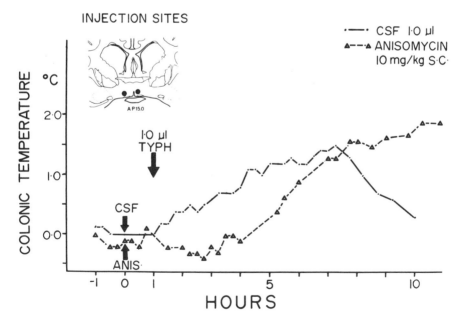

FIG. 6. Body temperature of the unanesthetized cat in two separate experiments. In the first, CSF was microinjected into the hypothalamus (1.0 μl), and in the second, 10 mg/kg anisomycin was infused intravenously. One hour later, in both cases, 1.0 μl of typhoid vaccine (1:10 dilution) was infused in a volume of 1.0 μl into the two injection sites depicted in the histological inset of AP 15.0.

Perhaps the most crucial issue revolves about the question of whether the protein factor operates in the diencephalic mediation of a fever. Therefore, in the next series of experiments with the cannulated cats, we first located bilateral hypothalamic sites that were reactive to a 1:10 dilution of *S. typhosa* infused in a 1.0 μl volume. Two days later a lower dose of anisomycin, 10 mg/kg, was injected intravenously 1 hr before the intrahypothalamic infusion of the typhoid bacteria. As illustrated in Fig. 6, anisomycin entirely prevented the development of a fever for over 3 hr. In contrast, the same concentration and volume of typhoid in the control, non-anisomycin-treated cat caused an almost immediate and sustained rise in the animal's core temperature (Fig. 6).

Taken together, these results suggest to us that a pyrogen acts locally within the anterior hypothalamic area to cause the synthesis of new protein material. Other experiments currently under way hopefully will delineate the effects of protein inhibition on the hyperthermia induced by other suspected intermediaries as well as on the lability of the ionic mechanism in the caudal hypothalamus.

CONCLUSION

There are difficult issues to contemplate in the evaluation of every putative fever factor, even those yet to evolve. The following questions underscore the nature of these issues.

Pharmacologically, what does a given factor do in the brain in terms of a central mechanism concerned with thermogenesis? Does the substance release 5-HT or acetylcholine? Does it alter the balance in amine activity? Does it block postsynaptic catecholamine receptors? Does it unbind, displace, release, or otherwise sequester calcium ions in the hypothalamus?

Anatomically, where does the substance act? In the anterior hypothalamic preoptic area within the thermosensitive zone? Or in the posterior hypothalamic thermally insensitive zone? Or in other structures in the brainstem?

Physiologically, does the substance really have anything to do with thermogenesis in terms of the principal mechanisms of heat production and conservation including vasoconstriction, increased metabolic rate, pilomotor response, shivering, and the reciprocal blockade of the heat loss pathway? Is the factor equally involved in heat production in the animal's defense against cold or only in a bacterial fever? If so, does an endotoxin or leukocyte pyrogen augment the metabolic synthesis, release, or accumulation of the intermediary substance? This latter functional consideration is of great importance, since the endogenous activity of the factor would clearly reflect its biological attribute.

In view of these questions, a provisional set of criteria for determining whether an amine, cation, peptide, amino acid, or other substance in the CNS plays a role in fever is presented.

1. The putative fever factor should act on the circumscribed area of nerve cells within the anterior hypothalamic preoptic area, which is the single most reactive structure to either leukocyte pyrogen (6) or endotoxin (20).

2. The potency of the fever factor on the cells of the hypothalamus should reflect a concentration (dose)-response relationship in terms of the induced pyrexia.

3. The factor-induced elevation in temperature should be attenuated or otherwise altered by an antipyretic which may itself exert a central action.

4. When a pyrogen is administered peripherally in a concentration sufficient to evoke fever, a change in the synthesis or accumulation or *in vivo* release of the factor ought to occur. If so, the magnitude of release should correlate with the magnitude and rate of rise in the animal's core temperature.

5. A pyrogen fever ought not to develop independently of the presence, synthesis, or release of the factor.

6. When synthesis of the putative fever factor is inhibited, the genesis of a fever ordinarily produced by a given endotoxin or leukocyte pyrogen should likewise be impaired.

7. The factor should exert one or more distinct effects *in vivo* on neurons, neuroglia, or pathways ostensibly involved in pathological thermogenesis or its amelioration. These would include serotonergic, cholinergic, or noradrenergic neurons as well as those cells which not only are sensitive to an ionic imbalance, but also exhibit calcium lability.

ACKNOWLEDGMENTS

This research was supported in part by Office of Naval Research Contract N00014–75–C–0203 and by National Science Foundation Grant BMS-18441 to R. D. Myers.

REFERENCES

1. Beleslin, D. B., Dimitrijević, M., and Samardžić, R. (1974): Hyperthermic effect of palmitate sodium, stearate sodium and oleate sodium injected into the cerebral ventricles of conscious cats. *Neuropharmacology*, 13:221–223.
2. Borsook, D., Laburn, H. P., Rosendorff, C., Willies, G. H., and Woolf, C. J. (1977): A dissociation between temperature regulation and fever in the rabbit. *J. Physiol.*, 266:423–433.
3. Clark, W. G. (1977): Emetic and hyperthermic effects of centrally injected methionine-enkephalin in cats. *Proc. Soc. Exp. Biol. Med.*, 154:540–542.
4. Clark, W. G., Lipton, J. M., and Said, S. I. (1978): Hyperthermic responses to vasoactive intestinal polypeptide (VIP) injected into the third cerebral ventricle of cats. *Neuropharmacology*, 17:883–885.
5. Cooper, K. E., and Veale, W. L. (1974): Fever, an abnormal drive to the heat-conserving and producing mechanism? In: *Recent Studies of Hypothalamic Function*, edited by K. Lederis and K. E. Cooper, pp. 391–398. S. Karger, Basel.
6. Cooper, K. E., Veale, W. L., and Pittman, Q. J. (1976): Pathogenesis of fever. In: *Brain Dysfunction in Infantile Febrile Convulsions*, edited by M. A. B. Brazier and F. Coceani, pp. 107–115. Raven Press, New York.

7. Feldberg, W. (1975): The Ferrier Lecture, 1974. Body temperature and fever: Changes in our views during the last decade. *Proc. R. Soc. Lond.* [*Biol.*], 191:199–229.
8. Feldberg, W., and Myers, R. D. (1965): Changes in temperature produced by microinjections of amines into the anterior hypothalamus of cats. *J. Physiol.*, 177:239–245.
9. Ferri, S., Arrigo Reina, A., Santagostino, A., Scoto, G. M., and Spadaro, C. (1978): Effects of met-enkephalin on body temperature of normal and morphine-tolerant rats. *Psychopharmacology*, 58:277–281.
10. Fleetwood, M. K., Gander, G. W., and Goodale, F. (1975): Effect of metabolic inhibitors on pyrogen production by rabbit leucocytes. *Proc. Soc. Exp. Biol. Med.*, 149:336–339.
11. Flood, J. F., Rosenzweig, M. R., Bennett, E. L., and Orme, A. E. (1974): Comparison of the effects of anisomycin on memory across six strains of mice. *Behav. Biol.*, 10:147–160.
12. Graham-Smith, D. G. (1972): The prevention by inhibitors of brain protein synthesis of the hyperactivity and hyperpyrexia produced in rats by monoamine oxidase inhibition and the administration of L-tryptophan or 5-methoxy-*N*, *N*-dimethyl-tryptamine. *J. Neurochem.*, 19:2409–2422.
13. Horita, A., Carino, M. A., and Chestnut, R. M. (1976): Influence of thyrotropin releasing hormone (TRH) on drug-induced narcosis and hypothermia in rabbits. *Psychopharmacology*, 49:57–62.
14. Metcalf, G. (1974): TRH: A possible mediator of thermoregulation. *Nature*, 252:310–311.
15. Myers, R. D. (1974): Ionic concepts of the set-point for body temperature. In: *Recent Studies of Hypothalamic Function*, edited by K. Lederis and K. E. Cooper, pp. 371–390. S. Karger, Basel.
16. Myers, R. D. (1980): Hypothalamic control of thermoregulation: Neurochemical mechanisms. In: *Handbook of the Hypothalamus*, edited by P. Morgane and J. Panksepp. Marcel Dekker, New York (*in press*).
17. Myers, R. D., and Waller, M. B. (1976): Is prostaglandin fever mediated by the presynaptic release of hypothalamic 5-HT or norepinephrine? *Brain Res. Bull.*, 1:47–56.
18. Myers, R. D., and Waller, M. B. (1977): Serotonin and thermoregulation. In: *Serotonin in Health and Disease, Vol. 11, Physiological Regulation and Pharmacological Action*, edited by W. B. Essman, pp. 1–68. Spectrum, New York.
19. Myers, R. D., Metcalf, G., and Rice, J. C. (1977): Identification by microinjection of TRH-sensitive sites in the cat's brainstem that mediate respiratory, temperature and other autonomic changes. *Brain Res.*, 126:105–115.
20. Myers, R. D., Rudy, T. A., and Yaksh, T. L. (1974): Fever produced by endotoxin injected into the hypothalamus of the monkey and its antagonism by salicylate. *J. Physiol.*, 243:167–193.
21. Myers, R. D., Simpson, C. W., Higgins, D., Nattermann, R. A., Rice, J. C., Redgrave, P., and Metcalf, G. (1976): Hypothalamic Na$^+$ and Ca^{++} ions and temperature setpoint: New mechanisms of action of a central or peripheral thermal challenge and intrahypothalamic 5-HT, NE, PGE$_1$ and pyrogen. *Brain Res. Bull.*, 1:301–327.
22. Nutik, S. L. (1971): Effect of temperature change of the preoptic region and skin on posterior hypothalamic neurons. *J. Physiol. (Paris)*, 63:368–370.
23. Otsuka, M., and Takahashi, T. (1977): Putative peptide neurotransmitters. *Annu. Rev. Pharmacol. Toxicol.*, 17:425–439.
24. Pestka, S. (1971): Inhibitors of ribosome functions. *Annu. Rev. Microbiol.* 25:487–562.
25. Siegert, R., Philipp-Dormston, W. K., Radsak, K., and Menzel, H. (1976): Mechanism of fever induction in rabbits. *Infect. Immun.*, 14:1130–1137.
26. Squire, L. R., and Barondes, S. H. (1974): Anisomycin, like other inhibitors of cerebral protein synthesis, impairs 'long-term' memory of a discrimination task. *Brain Res.*, 66:301–308.
27. Veale, W. L., Cooper, K. E., and Pittman, Q. J. (1977): Role of prostaglandins in fever and temperature regulation. In: *Prostaglandins, Vol. 3*, edited by P. W. Ramwell, pp. 145–167. Plenum Press, New York.
28. Villablanca, J., and Myers, R. D. (1964): Fever production by endotoxin injections in the cat. *Arch. Biol. Med. Exp.*, 1:102.
29. Villablanca, J., and Myers, R. D. (1965): Fever produced by microinjection of typhoid vaccine into hypothalamus of cats. *Am. J. Physiol.*, 208:703–707.

Fever, edited by James M. Lipton.
Raven Press, New York © 1980.

On the Central Protein Mediator of Fever

Christopher C. Barney, Melvin J. Fregly, Michael J. Katovich,
and Paul E. Tyler

*Department of Physiology, University of Florida College of Medicine,
Gainesville, Florida 32610*

Fever is a regulated increase in body temperature that occurs in response to exogenous pyrogens (25). These pyrogens, in turn, induce the formation of endogenous pyrogens that act on the brain (6,17). This observation has stimulated a number of investigators to consider the role of various neurochemical mediators in the genesis of fever. The possible central mediators of fever include the putative neurotransmitters 5-hydroxytryptamine, norepinephrine, epinephrine, and acetylcholine (25). More recently, it has also been suggested that central prostaglandins may be mediators of fever (10,22,30). Their role, however, is still in question (1,7,9,24,29). Other putative mediators of fever include cyclic AMP (21,23,31) and sodium and calcium ions (19).

Recently Siegert and his colleagues (27,28) proposed that the development of fever depends on the synthesis of a specific protein mediator. These investigators also suggested that several exogenous pyrogens may induce a fever by way of the same intermediate step, i.e., the synthesis of a specific protein. Our objective is to review some of the studies of Siegert and his colleagues, as well as some recent studies from our laboratory that are pertinent to the hypothesis that central protein synthesis is essential to fever.

EFFECT OF CYCLOHEXIMIDE ON THE DEVELOPMENT OF EXOGENOUS PYROGEN-INDUCED FEVER

Newcastle disease virus (NDV) produces fever when administered to rabbits (Fig. 1A) (27). Following pretreatment with saline, NDV (2,000 hemagglutination units/kg) gave rise to a long-lasting increase in body temperature which could be blocked by pretreatment with cycloheximide, an inhibitor of protein synthesis (20), at a dose of 5 mg/kg, (Fig. 1B). Following administration of cycloheximide, rectal temperature fell approximately 0.6°C. Subsequent administration of NDV 90 min later did not induce an early fever reaction, although rectal temperature did increase 7 hr later. This late febrile response could be blocked by a second administration of cycloheximide 4 hr after injection of NDV (Fig. 1C).

Fever due to NDV is not the only fever that can be blocked by cycloheximide.

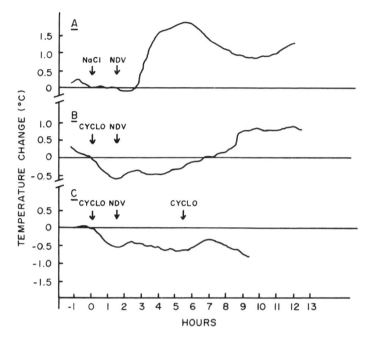

FIG. 1. Mean change in rectal temperature of rabbits administered Newcastle disease virus (NDV, 2,000 HAU/kg) with and without pretreatment with cycloheximide (CYCLO). Shown are data from rabbits pretreated with NaCl **(A)** and cycloheximide (5 mg/kg) **(B)** and rabbits administered cycloheximide (5 mg/kg) before and 2.5 mg/kg after the administration of NDV **(C)**. (Adapted from Siegert et al., ref. 27.)

Cycloheximide pretreatment (5 mg/kg) also prevented the febrile response of rabbits to *Escherichia coli* lipopolysaccharide (LPS, 5 μg/kg; Fig. 2I) and to polyinosinic:polycytidylic acid [Poly (I:C), 16.5 μg/kg; Fig. 2II], as well as to NDV (Fig. 2III) (28). In each case cycloheximide lowered baseline body temperature while control injections of saline had no effect (Fig. 2IV). These experiments by Siegert et al. (27,28) suggested that cycloheximide was an effective antipyretic in rabbits and that the synthesis and release of protein was required as a mediator of fever.

EFFECT OF CYCLOHEXIMIDE ON PRODUCTION AND PYROGENICITY OF ENDOGENOUS PYROGEN

Although cycloheximide prevented the rise in temperature following administration of exogenous pyrogens, it did not appear to do so by preventing the production of endogenous pyrogen. When the serum of rabbits given either LPS, Poly (I:C) or NDV was administered to nontreated rabbits, the recipient rabbits responded with rapid increases in body temperature. This response was observed even though the donor rabbits had been pretreated with cycloheximide

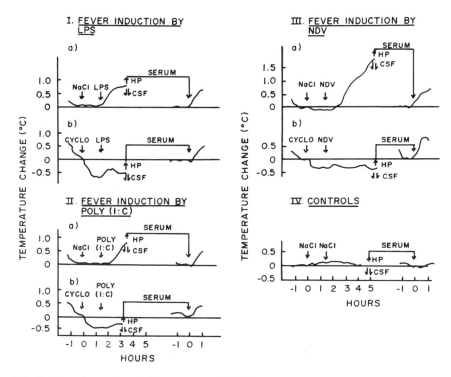

FIG. 2. Mean change in rectal temperature of rabbits administered *E. coli* lipopolysaccharide (5 μg/kg) **(I, LPS)**, double-stranded Poly (I:C) **[II, Poly (I:C)]** (16.5 μg/kg), or Newcastle disease virus (2,000 HAU/kg) **(III, NDV)** following NaCl **(a)** or cycloheximide (5 mg/kg; **b**) pretreatment. Also shown is the mean response to two control injections of NaCl **(IV)**. Heart puncture for serum to test for the presence of endogenous pyrogen performed at HP. Removal of cerebrospinal fluid from the cisterna magna for measurements of PGE and cyclic AMP levels performed at CSF. Second curve on each line is the mean rectal temperature response of untreated rabbits receiving serum from the treated rabbits. (Adapted from Siegert et al., ref. 28.)

(Fig. 2) (28). The finding that the febrile response of the recipient rabbits could be prevented by heating the donor serum samples (90°C for 30 min) indicates that there was endogenous pyrogen in the sera of both cycloheximide- and saline-pretreated rabbits. The serum of control animals was without effect on rectal temperatures of recipient rabbits (Fig. 2IV).

The endogenous pyrogens produced by LPS, Poly (I:C), and NDV appeared to be similar in that the magnitude of the febrile response to each was essentially the same (Fig. 3) (28). Pretreatment of recipient rabbits with saline did not prevent the increase in rectal temperature induced by serum from donor rabbits administered LPS, Poly (I:C), or NDV. On the other hand, pretreatment of recipient rabbits with cycloheximide (5 mg/kg) prevented the febrile effect of the endogenous pyrogen regardless of the exogenous pyrogen administered (Fig. 3). Thus cycloheximide appears to block fever induced in the rabbit by either exogenous or endogenous pyrogen. These findings of Siegert et al. (27,28) suggest

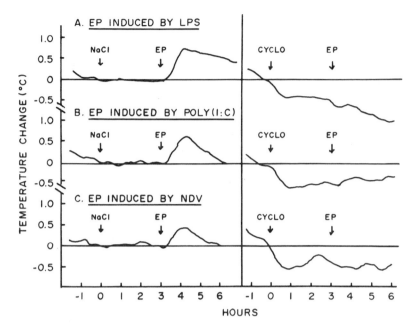

FIG. 3. Mean change in rectal temperature of rabbits administered endogenous pyrogen induced in separate rabbits by administration of LPS **(A),** Poly (I:C) **(B),** or NDV **(C)** following NaCl and cycloheximide (5 mg/kg) pretreatment. (Adapted from Siegert et al., ref. 28.)

that cycloheximide prevents fever by acting at a site beyond that at which endogenous pyrogen is produced.

EFFECT OF CYCLOHEXIMIDE ON PRODUCTION OF PGE AND CAMP DURING FEVER

Administration of pyrogens leads to an increase in the concentration of both prostaglandin (PG) and cyclic AMP in cerebrospinal fluid (CSF) obtained from the cerebral ventricles of rabbits (10,16,21,22). Phillip-Dormston and Siegert (22) showed that the increase in prostaglandin concentration following administration of pyrogens was specific to the hyperthermic prostaglandins, PGE, with no change occurring in the concentration of $PGF_{2\alpha}$. Other studies (4,8), including a recent study by Bernheim et al. (3), suggest that the increase in PGE concentration in the CSF is specific to fever and is not the result of increased metabolic rate, body temperature, or brain temperature. Siegert et al. (28) have shown that administration of LPS, Poly (I:C), and NDV to rabbits results in significant increase in PGE and cyclic AMP concentrations in the CSF (Fig. 4). The increases in PGE and cyclic AMP concentrations in the CSF induced by these three exogenous pyrogens were of similar magnitude. Thus the exogenous pyrogens all appear to have similar effects on two of the proposed central mediators

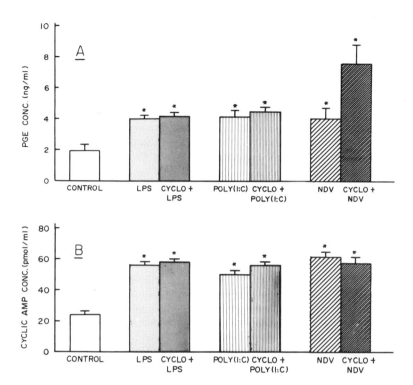

FIG. 4. Mean PGE **(A)** and cyclic AMP **(B)** concentrations in the CSF of rabbits administered LPS, poly (I:C), or NDV with and without cycloheximide pretreatment. Also shown are PGE and cyclic AMP concentrations in the CSF of control rabbits. One SEM is set off at each value. *, $p < 0.001$ as compared to control levels. (Data from Siegert et al., ref. 28.)

of pyrogen fever, PGE and cyclic AMP, as well as on the production of endogenous pyrogen. Siegert et al. (28) also showed that pretreatment of rabbits with cycloheximide (5 mg/kg), which prevented the febrile response to the exogenous pyrogens (Fig. 2), did not prevent increases in the level of PGE and cyclic AMP in the CSF (Fig. 4). Similar results were observed after administration of endogenous pyrogens induced by LPS, Poly (I:C), or NDV to either saline- or cycloheximide-pretreated rabbits. These data indicate that cycloheximide does not alter the effect of endogenous pyrogen on the production and/or release of the proposed central mediators of fever, PGE and cyclic AMP. According to Siegert et al. (28), the action of cycloheximide in preventing pyrogen-induced fever must, therefore, occur somewhere past the step involving the increase in cyclic AMP levels.

OTHER STUDIES WITH CYCLOHEXIMIDE

Young and Dowling (32) have shown that cycloheximide acts as an antipyretic agent in cancer patients with noninfectious fever. When cycloheximide was administered, either as a single injection (1 mg/kg) or as a 10-hr infusion (0.2 mg/kg/hr), to a patient with fever associated with Hodgkin's disease, body temperature decreased by 3°C and, in the case of the infusion, remained depressed throughout the infusion period. Cycloheximide (2.4 mg/kg/24 hr) was also effective in reducing body temperature over longer periods. Cycloheximide is thus an effective antipyretic in humans suffering from cancer-related increases in body temperature.

Cycloheximide has also been shown to have an antihyperthermic effect in rats administered a monoamine oxidase (MAO) inhibitor and L-tryptophan (15). When rats were pretreated with the MAO inhibitor tranylcypromine and then administered either L-tryptophan or 5-methoxy-N,N-dimethyltryptamine, they exhibited an increase in motor activity and an increase in colonic temperature. When the rats were pretreated with cycloheximide (10 mg/kg), which inhibited brain protein synthesis by 90%, both the increase in activity and the hyperthermia were attenuated (15). This effect of cycloheximide was dose dependent. These data suggest that the antihyperthermic action of cycloheximide is not limited to an effect on pyrogen-induced fever.

EFFECT OF CYCLOHEXIMIDE ON TEMPERATURE REGULATION IN RATS

We recently investigated the specificity of the effect of cycloheximide on body temperature (2). Since the thermoregulatory responses of mammals to cold exposure are similar to those induced by fever, the effect of cycloheximide on maintenance of body temperature by restained female rats exposed to a cold (15 ± 1°C) environment was tested. In addition, thermoregulatory responses of cycloheximide-treated rats to a neutral (25 ± 1°C) and a warm (34 ± 1°C) environment were tested. The methods used for this experiment have been described in detail elsewhere (2).

At all three ambient temperatures administration of cycloheximide was accompanied by a significant decrease in colonic temperature (Fig. 5). By 120 min after administration of the drug, mean colonic temperature of the cycloheximide-treated group decreased 1.8°C at ambient temperatures of 34 and 25°C and 3.0°C at an ambient temperature of 15°C. The corresponding changes in the colonic temperature of the control group were decreases of 0.8°C (34°C) and 0.2°C (25°C) and an increase of 0.2°C (15°C). At each ambient temperature the mean colonic temperature of the cycloheximide-treated group was significantly below that of the control group from 60 to 120 min after treatment. It should be noted, however, that although the rats appeared relatively healthy at the end of the experimental period at each ambient temperature, this dose of cycloheximide proved to be lethal to all treated rats within 48 hr of administration.

These data suggest that cycloheximide (5 mg/kg) has a significant effect on temperature regulation in rats. This finding confirms and extends the earlier

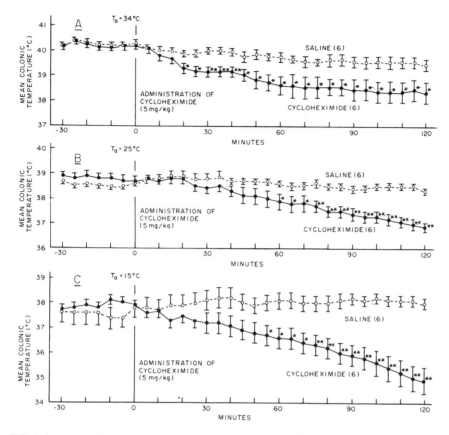

FIG. 5. Mean colonic temperature of six control *(open circles)* and six cycloheximide-treated *(solid circles)* rats at ambient temperatures of 34°C **(A)**, 25°C **(B)**, and 15°C **(C)**. Cycloheximide (5 mg/kg i.p.) administered at 0 time. One SE is set off at each mean. *, $p < 0.05$; **, $p < 0.01$. (From Barney et al., ref. 2, with permission.)

report of Grahame-Smith (15), who also observed reductions in the body temperature of rats administered cycloheximide. Although Siegert et al. (27,28) observed a decrease in body temperature of rabbits soon after administration of cycloheximide at an ambient temperature of 20°C, these authors did not feel that the fall in body temperature was significant since cycloheximide did not prevent an increase in body temperature when the rabbits were exposed to heat (35°C) (28). Their findings thus differ from ours with respect to the effects of cycloheximide on temperature regulation during exposure to heat. Differences in experimental protocol (transient versus steady-state heat exposure) or in species studied (rabbits versus rats) may account for the difference in results. Our observation that cycloheximide had a similar effect on colonic temperature at each ambient temperature, with the greatest decrease occurring at an ambient temperature of 15°C, indicates that cycloheximide has a general depressant effect on temperature regulation in the rat. To investigate this, we studied the effect of cycloheximide on the rate of heat production by rats exposed to cold.

The rate of heat production, estimated from oxygen consumption, was measured in 12 female rats. After a 30-min adjustment period, control measurements were made for 30 min and then half of the rats were administered cycloheximide (5 mg/kg i.p.) while the remaining half received the vehicle. During the control period and for 60 min thereafter, the temperature of the water bath in which the rat was immersed in an aluminum cylinder was maintained at $25 \pm 1°C$. The water bath temperature was then rapidly lowered to $15 \pm 1°C$ and measurements were continued for an additional 60 min.

Cycloheximide depressed both colonic temperature and rate of oxygen consumption (Fig. 6). During the control period there was no difference in either

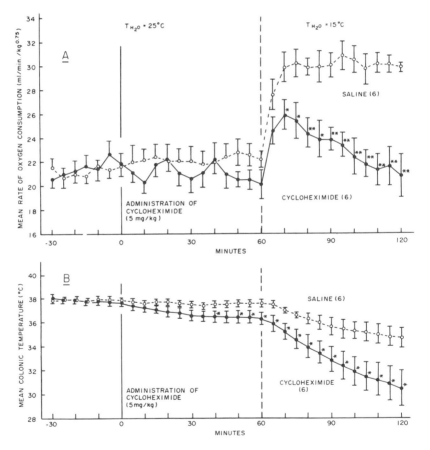

FIG. 6. Rates of oxygen consumption **(A)** and colonic temperatures **(B)** of six control *(open circles)* and six cycloheximide-treated *(solid circles)* rats. Cycloheximide (5 mg/kg i.p.) administered at 0 time. Water bath temperature decreased from 25 to 15°C at 60 min. Shown are the mean values $\pm$ 1 SEM. *, $p < 0.05$; **, $p < 0.01$. (From Barney et al., ref. 2, with permission.)

the mean rate of oxygen consumption (Fig. 6A) or the mean colonic temperature (Fig. 6B) between two groups. During the 60-min period immediately following administration of cycloheximide, the cycloheximide-treated group exhibited a decline in colonic temperature and a slight depression in the rate of oxygen consumption. By the end of the cold exposure, mean colonic temperature of the control decreased 2.9°C while that of the cycloheximide-treated group decreased 5.8°C ($p < 0.01$). This difference between mean colonic temperatures of the two groups can be related to the significant difference between the cold-induced increase in mean rate of oxygen consumption in the two groups. During the cold stress, the average rate of oxygen consumption increased 35% in the control group, but only 9% in the cycloheximide-treated group. Thus, in the rat, cycloheximide has a depressant effect on the cold-induced increase in rate of oxygen consumption.

A PROTEIN MEDIATOR OF FEVER?

The data of Siegert et al. (27,28) suggest that pretreatment with cycloheximide can prevent the febrile response to exogenous pyrogen without preventing the associated increases in the levels of endogenous pyrogen in serum or PGE and cAMP in CSF. These data support the concept of a protein synthesis-dependent mediator of fever as shown in Fig. 7. In this schema exogenous pyrogens give rise to endogenous pyrogen, a process that shows the phenomenon of tolerance (25). The endogenous pyrogen then acts on the brain to cause an increase in the levels of PGE and cyclic AMP in the CSF (10,21–23) which, in turn, leads in some way to the formation of a specific protein that results in an increased body temperature. As stated earlier, there is evidence both for and against a role of PGE in the genesis of fever (1,7,9,10,22,24,29,30). The role of a specific protein mediator of fever is also unproved. However, if it exists, it would appear to play a more general role in temperature regulation since cycloheximide decreased baseline body temperatures of both rabbits (27,28) and rats (2,15) and prevented pyrogen-induced fever in rabbits (27,28), fever associated with cancer in humans (32), and hyperthermia induced by MAO inhibition and administration of L-tryptophan in rats (15).

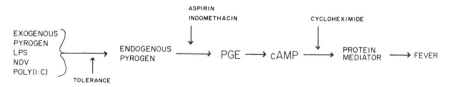

FIG. 7. Scheme showing the possible role of PGE, cyclic AMP, and a protein mediator in the genesis of fever. Antipyretics such as aspirin and indomethacin block the pyrogen-induced increases in PGE and cyclic AMP, whereas cycloheximide may prevent the formation of the protein mediator.

Our studies suggest that the decrease in body temperature accompanying administration of cycloheximide is associated with a reduction in the rate of heat production. The fall in body temperature with cycloheximide contrasts with the effects of the other well-known antipyretics which, with some exceptions, are generally without effect on body temperature of afebrile animals (30).

The schema in Fig. 7 suggests that inhibition of the synthesis of PGE prevents fever. In addition, very high doses of aspirin are reported to prevent the maintenance of body temperature of rats exposed to cold (12,18,26), although this is reported to be caused by increased heat loss rather than decreased heat production (18). We have recently shown that administration of indomethacin (2.5 mg/kg i.p.) to rats, a dose known to attenuate pyrogen-induced fever in rats (11), is without effect on colonic temperature at an ambient temperature of 15°C *(unpublished data)*. Since these results differ from those observed with cycloheximide, they suggest that cycloheximide may act at different levels of the central nervous system to affect both normal temperature regulation and the induction of fever. This could be either at the level of the synthesis of a neurotransmitter substance or at receptors involved in the central control of body temperature.

Alternatively, and perhaps more likely, cycloheximide may have a general debilitating effect on the organism as a whole, interfering with the ability to regulate body temperature. Cycloheximide is known to have many debilitating side effects including severe acidosis, lowered blood pressure, internal bleeding, irreversible changes in plasma and cell enzyme levels, changes in cell structure, and changes in hormone production and intermediary metabolism (5,13,14,33). In patients with cancer, cycloheximide caused vomiting, abdominal discomfort, diarrhea, anorexia, lassitude, and CNS depression (32). Grahame-Smith (15) reported that rats given cycloheximide were less responsive, less interested in their surroundings, and exhibited diarrhea. These adverse effects were, for the most part, dose dependent. The rats administered cycloheximide in our studies all died within 48 hr of administration. It is not yet known whether cycloheximide can alter temperature regulation and prevent fever at lower doses which do not have as many adverse effects. Siegert et al. (27,28) did not mention any adverse effects of treatment with cycloheximide. It may be possible, therefore, that rabbits are less sensitive to the inhibition of protein synthesis than rats.

A further puzzling aspect of the effect of cycloheximide in preventing fever in rabbits is that it was effective at doses that inhibited synthesis of protein in brain by only 30 to 50% (28). If the theory of a protein mediation of fever is correct, the fever-mediating protein must have been included in that 30 to 50%. In the case of the rat with tryptophan-induced hyperthermia, 90% inhibition of brain protein synthesis by cycloheximide (10 mg/kg) was required to prevent the hyperthermia (15). Since half of this dose was lethal in our studies, it seems clear that the question of the specificity of this compound for the fever-mediating protein, as well as its nonspecific toxicity, must somehow be solved before this theory can enjoy full support.

ACKNOWLEDGMENTS

We acknowledge the graphic illustrations of Miss Charlotte Wright and the technical assistance of Mr. Ronald Basch. This work was supported by Office of Naval Research Contract N0014–75–C–0199 with funds provided by the Naval Bureau of Medicine and Surgery. Dr. Barney is a postdoctoral Fellow, Institutional Endocrine Training Grant, National Institute of Arthritis and Metabolic Diseases Grant AM–07164–04. Dr. Katovich is a Fellow, American Heart Association, Suncoast Chapter.

REFERENCES

1. Baird, J. A., Hales, J. R. S., and Lang, W. T. (1974): Thermoregulatory responses to injection of monoamines, acetylcholine and prostaglandins into a lateral cerebral ventricle of the echidna. *J. Physiol.,* 236:539–548.
2. Barney, C. C., Katovich, M. J., and Fregly, M. J. (1979): The effect of cycloheximide on temperature regulations in rats. *Brain Res. Bull.,* 4:355–358.
3. Bernheim, H. A., Gilbert, T. M., Stitt, J. T., and Bodel, P. T. (1979): Cerebrospinal Fluid (CSF) levels of prostaglandin E (PGE) during various manipulations of brain and body temperature. *Fed. Proc.,* 38:1296.
4. Cammock, S., Dascombe, M. J., and Milton, A. S. (1976): Prostaglandins in thermoregulation. In: *Advances in Prostaglandin and Thromboxane Research, Vol. 1,* edited by B. Samuelsson and R. Paoletti, pp. 375–380. Raven Press, New York.
5. Ch'ih, J. J., Olszyna, D. M., and Devlin, T. M. (1976): Alterations in plasma and cellular enzyme and protein levels after lethal and non-lethal doses of cycloheximide in the rat. *Biochem. Pharmacol.,* 25:2407–2408.
6. Cooper, K. E., Cranston, W. I., and Honour, A. J. (1967): Observations on the site and mode of action of pyrogens in the rabbit brain. *J. Physiol.,* 191:325–337.
7. Cranston, W. I., Duff, G. W., Hellon, R. F., Mitchell, D., and Townsend, Y. (1976): Evidence that brain prostaglandin synthesis is not essential in fever. *J. Physiol.,* 259:239–249.
8. Cranston, W. I., Hellon, R. F., and Mitchell, D. (1975): Is brain prostaglandin synthesis involved in responses to cold? *J. Physiol.,* 249:425–434.
9. Cranston, W. I., Hellon, R. F., and Mitchell, D. (1975): A dissociation between fever and prostaglandin concentration in cerebrospinal fluid. *J. Physiol.,* 253:583–592.
10. Feldberg, W., Gupta, K. P., Milton, A. S., and Wendlandt, S. (1973): Effect of pyrogen and antipyretics on prostaglandin activity in cisternal C.S.F. of unanesthetized cats. *J. Physiol.,* 234:279–303.
11. Feldberg, W., and Saxena, P. N. (1975): Prostaglandins, endotoxin and lipid A on body temperature in rats. *J. Physiol.,* 249:601–615.
12. Francesconi, R. P., and Mager, M. (1975): Salicylate, tryptophan and tyrosine hypothermia. *Am. J. Physiol.,* 228:1431–1435.
13. Garcia-Sainz, J. A., Pina, E., and De Sanchez, V. C. (1978): Importance of the esterification process in adipose tissue metabolism as evidenced by cycloheximide. *Biochem. Pharmacol.,* 27:1577–1579.
14. Garren, L. D., Ney, R. L., and Davis, W. W. (1965): Studies on the role of protein synthesis in the regulation of corticosterone production by adrenocorticotropic hormones in vivo. *Proc. Natl. Acad. Sci. U.S.A.,* 53:1443–1450.
15. Grahame-Smith, D. G. (1972): The prevention by inhibitors of brain protein synthesis of the hyperactivity and hyperpyrexia produced in rats by monoamine oxidase inhibition and the administration of L-tryptophan or 5-methoxy–N,N-diamethyltryptamine. *J. Neurochem.,* 19:2409–2422.
16. Harvey, C. A., Milton, A. S., and Straughan, D. W. (1975): Prostaglandin E levels in cerebrospinal fluid of rabbits and the effects of bacterial pyrogen and antipyretic drugs. *J. Physiol.,* 248:26–27P.

17. Jackson, D. L. (1967): A hypothalamic region response to localized injection of pyrogens. *J. Neurophysiol.,* 30:586–602.
18. Lin, M. T. (1978): Effects of sodium acetylsalicylate on thermoregulatory responses of rats to different ambient temperatures. *Pfluegers Arch.,* 378:181–184.
19. Myers, R. D., and Tytell, M. (1972): Fever: Reciprocal shift in brain sodium to calcium ratio as the set-point temperature rises. *Science,* 178:765–767.
20. Pestka, S. (1971): Inhibitors of ribosome functions. *Annu. Rev. Microbiol.,* 25:487–562.
21. Philipp-Dormston, W. K. (1976): Evidence for the involvement of adenosine 3′,5′-cyclic monophosphate in fever genesis. *Pfluegers Arch.,* 362:223–227.
22. Philipp-Dormston, W. K., and Siegert, R. (1974): Prostaglandins of the E and F series in rabbit cerebrospinal fluid during fever induced by Newcastle disease virus, *E. coli*-endotoxin or endogenous pyrogen. *Med. Microbiol. Immunol.,* 159:279–284.
23. Philipp-Dormston, W. K., and Siegert, R. (1975): Adenosine 3′,5′-cyclic monophosphate in rabbit cerebrospinal fluid during fever induced by *E. coli*-endotoxin. *Med. Microbiol. Immunol.,* 161:11–13.
24. Pittman, Q. J., Veale, W. L., and Cooper, K. E. (1975): Temperature responses of lambs after centrally injected prostaglandins and pyrogens. *Am. J. Physiol.,* 228:1034–1038.
25. Rosendorff, C. (1976): Neurochemistry of fever. *S. Afr. J. Med. Sci.,* 41:23–48.
26. Satinoff, E. (1972): Salicylate: Action on body temperature in rats. *Science,* 176:532–533.
27. Siegert, R., Phillip-Dormston, W. K., Radsak, K., and Menzel, H. (1975): Inhibition of Newcastle disease virus-induced fever in rabbits by cycloheximide. *Arch. Virol.,* 48:367–373.
28. Siegert, R., Phillip-Dormston, W. K., Radsak, K., and Menzel, H. (1976): Mechanism of fever induction in rabbits. *Infect. Immun.,* 14:1130–1137.
29. Veale, W. L., and Cooper, K. E. (1975): Comparison of sites of action of prostaglandin E and leucocyte pyrogen in brain. In: *Temperature Regulation and Drug Action,* edited by P. Lomax, E. Schonbaum, and J. Jacob, pp. 310–318. S. Karger, Basel.
30. Veale, W. L., Cooper, K. E., and Pittman, Q. J. (1977): Role of prostaglandin in fever and temperature regulation. In: *The Prostaglandins, Vol. 3,* edited by P. Ranwell, pp. 145–167. Plenum Press, New York.
31. Woolf, C. J., Willies, G. H., Laburh H., and Rosendorff, C. (1975): Pyrogen and prostaglandin fever in the rabbit. I. Effects of salicylate and the role of cyclic AMP. *Neuropharmacology,* 14:397–403.
32. Young, C. W., and Dowling, M. D., Jr. (1975): Antipyretic effect of cycloheximide, an inhibitor of protein synthesis, in patients with Hodgkin's disease or other malignant neoplasms. *Cancer Res.,* 35:1218–1224.
33. Young, C. W., Robinson, P. F., and Sacktor, B. (1963): Inhibition of the synthesis of protein in intact animals by acetoxycycloheximide and a metabolic derangement concomitant with this blockade. *Biochem. Pharmacol.,* 12:855–865.

Fever, edited by James M. Lipton.
Raven Press, New York © 1980.

A Possible Site of Action and Mechanism Involved in Peptidoglycan Fever in Rats

K. Mašek, O. Kadlecová, and *P. Petrovický

*Institute of Pharmacology, Czechoslovak Academy of Sciences; and *Institute of Anatomy, Charles University Medical School, 120 00 Prague 2, Czechoslovakia*

A large body of information over the past two decades has accumulated on the biological activity of peptidoglycan, a basic structure of the cell wall of Gram-positive and Gram-negative bacteria (14,28). Pyrogenicity is one of the most striking properties of peptidoglycans from different bacteria, and this property has been the subject of our studies over the past 10 years. A growing body of data supports the opinion that bacterial pyrogens affect temperature regulation not only by influencing thermosensitive neurons in the preoptic region and anterior hypothalamus, but also by altering neuronal activity at other brain sites. Thermosensitive neurons have been found in the brainstem (4,13,16), and animals with large anterior hypothalamic/preoptic region lesions have responded with fever to i.v. injection of leukocyte pyrogen (6). Lipton and co-workers (17–19) suggested that the integrity of the preoptic/anterior hypothalamic junction and of the thermosensitive region of the medulla oblongata is necessary for regulation of body temperature.

One of the aims of our study was, therefore, to clarify further the possible cerebral site of action of peptidoglycan with particular attention to brainstem. The other objective was to investigate the possible involvement of different mediators, particularly monoamines, in peptidoglycan-induced fever. Noradrenergic and 5-hydroxytryptaminergic pathways are located in the brainstem, and, although the evidence for their involvement in fever is, so far, conflicting, their physical proximity to thermosensitive sites suggests that they may have a role in thermoregulatory functions. Finally, in a study which compared pyrogenic effects of synthetically prepared peptides and glycopeptides, we determined the minimal structure of these bacterial components that is required to produce fever.

MATERIAL AND METHODS

Male albino rats of the Wistar strain weighing 200 to 250 g were used. All experiments were performed at a constant environmental temperature of 22 to 24°C. Rectal temperature was measured with a thermistor thermometer. In the pyrogen tests either the product of cell wall of group A streptococcus peptidoglycan (21) or synthetic peptides and glycopeptides (32) were used. Brain lesions were produced using stereotaxic coordinates of Fifková and Maršala (11). Direct current of 2 mA intensity was applied for 2 sec. With this method, lesions of about 0.5 to 2.0 mm in diameter were produced. After the rats were sacrified, the brains were perfused with saline solution followed by formalin and fixed in 10% formalin solution for 2 to 12 months. They were then serially sectioned at 25 μm on a freezing microtome. Some brains were impregnated using the method of Nauta (23) to study degeneration of fibers. For the determination of turnover rates of norepinephrine (NE) and 5-hydroxytryptamine, the brains were carefully removed, blotted, and chilled. The turnover rate of brain NE was determined from the rate of disappearance of endogenous NE after blockade of synthesis with α-methyl-*p*-tyrosine (200 mg/kg) (3). The fluorometric method of Chang (5) was used to measure NE level. The turnover rate of brain 5-hydroxytryptamine was calculated, as described by Neff and Tozer (24), from the initial linear increase of 5-hydroxytryptamine after i.p. administration of 75 mg/kg nonreversible monoamine oxidase inhibitor pargyline. The fluorometric method of Bogdanski et al. (2), with the modification of Snyder et al. (30), was used to measure the level of tissue 5-hydroxytryptamine. Drugs used were α-methyl-*p*-tyrosine (Merck Sharp & Dohme), pargyline (Abbot Laboratories), indomethacin (Sigma Chemical Co.), and theophylline (Spofa).

RESULTS

Figure 1 shows the damage to medulla oblongata, pons, and mesencephalon which led either to total inhibition or to marked inhibition of fever after peptidoglycan in the rat. It is clear that destruction of the raphe nuclei and closely related peripheral structures effectively inhibited the pyrogenic reaction. Lesion at the level of medulla oblongata and pons involved nucleus raphe parvus et magnus, nucleus centralis superior, nucleus ventralis et dorsalis, tegmenti Guddeni, and nucleus linearis caudalis. Throughout the brainstem there were small lesions in the medial portion of the nucleus reticularis ventralis, gigantocellularis, and reticularis pontis caudalis et oralis. Like the raphe nuclei, this part of the brainstem contains serotonergic neurons. In the mesencephalon some lesions were located in cellular structures (nucleus linearis intermedius and rostralis), but mainly they were situated in the neighboring fiber systems. It is interesting that many lesions which decreased the pyrogenic response were located in the substantia grisea centralis. This region includes the periventricular system, which contains the ascending and descending connection of the hypothalamus. The other structures which are necessary to the pyrogenic effect of peptidoglycan and glycopeptide are the nucleus dorsalis nervi vagi and nucleus parabrachialis.

Experiments in which the turnover rate of 5-hydroxytryptamine and NE in brainstem were measured are summarized in Tables 1 and 2. From this information it is evident that although there was a marked increase of turnover rate of 5-hydroxytryptamine during peptidoglycan-induced fever, there were no

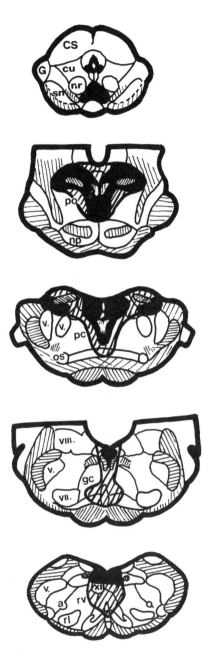

FIG. 1. Regional brain damage which led to marked changes in the fever reaction to peptidoglycan. *Black areas,* total inhibition; *hatched areas,* marked inhibition of fever; febrile response was less than one-third of normal. Abbreviations: a, nucleus ambiguus; CS, colliculus superior; cu, nucleus cuneiformis; G, corpus geniculatum; gc, nucleus gigantocellularis; np, nuclei pontis; nr, nucleus ruber; OS, oliva superior; Pc, nucleus reticularis pontis caudalis; po, nucleus reticularis pontis oralis; rl, nucleus reticularis lateralis; rv, nucleus reticularis ventralis; sn, substantia nigra; V., nucleus terminationis et motorius nervi trigemini; VIII., nucleus nervi facialis; VIII., nucleus nervi vestibulo-cochlearis; XII., nucleus nervi hypoglossi.

changes in NE turnover. This strongly suggests the activation of 5-hydroxy-tryptamine-containing structures, but not NE-containing cells in the production of fever.

The administration of indomethacin (3 mg/kg i.p.), a potent inhibitor of

TABLE 1. *Turnover rate of 5-hydroxytryptamine in brainstem measured from the accumulation after inhibition of MAO[a]*

| Treatment | 5-HT level (μg/g) at | | Turnover rate (μg/g/hr) |
	0 min	30 min	
Saline	0.54 ± 0.03	0.96 ± 0.05	0.84
Peptidoglycan	0.61 ± 0.02	1.62 ± 0.06	2.02

[a] Numbers represent mean value of six animals with fiducial limits.

TABLE 2. *Turnover rate of norepinephrine in brainstem measured from amine decline after blockade of synthesis[a]*

Treatment	Steady-state NE level (μg/g)	Rate constant of amine loss k (hr^{-1})	Turnover rate (μg/g/hr)
Saline	0.62 ± 0.02	0.21	0.130
Peptidoglycan	0.65 ± 0.03	0.17	0.110

[a] Numbers represent mean value of six animals with fiducial limits.

prostaglandin synthetase, markedly reduced the peptidoglycan-induced fever. This suggests that prostaglandin release is necessary for temperature elevation induced by peptidoglycan. The effect of this bacterial cell wall component, however, seems also to be related to the level of cyclic AMP since the administration of theophylline (250 mg/kg) markedly potentiated the fever elicited by peptidoglycan. The effect of theophylline was, however, apparent only when the normal level of prostaglandins was present, since the administration of indomethacin completely prevented the effect of theophylline (Fig. 2).

Table 3 summarizes the results of synthetically prepared peptides and glycopeptides. From the results it is evident that the tetrapeptide subunit composed of L-alanyl-D-isoglutamyl-L-lysyl-D-alanine is pyrogenic. However, the character of the pyrogenic response produced by this tetrapeptide is different in that the time to peak fever is delayed. The addition of N-acetylmuramic acid to the

TABLE 3. *Pyrogenicity of synthetic peptides and glycopeptides[a]*

Compound tested	Dose (μg/kg)	Pyrogenicity ΔT (°C)
L-Ala-D-Glu-NH$_2$	200	0.6
L-Ala-D-isoGlu-L-Lys-D-Ala-OH	200	0.9 [b]
NAM-L-Ala-D-isoGlu-L-Lys-D-Ala-OH	200	1.5 [b]
NAM-L-Ala-D-Glu-NH$_2$	200	1.4 [b]

[a] Values represent means from six animals; NAM, N-acetylated muramic acid.
[b] Statistically significant results, $p < 0.05$.

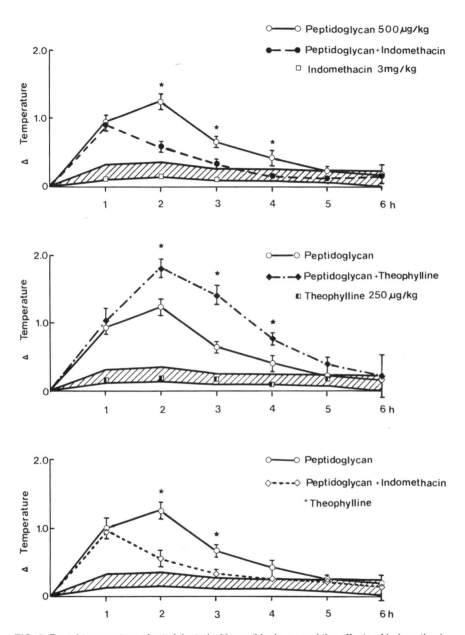

FIG. 2. Rectal temperature of rats injected with peptidoglycan and the effects of indomethacin **(top)**, theophylline **(middle)**, and indomethacin and theophylline **(bottom)** on peptidoglycan fever. Each point represents the mean value of six animals with fiducial limits ($p = 0.95$); *asterisk* denotes statistically significant difference.

molecule reduced the period of latency, and the resulting pyrogenic response was similar to that noted after the administration of bacterial peptidoglycan polymer. Two terminal amino acids, L-lysine and D-alanine, could be omitted and the remaining muramyl dipeptide was still equally pyrogenic. Finally, we have investigated with the aid of electrolytic lesions whether the site of action of synthetic N-acetylmuramyl-L-alanyl-D-isoglutamine is the same as in the case of the natural product. The results of these experiments clearly indicate that this synthetic low molecular weight product acts on the same central structures as the bacterial peptidoglycan polymer.

DISCUSSION

During the past decade an increasing amount of evidence has suggested that there is a component of fever that is mediated outside the anterior hypothalamus/preoptic region. Several groups have proposed that brainstem reticular formation (4,7,13,16) is important to body temperature regulation, and our results support the opinion. Moreover, our findings suggest that the serotonergic neurons of the brainstem are involved in the peptidoglycan-induced fever in rats since destruction of raphe nuclei (except nucleus raphe dorsalis, which was never completely destroyed) and neighboring reticular formation effectively inhibited fever. The peripheral structures destroyed included nucleus reticularis ventralis, gigantocellularis, and reticularis pontis caudalis et oralis, which, like nuclei raphe, contain serotonergic neurons (25).

The marked increase in turnover rate of serotonin in brainstem during peptidoglycan fever further supports the idea of serotonin participation in the mediation of fever. The evidence concerning involvement of monoaminergic structures in fever is conflicting (9,10,12,20,31). Lesions in the mesencephalon also inhibited fever. There lesions involved not only definite nuclear structures, but also parts of the fiber systems of cerebellum, nucleus ruber, hypothalamus, and reticular formation. It is also interesting that many of the successful lesions which depressed the fever response were located in the substantia grisea centralis. Both warm-sensitive neurons and serotonin (8) have been found in this region. This brain region contains a periventricular system of ascending and descending connection of the hypothalamus. These observations suggest that in addition to serotonergic structures, nonserotonergic systems are also involved. Moreover, the results support the idea of Lipton, who assumed that the integrity of the preoptic/anterior hypothalamic region with other brainstem areas, particularly those in the medulla oblongata, is necessary for regulation of body temperature and hyperthermic responses (17,19).

The first evidence that prostaglandins might be released during fever was provided by Milton and Wendlandt (22) and was confirmed later by Feldberg et al. (10). Our results with indomethacin suggest that prostaglandin release is necessary for fever response induced by peptidoglycan in rats. However, the site of prostaglandin release during fever is not completely clear, since these autacoids seem to have opposite effects on body temperature when injected into the preoptic/anterior hypothalamic region and the medulla oblongata (19)

The effect of peptidoglycan on temperature seems also to be related to the level of cyclic AMP, since the administration of theophylline, an inhibitor of phosphodiesterase, enhanced peptidoglycan fever when a normal level of prostaglandins was present. Cyclic AMP is present in nervous tissue (1), and considerable evidence supports a role of this compound in the mediation of synaptic transmission in the brain (15).

The general structure of bacterial peptidoglycan is well established. The compound consists of repeating units of N-acetyl glucosamine and N-acetyl muramic acid, to which are attached chains of amino acid units (peptides). In the case of streptococcal peptidoglycan, tetrapeptide is composed of L-alanine, D-glutamic acid, L-lysine, and D-alanine. These peptides, linked together by dialanine bridges, cross-link the polysaccharide chains (26,27,29). Our comparative study with several synthetically prepared peptidoglycan subunits, peptides and glycopeptides, clearly demonstrated that even the tetrapeptide (L-alanyl-D-isoglutamyl-L-lysyl-D-alanine) had some pyrogenic potency. However, the fever produced by the tetrapeptide was slow in onset and took a long time to reach maximum. The introduction of N-acetyl muramic acid into the subunit shortened the period of latency, and the fever response was more pronounced. If two terminal amino acids, L-lysine and D-alanine, were omitted, the resulting product, muramyl dipeptide, was equally as pyrogenic as muramyl tetrapeptide. Therefore, the smallest subunit of bacterial peptidoglycans that is required for pyrogen potency appears to be the muramyl dipeptide.

REFERENCES

1. Bloom, F. E. (1972): Adenosine 3',5'-monophosphate is localized in cerebellar neurons: Immunofluorescence evidence. *Science,* 177:436.
2. Bogdanski, D. F., Pletscher, A., Brodie, B. B., and Udenfriend, S. (1956): Identification and assay of serotonin in brain. *J. Pharmacol. Exp. Ther.,* 117:82–88.
3. Brodie, B. B., Costa, E., Dlabač, A., Neff, N. H., and Smookler, H. H. (1966): Application of steady-state kinetics to the estimation of synthesis rate and turnover time of tissue catecholamines. *J. Pharmacol. Exp. Ther.,* 154:493–498.
4. Chai, C. Y., and Lin, M. T. (1972): Effects of heating and cooling of the spinal cord and medulla oblongata on thermoregulation in monkeys. *J. Physiol. (Lond.),* 225:297–308.
5. Chang, C. C. (1964): A sensitive method for spectrofluorometric assay of catecholamines. *Int. J. Neuropharmacol.,* 3:643–649.
6. Cooper, K. E., Veale, W. L., and Pittman, Q. J. (1976): Pathogenesis of fever. In: *Brain Dysfunction in Infantile Febrile Convulsions,* edited by M. A. B. Brazier and F. Coceani, pp. 107–115. Raven Press, New York.
7. Cranston, W. J., and Rawlins, M. D. (1972): Effects of intracerebral micro-injection of sodium salicylate on temperature regulation in the rabbit. *J. Physiol. (Lond.),* 222:257–266.
8. Dahlström, A., and Fuxe, K. (1965): Evidence for the existence of monoamine neurons in the central nervous system. *Acta Physiol. Scand. [Suppl.],* 64:247.
9. Des Prez, R., Helman, R., and Oates, J. A. (1966): Inhibition of endotoxin fever by reserpine. *Proc. Soc. Exp. Biol. Med.,* 122:746–749.
10. Feldberg, W., Gupta, K. P., Milton, A. S., and Wendlandt, S. (1973): Effect of pyrogen and antipyretics on prostaglandin activity in cisternal c.s.f. of unanesthetized cats. *J. Physiol. (Lond.),* 234:279.

11. Fifková, E., and Maršala, J. (1960): Stereotaxie podkorových struktur mozku krysy, králíka a kočky. In: *Babákova Sbírka, Vol. 17*, pp. 7–126. Státní Zdravotnické Nakladatelství, Prague.

12. Giarman, N. J., Tanaka, C., Mooney, J., and Atkins, E. (1968): Serotonin, norepinephrine and fever. In: *Advances in Pharmacology, Vol. 6A*, edited by S. Garattini and P. A. Shore, pp. 307–317. Academic Press, New York.

13. Hardy, J. D. (1971): Posterior hypothalamus and the regulation of body temperature. *Fed. Proc.*, 32:1564–1571.

14. Heymer, B. (1975): Biological properties of the peptidoglycan. *Z. Immunitaets-forsch.*, 149:245–257.

15. Hoffer, B. J., Siggins, G. R., Olivier, A. P., and Bloom, F. E. (1971): Cyclic AMP mediation of norepinephrine inhibition in rat cerebellar cortex: A unique class of synaptic response. *Ann. N.Y. Acad. Sci.*, 185:531.

16. Holmes, R. L., Newman, P. P., and Wolstencroft, J. H. (1960): A heat-sensitive region in the medulla. *J. Physiol. (Lond.)*, 152:93–98.

17. Lipton, J. M. (1973): Thermosensitivity of medulla oblongata in control of body temperature. *Am. J. Physiol.*, 224:890–897.

18. Lipton, J. M., Dwyer, P. E., and Fossler, D. E. (1974): Effect of brainstem lesions on temperature regulation in hot and cold environments. *Am. J. Physiol.*, 226:1356–1365.

19. Lipton, J. M., Welch, J. P., and Clark, W. G. (1973): Changes in body temperature produced by injecting prostaglandin E_1, EGTA and bacterial endotoxins into the PO/AH region and the medulla oblongata of the rat. *Experientia*, 29:806–808.

20. Mašek, K., Rašková, H., and Rotta, J. (1968): The mechanism of the pyrogenic effect of group A streptococcus cell wall mucopeptide. *J. Physiol. (Lond.)*, 198:345–353.

21. Mašek, K., Rašková, H., and Rotta, J. (1972): On the mechanism of fever caused by the mucopeptide of group A streptococcus. *Naunyn Schmiedebergs Arch. Pharmacol.*, 274:138–145.

22. Milton, A. S., and Wendlandt, S. (1971): Effects on body temperature of prostaglandins of the A, E and F series on injection into the third ventricle of unanesthetized cats and rabbits. *J. Physiol. (Lond.)*, 218:325–336.

23. Nauta, W. J. H. (1957): Silver impregnation of degenerating axons. In: *New Research Technique of Neuroanatomy*, edited by W. F. Windle, pp. 17–26. Charles C Thomas, Springfield, Ill.

24. Neff, N. H., and Tozer, T. N. (1968): In vivo measurement of brain serotonin turnover. In: *Advances in Pharmacology, Vol. 6A*, edited by S. Garattini and P. A. Shore, pp. 97–109. Academic Press, New York.

25. Palkovits, M., Brownstein, M., and Saavedra, J. M. (1974): Serotonin content of the brainstem nuclei in the rat. *Brain Res.*, 80:237–249.

26. Park, J. T. (1967): The mechanism by which penicillin causes conversion of bacterial cells to spheroplasts. In: *Microbial Protoplasts, Spheroplasts, and L-Forms*, edited by L. B. Gruze, pp. 52–74. Williams & Wilkins, Baltimore.

27. Perkins, H. R. (1963): Chemical structure and biosynthesis of bacterial cell walls. *Bacteriol. Rev.*, 27:18.

28. Rotta, J. Rýc, M., Mašek, K., and Zaoral, M. (1978): The activity of synthetic analogues of streptococcal peptidoglycan in biological experiments and the potentiation of the peptidoglycan effect by other streptococcal products. Presented at VIIth International Symposium on *Streptococcus pyrogenes*. Oxford, September 12–16.

29. Salton, M. R. J. (1964): *The Bacterial Cell Wall*. Elsevier, Amsterdam.

30. Snyder, S. H., Axelrod, J., and Zweig, M. (1965): A sensitive and specific fluorescence assay for tissue serotonin. *Biochem. Pharmacol.* 14:831–835.

31. Takagi, H., and Kuruma, I. (1966): Effect of bacterial lipopolysaccharide on the content of serotonin and norepinephrine in rabbit brain. *Jpn. J. Pharmacol.*, 16:478–479.

32. Zaoral, M., Ježek, J., Straka, R., Mašek, K. (1978): Glycopeptides in bacterial walls. A novel method of removal benzyl and bezylidene residues. *Coll. Czech. Chem. Commun.*, 43:1797–1802.

Fever, edited by James M. Lipton.
Raven Press, New York © 1980.

Antipyretics: Mechanisms of Action

Wesley G. Clark

Department of Pharmacology, University of Texas Health Science Center at Dallas, Dallas, Texas 75235

Antipyretic drugs act within the central nervous system to oppose pyrogen-induced increases in the level about which body temperature is regulated. They lower temperature of febrile subjects in doses which do not appreciably reduce the temperature of afebrile subjects. This observation indicates that antipyretics do not exert their primary action directly on the thermoregulatory system, although, theoretically, they might decrease body temperature by several actions on this system (9): (a) Lowering of the thermoregulatory set-point, reduction of input from cold receptors, or enhancement of input from warmth receptors (Fig. 1b) decreases the level about which body temperature is regulated, an effect opposite to that caused by pyrogens. If any of these mechanisms were their primary action, antipyretics would lower body temperature equally well in both febrile and afebrile subjects. (b) General depression of thermoregulatory control (Fig. 1c) allows body temperature to passively decrease in a cool environment. However, recovery from fever after antipyretic administration is an active response as indicated by sweating, tachypnea, etc. (3,32,44,51). General depression of thermoregulatory function would also lower temperature of afebrile subjects in a cool environment. (c) Antipyretics might act on specific effectors or neuroeffector pathways to cause sweating, tachypnea, decreased cutaneous vasomotor tone, or decreased heat production (Fig. 1d). However, with the remainder of the thermoregulatory system intact, compensatory mechanisms would be activated to correct the temperature deviation produced by the drug, and a mixture of opposing thermoregulatory effector activities would occur. To the contrary, antipyresis is a coordinated recovery from fever (51). Evidence against a direct action on effectors is a report that salicylate did not alter peripheral heat elimination in afebrile subjects (54). Furthermore, when afebrile people take aspirin or acetaminophen for analgesia, these drugs do not evoke sweating as they do in febrile subjects.

The point here is that, since fever represents a coordinated response in which body temperature is regulated at a higher than normal level (21,46), any agent which acts directly on the thermoregulatory system to lower fever should also lower normal temperature (Fig. 1b to d, *bottom*). Yet antipyretics do not even lower body temperature under all conditions when it is elevated; for instance, during exercise (28,35), during exposure to a hot environment (32), during cool-

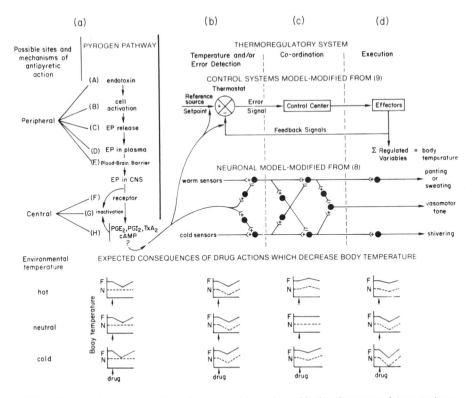

FIG. 1. Schematic representation of pyrogen interaction with the thermoregulatory system. Antipyretics inhibit the series of events **(a)** initiated by pyrogens, which causes an adjustment of the thermoregulatory system so that body temperature is regulated at a higher level. A direct action of antipyretics on the thermoregulatory system **(b–d)** would alter body temperature in both febrile and afebrile subjects. The charts at the bottom indicate the expected qualitative changes in temperature of febrile (F) and normothermic (N) subjects at various environmental temperatures if drugs were administered which acted on the specific component **(a–d)** to lower body temperature.

ing of the hypothalamus (23), or when temperature is regulated at a higher level after administration of prostaglandins (10) or morphine (15,55). If, however, antipyretics interrupt the specific series of events by which pyrogens raise the level of thermoregulation (Fig. 1a), it is easy to understand why they would reduce fever without altering normal body temperature. For the past 10 years, a primary aim in antipyretic research has been to determine where antipyretics act within this pathway. Although antipyretics do appear to "lower the set-point," do cause sweating, vasodilation, etc., these changes are subsequent to their primary action, which can be demonstrated only in the presence of pyrogen. Depending on the specific mechanism of their antipyretic action, antipyretics may also block hyperthermic responses to agents which are not required for pyrogen-induced fever but which use the same "final common pathway" prior to the thermoregulatory system. Behavioral activity can also contribute to the development of fever (57,58) and to antipyresis, even in ectotherms. For instance, lizards given *Aeromonas hydrophila* varied their positions in relation to heat lamps to increase their temperature (6). Injections of salicylate inhibited the pyrogenic response. Likewise, acetaminophen added to water in chambers containing sunfish prevented or reversed a behaviorally induced increase in water temperature evoked by injection of *A. hydrophila* (53). The antipyretics did not alter behavior in the absence of pyrogen. These results further indicate the independence of antipyretic action from physiological thermoregulatory mechanisms and reinforce the concept that antipyretics more specifically antagonize pyrogens.

It is correct that antipyretics reduce temperature during fever in doses which do not appreciably lower normal temperature, although there have been many reports of hypothermic responses of afebrile experimental animals to antipyretics and a report (39) that aspirin reduced the rise in temperature of monkeys exposed to a hot environment. A survey of the literature published primarily since 1965 (Table 1) indicates that in 93% of 59 reports in which the effect of various agents was studied in both febrile and afebrile animals, antipyresis was produced by doses which did not cause hypothermia (arbitrarily defined as a mean decrease in body temperature greater than $0.5°C$) in afebrile animals. In the four studies in which hypothermia did develop with antipyretic doses, the decrease in temperature of afebrile animals was less than half that in febrile animals. If, in addition, studies are included in which the effect of antipyretics was determined only in afebrile animals, hypothermia was obtained in a higher percentage (Table 1, Totals). There was considerable variation depending on the antipyretic and species used. Rats and mice often developed hypothermia. A contributing factor may have been the use of restraint, which by itself has been reported to cause hypothermia in these species (1,4) and to alter thermal responses to certain drugs, such as morphine (40,41,63). However, even in the rat, in which a salicylate dose–hypothermic response relationship has been established in several reports (7,31,33,52,56), hypothermia was noted in only 9 of 19 studies with this antipyretic. Of the antipyretics, phenacetin and aminopyrine were especially likely to cause hypothermia. In contrast, even at cool environmental temperatures, salicylate in the rabbit (51) and salicylate, acetaminophen, and indomethacin in the cat (24) did not appreciably reduce normal temperature.

Thus the most commonly used antipyretics act prior to involvement of the thermoregulatory system in fever and are appropriately classified as antipyretics. These agents have the advantage of not causing hypothermia, at least within a certain dosage range. Agents that act directly on the thermoregulatory system and can lower body temperature in both febrile and afebrile subjects would better be classified as "hypothermogenic" agents since their action is not specific for fever. As shown in Table 1, certain agents, in particular phenacetin and aminopyrine, may be both antipyretic and, at higher doses, hypothermogenic. Hypothermogenic agents have the disadvantage of necessitating more careful

TABLE 1. *Reports of hypothermic responses to antipyretics*[a]

Antipyretic	Cat	Guinea pig	Mouse	Rabbit	Rat	Misc.	Subtotal	Total[c]
				Species[b]				
Acetaminophen	0/3		0/1			0/1	0/5	4/14
Aminopyrine		0/1	1/2	0/1			1/4	9/13
Indomethacin	0/2		0/2	1/3	0/1		1/8	2/15
Phenacetin	1/1				0/1		1/2	8/10
Phenylbutazone		0/1	0/3		0/1		0/5	0/6
Salicylate	0/2	0/1	0/1	0/7	1/5	0/5	1/21	10/46
Miscellaneous	0/2	0/1	0/3	0/4	0/2	0/2	0/14	6/22
Subtotal	1/10	0/4	1/12	1/15	1/10	0/8	4/59	
Total[c]	3/15	1/6	6/19	6/29	23/41	0/16		39/126

[a] Each report deals with a specific antipyretic in a given species.
[b] Ratio of reports of both hypothermia and antipyresis to reports of antipyresis.
[c] Ratio of reports of hypothermia to total no. of reports including reports in which antipyretic doses were not determined.

control of dosage to avoid lowering the temperature of febrile subjects to hypothermic levels. Furthermore, if their action were to depress thermoregulatory control, fever might be enhanced in patients in a hot environment. Thus the use of agents which interfere relatively specifically with the febrile process and not with thermoregulation *per se* will most likely remain the chief pharmacologic approach to antipyresis.

Figure 1a indicates a presumed sequence of reactions elicited by pyrogen and leading to regulation of body temperature at an elevated level and also indicates points within this sequence (A to H) at which antipyretics might interfere. Evidence summarized elsewhere (10) indicates that a peripheral action is unlikely to contribute much to antipyresis. Antipyretics have antagonized endotoxin in many studies, but since they can also antagonize endogenous pyrogens in a dose-related fashion, a direct interaction with exogenous pyrogen is unlikely. There have been reports that antipyretics in the rabbit and chicken were ineffective when given before administration of pyrogen (25,30,43,44). Most reports, however, indicate antipyretic effectiveness of drugs given prior to endogenous pyrogen administration to the rabbit (5,38,47,64,66,69), cat (11–13,19,59), goat (64), and monkey (47). Therefore, it is clear than when submaximal doses of pyrogen are given, pretreatment with antipyretics usually diminishes the response. For the most part, antipyretics have not been demonstrated to inhibit release of endogenous pyrogens, either by comparison of release from leukocytes incubated with and without antipyretics *in vitro* or by assessing pyrogen release *in vivo* by transferring to recipients plasma from endotoxin-treated donors also given antipyretic or vehicle. Antipyretics do not interact chemically with endogenous pyrogen to inactivate it, at least in an irreversible fashion. They inhibit the pyrogenic activity of endogenous pyrogen given centrally so they apparently do not block access of the pyrogen to a central site of action. Antipyretics are also effective when injected directly into the central nervous system, regardless of the route of pyrogen administration. Antagonism of endogenous pyrogen has been produced by injections of salicylate directly into specific brain regions, in particular the preoptic/anterior hypothalamus (PO/AH) (26,38,60,61), but also the midbrain (26).

It is thus well established that antipyretics act within the brain, and the primary unresolved question is the specific mechanism by which they antagonize pyrogen within the central nervous system. Two explanations for the central action of antipyretics have received the most attention (10): competition of antipyretics with endogenous pyrogen for a receptor and inhibition of prostaglandin synthesis. The former mechanism is indicated by production of a parallel shift to the right of the log dose-response curve for leukocytic pyrogen which has been demonstrated for indomethacin (13), acetaminophen, and salicylate (12).

Prostaglandin synthesis inhibition is thought to be a mechanism of antipyretic action based on evidence that prostaglandins are required for fever (Milton, *this volume*) and the observation that when antipyretics reduce fever they also lower the concentration of prostaglandins in the cerebrospinal fluid toward normal (42). Although there is no doubt that nonsteroidal anti-inflammatory agents can inhibit prostaglandin synthesis, such inhibition does not necessarily account for their antipyretic effect. Against such an action is evidence that prostaglandins are not required for fever (Hellon et al., *this volume*). This includes the report that doses of prostaglandin antagonists SC 19220 and HR 546 that reduced prostaglandin-induced hyperthermia did not alter endogenous pyrogen-induced fever (22). One explanation may be that an arachidonic acid derivative other than prostaglandin is involved (37). Central administration of prostacyclin can cause hyperthermia (17), whereas the endoperoxide intermediates may not (34). An unpublished observation indicated that administration of bacterial pyrogen to echidnas caused fever which was antagonized by acetaminophen (2), even though this species responded primarily with hypothermia to intraventricular administration of prostaglandins.

Even if prostaglandins or other derivatives of arachidonic acid are required for fever, there is evidence that antipyretics act prior to the cyclo-oxygenase responsible for formation of the cyclic endoperoxide intermediates which are converted into prostaglandins, prostacyclin, and thromboxanes. If endotoxin causes fever by release of an arachidonic acid derivative, then comparable increases in temperature after endotoxin and arachidonate injection should reflect comparable concentrations of the active derivative at its site of action. Antipyretics which inhibit cyclo-oxygenase would be expected to inhibit endotoxin and arachidonate about equally, and a high correlation between blockade of the two hyperthermogenic agents should also result. Yet when comparisons were made of the relative abilities of antipyretics to antagonize hyperthermic responses to central administration of endotoxin and arachidonate in the cat, a wide variation in relative effectiveness occurred. The acidic antipyretics acetaminophen and indomethacin blocked endotoxin to a much greater extent than they blocked arachidonate (14), with little or no correlation. On the other hand, tilorone, a basic antipyretic, blocked both endotoxin and arachidonate approximately equally (20), but the correlation was negative whereas another basic antipyretic, L 8027, was intermediate in blocking arachidonate relative to endotoxin (18). Thus antagonism of arachidonate did not correlate well with antipyretic activity against endotoxin, and different antipyretics showed considerable variability in relative ability to antagonize pyrogen and arachidonate. If arachidonic acid derivatives are required for fever and if antipyretics do not compete specifically with endogenous pyrogen, it is conceivable that antipyretics antagonize pyrogen-induced release of arachidonic acid from phospholipids in plasma membranes and that such an action combined with varying degrees of inhibition of cyclo-oxygenase or subsequent synthetases might account for the different relative antagonisms of endotoxin and arachidonate noted above. There has been a recent report that low concentrations of indomethacin can inhibit phospholipase A_2 from rabbit polymorphonuclear leukocytes (36).

Two other hypothetical mechanisms for drug-induced antipyresis should be mentioned. Like prostaglandins of the E series, the concentration of cyclic AMP in cerebrospinal fluid approximately doubles during endotoxin-induced fever (27,48,50,62). Cholera toxin activates adenylate cyclase in a wide variety of systems (29,65), and central administration of this toxin to the cat (16) and chick (45) caused hyperthermia, presumably due to endogenous cyclic AMP formation, which was antagonized by indomethacin, acetaminophen, and salicylate (16). Central injections of dibutyryl-cyclic AMP also caused hyperthermic responses (16,49,67–69), which were reduced by antipyretics in the cat (16) but not in the rabbit (67). Such evidence is suggestive, but inconclusive at the present time, of a contribution of cyclic AMP to fever and possibly to antipyresis. Although there is as yet no evidence for a major action of classic antipyretics on pyrogen transport, a new area for study derives from the evidence discussed by Dr. Lipton that the action of endogenous pyrogen and prostaglandins may be terminated by active transport from their sites of action or into the cerebrospinal fluid.

SUMMARY

Antipyretics interact within the central nervous system specifically with the febrile process rather than with the thermoregulatory system *per se.* It is unlikely that they act primarily by inhibiting prostaglandin synthesis. Although antipyretics appear to compete with endogenous pyrogen, or possibly some other mediator specifically required for fever production, interactions with cyclic nucleotides or mechanisms which transport pyrogen from its site of action may present new approaches to understanding antipyresis.

REFERENCES

1. Antoon, J. W., and Gregg, R. V. (1976): The influence of body temperature on the production of ulcers of restraint in the rat. *Gastroenterology*, 70:747–750.
2. Baird, J. A., Hales, J. R. S., and Lang, W. J. (1974): Thermoregulatory responses to the injection of monoamines, acetylcholine and prostaglandins into a lateral cerebral ventricle of the echidna. *J. Physiol. (Lond.)*, 236:539–548.
3. Barbour, H. G. (1919): Antipyretics. III. Acetylsalicylic acid and heat regulation in fever cases. *Arch. Intern. Med.*, 24:624–632.
4. Beaton, J. M., Benington, F., Bradley, R. J., Kuhlemeier, K. V., and Morin, R. D. (1976): Stereospecific actions of 2,5-dimethoxy-4-methylamphetamine (DOM) on colonic temperature in the rat at various ambient temperatures. *Br. J. Pharmacol.*, 57:547–550.
5. Bennett, I. L., Jr., and Beeson, P. B. (1953): Studies on the pathogenesis of fever. II. Characterization of fever-producing substances from polymorphonuclear leukocytes and from the fluid of sterile exudates. *J. Exp. Med.*, 98:493–508.
6. Bernheim, H. A., and Kluger, M. J. (1976): Fever and antipyresis in the lizard *Dipsosaurus dorsalis. Am. J. Physiol.*, 231:198–203.
7. Bizzi, A., Garattini, S., and Veneroni, E. (1965): The action of salicylate in reducing plasma free fatty acids and its pharmacological consequences. *Br. J. Pharmacol.*, 25:187–196.
8. Bligh, J. (1972): Neuronal models of mammalian temperature regulation. In: *Essays on Temperature Regulation*, edited by J. Bligh and R. Moore, pp. 105–120. North-Holland, Amsterdam.
9. Borison, H. L., and Clark, W. G. (1967): Drug actions on thermoregulatory mechanisms. *Adv. Pharmacol.*, 5:129–212.

10. Clark, W. G. (1979): Mechanisms of antipyretic action. *Gen. Pharmacol.*, 10:71–77.
11. Clark, W. G., and Alderdice, M. T. (1972): Inhibition of leukocytic pyrogen-induced fever by intracerebroventricular administration of salicylate and acetaminophen in the cat. *Proc. Soc. Exp. Biol. Med.*, 140:399–403.
12. Clark, W. G., and Coldwell, B. A. (1972): Competitive antagonism of leukocytic pyrogen by sodium salicylate and acetaminophen. *Proc. Soc. Exp. Biol. Med.*, 141:669–672.
13. Clark, W. G., and Cumby, H. R. (1975): The antipyretic effect of indomethacin. *J. Physiol. (Lond.)*, 248:625–638.
14. Clark, W. G., and Cumby, H. R. (1976): Antagonism by antipyretics of the hyperthermic effect of a prostaglandin precursor, sodium arachidonate, in the cat. *J. Physiol. (Lond.)*, 257:581–595.
15. Clark, W. G., and Cumby, H. R. (1978): Hyperthermic responses to central and peripheral injections of morphine sulphate in the cat. *Br. J. Pharmacol.*, 63:65–71.
16. Clark, W. G., Cumby, H. R., and Davis, H. E., IV (1974): The hyperthermic effect of intracerebroventricular cholera enterotoxin in the unanaesthetized cat. *J. Physiol. (Lond.)*, 240:493–504.
17. Clark, W. G., and Lipton, J. M. (1979): Hyperthermic effect of prostacyclin injected into the third cerebral ventricle of the cat. *Brain Res. Bull.*, 4:15–16.
18. Clark, W. G., and Lipton, J. M. (1979): Antagonism of hyperthermogenic agents by L 8027, an inhibitor of prostaglandin and thromboxane synthetase. *Proc. Soc. Exp. Biol. Med.*, 160:473–476.
19. Clark, W. G., and Moyer, S. G. (1972): The effects of acetaminophen and sodium salicylate on the release and activity of leukocytic pyrogen in the cat. *J. Pharmacol. Exp. Ther.*, 181:183–191.
20. Clark, W. G., and Robins, J. A. (1978): The antipyretic effect of tilorone hydrochloride in the cat. *Br. J. Pharmacol.*, 62:281–287.
21. Cranston, W. I., Duff, G. W., Hellon, R. F., and Mitchell, D. (1976): Thermoregulation in rabbits during fever. *J. Physiol. (Lond.)*, 257:767–777.
22. Cranston, W. I., Duff, G. W., Hellon, R. F., Mitchell, D., and Townsend, Y. (1976): Evidence that brain prostaglandin synthesis is not essential in fever. *J. Physiol. (Lond.)*, 259:239–249.
23. Cranston, W. I., Hellon, R. F., Luff, R. H., Rawlins, M. D., and Rosendorff, C. (1970): Observations on the mechanism of salicylate-induced antipyresis. *J. Physiol. (Lond.)*, 210:593–600.
24. Cranston, W. I., Hellon, R. F., and Mitchell, D. (1975): Is brain prostaglandin synthesis involved in responses to cold? *J. Physiol. (Lond.)*, 249:425–434.
25. Cranston, W. I., Luff, R. H., Rawlins, M. D., and Wright, V. A. (1971): Influence of the duration of experimental fever on salicylate antipyresis in the rabbit. *Br. J. Pharmacol.*, 41:344–351.
26. Cranston, W. I., and Rawlins, M. D. (1972): Effects of intracerebral micro-injection of sodium salicylate on temperature regulation in the rabbit. *J. Physiol. (Lond.)*, 222:257–266.
27. Dascombe, M. J., and Milton, A. S. (1976): Cyclic adenosine 3',5'-monophosphate in cerebrospinal fluid during thermoregulation and fever. *J. Physiol. (Lond.)*, 263:441–463.
28. Downey, J. A., and Darling, R. C. (1962): Effect of salicylates on elevation of body temperature during exercise. *J. Appl. Physiol.*, 17:323–325.
29. Finkelstein, R. A. (1973): Cholera. *CRC Crit. Rev. Microbiol.*, 2:553–623.
30. Gander, G. W., Chaffee, J., and Goodale, F. (1967): Studies on the antipyretic action of salicylates. *Proc. Soc. Exp. Biol. Med.*, 126:205–209.
31. Green, M. D., and Lomax, P. (1973): The effects of sodium salicylate on body temperature in the normothermic rat. *Proc. West. Pharmacol. Soc.*, 16:257–261.
32. Guerra (Perez-Carral), F., and Barbour, H. G. (1943): The mechanism of aspirin antipyresis in monkeys. *J. Pharmacol. Exp. Ther.*, 79:55–61.
33. Hart, J. L. (1975): Salicylate hypothermia in rats exposed to hyperbaric air and helium. *J. Appl. Physiol.*, 39:575–579.
34. Hawkins, M., and Lipton, J. M. (1977): Analogs of endoperoxide precursors of prostaglandins: Failure to affect body temperature when injected into primary and secondary central temperature controls. *Prostaglandins*, 13:209–218.
35. Jacobson, E. D., and Bass, D. E. (1964): Effects of sodium salicylate on physiological responses to work in heat. *J. Appl. Physiol.*, 19:33–36.
36. Kaplan, L., Weiss, J., and Elsbach, P. (1978): Low concentrations of indomethacin inhibit

phospholipase A_2 of rabbit polymorphonuclear leukocytes. *Proc. Natl. Acad. Sci. U.S.A.*, 75:2955–2958.
37. Laburn, H., Mitchell, D., and Rosendorff, C. (1977): Effects of prostaglandin antagonism on sodium arachidonate fever in rabbits. *J. Physiol. (Lond.)*, 267:559–570.
38. Lin, M. T., and Chai, C. Y.(1972): The antipyretic effect of sodium acetylsalicylate on pyrogen-induced fever in rabbits. *J. Pharmacol. Exp. Ther.*, 180:603–609.
39. Lin, M. T., and Chai, C. Y. (1975): Effects of sodium acetylsalicylate on body temperature of monkeys under heat exposure. *J. Pharmacol. Exp. Ther.*, 194:165–170.
40. Martin, G. E., and Morrison, J. E. (1978): Hyperthermia evoked by the intracerebral injection of morphine sulphate in the rat: The effect of restraint. *Brain Res.*, 145:127–140.
41. Martin, G. E., Pryzbylik, A. T., and Spector, N. H. (1977): Restraint alters the effects of morphine and heroin on core temperature in the rat. *Pharmacol. Biochem. Behav.*, 7:463–469.
42. Milton, A. S. (1976): Modern views on the pathogenesis of fever and the mode of action of antipyretic drugs. *J. Pharm. Pharmacol.*, 28:393–399.
43. Nistico, G., De Girolamo, G., and Preziosi, P. (1976): Intraventricular antipyretics and bacterial pyrogen fever. *Arch. Int. Pharmacodyn. Ther.*, 220:339–343.
44. Nistico, G., and Rotiroti, D. (1978): Antipyretics and fever induced in adult fowls by prostaglandins E_1, E_2 and O somatic antigen. *Neuropharmacology*, 17:197–203.
45. Nistico, G., Stephenson, J. D., and Preziosi, P. (1976): Behavioural, electrocortical and body temperature effects of cholera toxin. *Eur. J. Pharmacol.*, 36:459–462.
46. Palmes, E. D., and Park, C. R. (1965): The regulation of body temperature during fever. *Arch. Environ. Health*, 11:749–759.
47. Perlow, M., Dinarello, C. A., and Wolff, S. M. (1975): A primate model for the study of human fever. *J. Infect. Dis.*, 132:157–164.
48. Philipp-Dormston, W. K. (1976): Evidence for the involvement of adenosine 3',5'-cyclic monophosphate in fever genesis. *Pfluegers Arch.*, 362:223–227.
49. Philipp-Dormston, W. K., and Siegert, R. (1975): Fever produced in rabbits by N^6,O^{2-}dibutyryl adenosine-3',5'-cyclic monophosphate. *Experientia*, 31:471–472.
50. Philipp-Dormston, W. K., and Siegert, R. (1975): Adenosine 3',5'-cyclic monophosphate in rabbit cerebrospinal fluid during fever induced by *E. coli*-endotoxin. *Med. Microbiol. Immunol. (Berl.)*, 161:11–13.
51. Pittman, Q. J., Veale, W. L., and Cooper, K. E. (1976): Observations on the effect of salicylate in fever and the regulation of body temperature against cold. *Can. J. Physiol. Pharmacol.*, 54:101–106.
52. Polk, D. L., and Lipton, J. M. (1975): Effects of sodium salicylate, aminopyrine and chlorpromazine on behavioral temperature regulation. *Pharmacol. Biochem. Behav.*, 3:167–172.
53. Reynolds, W. W. (1977): Fever and antipyresis in the bluegill sunfish, *Lepomis macrochirus*. *Comp. Biochem. Physiol. [C]*, 57:165–167.
54. Rosendorff, C., and Cranston, W. I. (1968): Effects of salicylate on human temperature regulation. *Clin. Sci.*, 35:81–91.
55. Rudy, T. A., and Yaksh, T. L. (1977): Hyperthermic effects of morphine: Set point manipulation by a direct spinal action. *Br. J. Pharmacol.*, 61:91–96.
56. Satinoff, E. (1972): Salicylate: Action on normal body temperature in rats. *Science*, 176:532–533.
57. Satinoff, E., and Hendersen, R. (1977): Thermoregulatory behavior. In: *Handbook of Operant Behavior*, edited by W. K. Honig and J. E. R. Staddon, pp. 153–173. Prentice-Hall, Englewood Cliffs, N.J.
58. Satinoff, E., McEwen, G. N., Jr., and Williams, B. A. (1976): Behavioral fever in newborn rabbits. *Science*, 193:1139–1140.
59. Schoener, E. P., and Wang, S. C. (1974): Sodium acetylsalicylate effectiveness against fever induced by leukocytic pyrogen and prostaglandin E_1 in the cat. *Experientia*, 30:383–384.
60. Schoener, E. P., and Wang, S. C. (1975): Leukocytic pyrogen and sodium acetylsalicylate on hypothalamic neurons in the cat. *Am. J. Physiol.*, 229:185–190.
61. Schoener, E. P., and Wang, S. C. (1975): Observations on the central mechanism of acetylsalicylate antipyresis. *Life Sci.*, 17:1063–1068.
62. Siegert, R., Philipp-Dormston, W. K., Radsak, K., and Menzel, H. (1976): Mechanism of fever induction in rabbits. *Infect. Immun.*, 14:1130–1137.
63. Trzcinka, G. P., Lipton, J. M., Hawkins, M., and Clark, W. G. (1977): Effects on temperature

of morphine injected into the preoptic/anterior hypothalamus, medulla oblongata, and peripherally in unrestrained and restrained rats. *Proc. Soc. Exp. Biol. Med.,* 156:523–526.

64. van Duin, C. Th. M., van Essen, J. A., and van Miert, A. S. J. P. A. M. (1975): Mechanism of the antipyretic action of salicylates and pyrazolone derivates. *Zentralbl. Veterinaermed. [A],* 22:510–519.
65. Van Heyningen, S. (1977): Cholera toxin. *Biol. Rev.,* 52:509–549.
66. van Miert, A. S. J. P. A. M., and van Duin, C. Th. M. (1977): The antipyretic effect of flurbiprofen. *Eur. J. Pharmacol.,* 44:197–204.
67. Willies, G. H., Woolf, C. J., and Rosendorff, C. (1976): The effect of sodium salicylate on dibutyryl cyclic AMP fever in the conscious rabbit. *Neuropharmacology,* 15:9–10.
68. Willies, G. H., Woolf, C. J., and Rosendorff, C. (1976): The effect of an inhibitor of adenylate cyclase on the development of pyrogen, prostaglandin and cyclic AMP fevers in the rabbit. *Pfluegers Arch.,* 367:177–181.
69. Woolf, C. J., Willies, G. H., Laburn, H., and Rosendorff, C. (1975): Pyrogen and prostaglandin fever in the rabbit. I. Effects of salicylate and the role of cyclic AMP. *Neuropharmacology,* 14:397–403.

Fever, edited by James M. Lipton.
Raven Press, New York © 1980.

Evidence for the Involvement of Prostaglandins in Pyrogen Fever

Anthony S. Milton

Department of Pharmacology, Marischal College, University of Aberdeen, Aberdeen AB9 1AS, Scotland

Nine years ago Milton and Wendlandt (14) provided the first intimation that prostaglandins might be involved in pyrogen fever and that antipyretic drugs might act by inhibiting the release of prostaglandins. Since that time considerable evidence has been obtained which supports this proposition, and this chapter summarizes results which the author and his colleagues have obtained in the intervening years. This chapter does not deal with the work of other authors and is not a full review of the subject. For a more complete discussion, readers are invited to read the more comprehensive reviews by Feldberg and Milton (6) and Milton (10).

THERMOREGULATORY RESPONSES TO PROSTAGLANDINS

The main observation of Milton and Wendlandt (14) was that minute amounts of prostaglandin E_1 (PGE_1) produced vigorous shivering and ear vasoconstriction when injected directly into the third cerebral ventricle of the conscious cat. The animals became sedated, curled up in a ball, and their rectal temperature rapidly rose. The threshold dose required to produce a rise in deep body temperature was approximately 3×10^{-11} moles, and the duration of the response was short, particularly when compared with the long-lasting fever produced by intraventricular injection of bacterial pyrogens. Other than this difference in the duration of action of PGE_1, the effects seen with PGE_1 were similar both behaviorally and autonomically to those produced by bacterial pyrogen. Prostaglandins A_1, $F_{1\alpha}$, and $F_{2\alpha}$ when given in the same dose ranges as PGE_1 were without effect on deep body temperature.

The second significant observation was that the antipyretic drug 4-acetamidophenol (paracetamol, acetaminophen) had no effect on hyperthermia produced by PGE_1. This was in direct contrast to the antipyresis seen when 4-acetamidophenol was administered during fever produced by intraventricular (i.c.v.) injection of bacterial pyrogen (13). As a result of these observations Milton and Wendlandt (14) proposed that "PGE_1 may be a modulator in temperature regulation and the action of antipyretics may be to interfere with the release of PGE_1 by pyrogens."

Subsequent experiments published by Milton and Wendlandt in 1971 (15,16) showed that prostaglandin E_2 (PGE$_2$) had an effect on body temperature identical to that of PGE$_1$, and that it was active in the same dose range. It was also found that PGE$_1$ was hyperthermogenic in the rabbit and rat.

Because of the observation that PGE$_1$ was hyperthermogenic in all mammalian species tested and, in contrast, monoamines produced inconsistent changes in body temperature when administered centrally to different species, it seemed that PGE$_1$ would be an ideal substance for modulating increases in deep body temperature, particularly the hyperthermia occurring during fever. In order to determine the physiological responses to PGE$_1$ which were involved in the increase in deep body temperature, Bligh and Milton (1) studied the effects of i.c.v. infusions of PGE$_1$ in the Welsh mountain sheep. The sheep was chosen as the experimental animal because it is able to maintain a constant deep body temperature when exposed to a wide range of ambient air temperatures. It does this by regulating both heat loss and heat gain responses, and these responses can be readily monitored. Bligh and Milton recorded deep body temperature, ear skin temperature, respiratory rate, and shivering.

When the ambient air temperature was 10°C, the respiratory rate was low, the ear skin temperature was the same as the air temperature, indicating vasoconstriction; and occasional bursts of activity were observed from electrical recordings of the thigh muscle, indicating shivering. These measurements showed that the animals maintained deep body temperature by minimizing heat loss and by occasionally increasing heat production. When PGE$_1$ was infused i.c.v. at the rate of 1 µg/min, the respiratory rate dropped slightly. There was no change in ear skin temperature, but violent shivering was observed and deep body temperature began to rise immediately. As soon as the infusion was stopped, shivering ceased and the animals began to pant and continued to do so until deep body temperature had returned to normal. In contrast, when the ambient air temperature was 45°C, well above normal deep body temperature, the animals panted vigorously, the ear vessels were dilated, and no shivering was seen at all, indicating that the animals were actively preventing body temperature from rising, primarily through increased evaporative heat loss. When the PGE$_1$ infusion was started, the respiratory rate dropped dramatically but there were no effects on the ear skin temperature and no shivering was observed. As a result of the decrease in respiratory rate, evaporative heat loss by panting was suppressed and deep body temperature rose rapidly. When the PGE$_1$ infusion was stopped, panting resumed and the respiratory rate rose well above preinfusion level. This elevated level was maintained until body temperature had returned to normal. When the animals were maintained at room temperature (18°C), the ear skin temperature was between ambient temperature and deep body temperature and the animals did not shiver. At this ambient temperature PGE$_1$ infusion produced a fall in respiratory rate, a decrease in ear skin temperature, indicating vasoconstriction, and occasional bursts of shivering. When the PGE$_1$

infusion was stopped, shivering ceased, ear temperature increased, and the respiratory rate rose. The deep body temperature quickly fell to normal.

These experiments on the Welsh mountain sheep showed that prostaglandin E_1 increased deep body temperature by inhibiting heat loss mechanisms including evaporative heat loss (panting) and surface heat loss (vasomotor) and by stimulating heat gain mechanisms such as shivering (metabolic heat production). The predominant pattern of thermoeffector activity depended on the ambient air temperature and therefore on the thermoregulatory pathways being driven at the time. Of particular interest was the observation that as soon as the PGE_1 infusions were stopped, the animals actively lost the heat they had gained during the infusion and deep body temperature was quickly restored to normal. This is reminiscent of the effects of antipyretic drugs in reducing fever produced by bacterial pyrogens.

In the cat at an ambient temperature of 18 to 22°C, PGE_1 and PGE_2 both increase deep body temperature by producing shivering and ear skin vasoconstriction and by promoting adoption of heat-conserving postures. Body temperature returns to normal after the PGE_1 hyperthermia through an active increase in heat loss brought about by ear vasodilatation, occasional sweating from the paw pads, occasional panting, and the resumption of normal body posture (16).

PROSTAGLANDINS AND NORMAL THERMOREGULATION

In order to determine whether central prostaglandins are involved in the maintenance of deep body temperature in normal as opposed to pathological conditions, Cammock et al., (2) subjected cats to different ambient temperatures, collected cerebrospinal fluid from the cisterna magna, and assayed the CSF for PGE_2 using radioimmunoassay.

During exposure to cold (0°C) the animals exhibited autonomic and behavioral thermoregulatory responses and deep body temperature rose slightly. During exposure to a high ambient temperature (45°C) the animals were unable to control deep body temperature, and although panting, sweating from the paw pads, and ear skin vasodilatation were observed, deep body temperature rose. The experiments were stopped after a short time to prevent convulsions and death. Whether the animals were exposed to cold or heat stress, PGE_2 content of the CSF was found not to be significantly different from that when the animals were maintained at 25°C. There is no evidence, therefore, that the prostaglandins are involved in normal thermoregulation. However, it is important to realize that any changes in PGE_2 release would probably occur in the region of the thermoregulatory area of the anterior hypothalamus, and such changes might be too small to produce significant changes in PGE_2 levels found in cisternal CSF.

It is known that deep body temperature rises if the cerebroventricular system of the cat is perfused with artificial CSF containing no calcium. In 1974 Dey et al. (4) investigated this hyperthermia to determine whether there was any evidence of PGE release which could account for the rise in deep body temperature. They found no increases in PGE levels when the ventricles of the conscious cat were perfused from the third ventricle to the cisterna magna with artificial CSF containing no calcium. During perfusion with calcium-free CSF there was violent shivering and initial vasoconstriction and the deep body temperature rose rapidly. Subsequently, however, panting and vasodilatation were observed as the animals apparently attempted to dissipate the heat gained. The shivering continued throughout the perfusion but ceased when the perfusion was terminated. Neither 4-acetamidophenol nor indomethacin reduced the hyperthermia produced by calcium-free CSF perfusion.

In 1975 Milton (9) investigated the hyperthermia produced by intravenous and i.c.v. injection of morphine in the conscious cat. The hyperthermia produced was unaffected by prostaglandin synthesis inhibitors, although it was completely blocked by the specific morphine antagonist naloxone; it was concluded that the prostaglandins were not involved in morphine hyperthermia.

RELEASE OF PROSTAGLANDINS DURING PYROGEN FEVER

In 1970 Milton and Wendlandt (14) reported that a prostaglandin-like substance had been found in CSF of the cat during pyrogen fever. In 1973 Feldberg et al. (5) collected CSF from the cisterna magna of the consicous cat and assayed it for PGE-like activity using a bioassay method. They found that the O-somatic antigen of *Shigella dysenteriae* produced fever when administered into both the third ventricle and the cisterna magna and also when given intravenously. In all cases, during the febrile response the PGE-like activity of the CSF increased and the three antipyretic drugs acetylsalicylic acid (aspirin), 4-acetamidophenol, and indomethacin all abolished the fever and at the same time the PGE content of the CSF fell. Thin-layer chromatography of the CSF samples followed by bioassay and radioimmunoassay indicated that the prostaglandin present in the CSF of the cat during fever was PGE_2 and not PGE_1. Harvey et al. (8) in 1975 obtained similar results in rabbits made febrile with O-somatic antigen of *S. dysenteriae* or with a purified pyrogen prepared from *Proteus vulgaris*. In addition, they found that if the rabbits were made tolerant to the fever-producing effect of the pyrogen by injecting it intravenously every day for 10 days, then on the tenth day, when the animals were refractory to the pyrogenic action, no increase in the PGE_2 content of the CSF was found.

It is now generally considered that bacterial pyrogens activate neutrophils and possibly monocytes and other cells within the body to synthesize and release a low molecular weight protein known as endogenous pyrogen (or leukocytic pyrogen). Harvey and Milton (7) prepared endogenous pyrogen from cat peritoneal exudate and found that when this material was infused i.v. into the conscious cat it produced fever associated with an increase in the PGE_2 content of the cisternal CSF. This fever and the increase in PGE_2 were inhibited by antipyretic agents. They also found that plasma obtained from a donor cat made febrile by i.v. *S. dysenteriae* and injected into a recipient cat previously made refractory to the pyrogen produced fever accompanied by an increase in cisternal CSF levels of PGE_2. These experiments showed that during bacterial pyrogen fever there was a circulating pyrogenic material in the plasma which differed from bacterial pyrogen and which was itself capable of producing PGE_2 release. It was concluded that this circulating pyrogen was endogenous pyrogen. In contrast, when fever was produced by injecting bacterial pyrogen i.c.v. in the cat, no circulating pyrogenic material could be detected in the plasma. These results indicated that centrally administered bacterial pyrogen does not activate the synthesis and release of endogenous pyrogen peripherally and that it must therefore produce fever by acting on cells within the central nervous system.

THERMOREGULATORY EFFECTS OF PROSTACYCLIN AND PROSTAGLANDIN ENDOPEROXIDE ANALOGS

Recently, experiments have been undertaken to determine if some other metabolites of arachidonic acid can produce rises in deep body temperature similar to those caused by prostaglandin E_2 (3,11). The unstable, highly potent vasodilator compound prostacyclin (PGI_2), its stable degradation product 6-oxo-$PGF_{1\alpha}$, and two stable methylene derivatives of the prostaglandin endoperoxide PGH_2 have been studied, and their effects on body temperature of conscious cats and rabbits when injected directly into the third ventricle have been determined. The two endoperoxide analogs which have been studied are isomers with the following structures: (15s)-hydroxy-11α,9α-(epoxymethano)prosta-5$_3$,13-edienoic acid and (15s)-hydroxy-11α,9α-(methanoepoxy)prosta-5$_3$,13-edienoic acid. These are referred to as 9α-PGM_2 and 11α-PGM_2, respectively. The responses of cats and rabbits to these two analogs and also to arachidonic acid have been studied following the administration of imidazole, a selective inhibitor of thromboxane synthesis which does not affect cyclo-oxygenase.

PGI_2 was administered i.c.v. to cats in doses of 50, 100, and 200 μg. The two higher doses caused rises in body temperature within a few minutes of injection, and these rises were associated with vigorous shivering, ear skin vasoconstriction, and piloerection. Some shivering was also observed after the lower dose although no effect on body temperature was seen. Sedation was a constant feature after all three doses.

6-Oxo-$PGF_{1\alpha}$ was given in the same doses. The lower dose had no effect on body temperature or on behavior of the animals. At 100 μg the temperature responses produced were similar to those seen after 100 μg PGI_2. However, the behavioral effects were different in that restlessness and an increase in the frequency of respiration often accompanied the rises in deep body temperature. In addition, the vigorous shivering and vasoconstriction seen with PGI_2 did not appear to be essential to the rises in body temperature produced by this compound. In rabbits, dose-related increases in deep body temperature were produced by doses of 10, 50, and 100 μg of PGI_2. The hyperthermic response to 100 μg of PGI_2 was found to be similar in magnitude to that produced by 5 μg PGE_2. The duration of the response was longer after PGI_2 than after PGE_2. Behavioral effects of PGI_2 also differed from those of PGE_2 in that the rabbits became active immediately after the injection of PGI_2.

9α-PGM_2 in doses of 10 and 20 μg produced hypothermic responses after an average latency of about 10 min. This hypothermia was found to last approximately 3 hr. The onset of the response was associated with vomiting, defecation, and ear skin vasodilatation. This was followed by a period of heat dissipation during which the frequency of respiration increased and the animals were observed to be lying down quietly with legs outstretched. Sedation, panting, and sweating from the paw pads occurred in some animals during these experiments. In contrast, 11α-PGM_2 in doses of 10 and 20 μg produced a rise in deep body temperature similar to that caused by low doses of PGE_2. A maximal response to 11α-PGM_2 was reached within 2 hr of injection. 4-Acetamidophenol had no effect on the hypo-or hyperthermia produced by the 9α- and 11α-PGM_2 compounds.

In the rabbit neither 9α-PGM_2 nor 11α-PGM_2 had any effect on deep body temperature. However, other effects such as ear skin vasodilatation, increased frequency of respiration, and sedation were often seen with both compounds. In over 50% of rabbits receiving a dose of 20 μg of either compound, death occurred immediately after the injection.

Arachidonic acid is a dose of 100 μg administered i.c.v. to rabbits produced a rise in body temperature of approximately 1°C. This hyperthermia was associated with increased motor activity immediately after injection followed by ear vasoconstriction until maximal temperature was attained. Imidazole (100 μg i.c.v.) administered to the rabbit 15 min prior to arachidonic acid had no significant effect on the temperature response.

PROTEIN SYNTHESIS INHIBITORS AND PROSTAGLANDIN FEVER

The effects of cycloheximide, a protein synthesis inhibitor, on fever produced by prostaglandins, arachidonic acid, and pyrogens have been studied in the rabbit (Milton and Sawhney, *unpublished observations*). In a dose of 5 mg/kg i.v., cycloheximide produced a slight but significant fall in deep body temperature when administered 90 min before i.v. injection of the pyrogen from *S. dysenteriae* (1 μg/kg). The temperature response to the pyrogen was completely abolished. In contrast, the hyperthermic response to i.c.v. injection of either pyrogen (1 μg/kg) or PGE_2 (1 μg) was unaffected. Similarly, the hyperthermic response to arachidonic acid, a precursor of prostaglandin E_2, was unaffected by cycloheximide. However, the nonsteroidal anti-inflammatory drug ketoprofen administered s.c. in a dose of 3 mg/kg completely abolished the hyperthermic response to arachidonic acid.

DISCUSSION

The most convincing evidence that prostaglandin E_2 is a mediator of pyrogen fever and that antipyretic drugs act by interfering with the release of PGE_2 is provided by three separate observations. First, the intraventricular or intrahypothalamic application of PGE_2 produces hyperthermia with accompanying autonomic and behavioral actions identical to that produced by bacterial pyrogen. Second, in all instances in which bacterial pyrogens have produced fever, a rise in the CSF level of PGE_2 has been found. Third, during antipyresis produced by a variety of nonsteroidal anti-inflammatory antipyretic drugs, a decrease in the elevated levels of PGE_2 in the CSF accompanies the fall in deep body temperature. This final observation is particularly important in the light of our present knowledge that these drugs are all potent inhibitors of the enzyme fatty acid cyclo-oxygenase, which is responsible for the first step in the conversion of the prostaglandin precursors to the prostaglandins. Since little preformed prostaglandin is present in tissues, one can equate inhibition of prostaglandin synthesis with inhibition of prostaglandin release. The evidence for the involvement in fever of prostaglandins other than PGE_2, the endoperoxides, and the thromboxanes is tenuous. Certainly changes in $PGF_{2\alpha}$ levels have been observed during pyrogen fever. However, the levels of $PGF_{2\alpha}$ found in the CSF of the cat have been small (12). If the concentration of PGE_2 found in the CSF during fever were applied to the hypothalamus, it would produce a rise in deep body temperature. However, the amounts of $PGF_{2\alpha}$ found in the CSF after pyrogen fever would have no effect. The results obtained with prostacyclin (PGI_2), its metabolite 6-oxo-$PGF_{1\alpha}$, and the hyperthermogenic endoperoxide 11α-PGM_2 indicate that they are considerably less potent than prostaglandin E_2, suggesting that they are unlikely to have a role in pyrogen fever. However, it should be realized that since 9α-PGM_2 and 11α-PGM_2 have opposite effects on deep body temperature, one cannot at this stage equate the action of these two analogs with the labile naturally occurring PGE_2.

The results obtained with arachidonic acid and imidazole in rabbits failed to support the hypothesis that the thromboxanes are pyrogenic. Imidazole, a selective inhibitor of thromboxane synthetase, would be expected to reduce arachidonic acid fever if the thromboxanes were pyrogenic, and this was not shown to be the case in the experiments described above. However, the observation that antipyretic drugs abolish the hyperthermic response to arachidonic acid is evidence that arachidonic acid is converted to a hyperthermic prostaglandin.

CONCLUSION

There is considerable support for the proposal that a prostaglandin, probably prostaglandin E_2, is a mediator of pyrogen fever, and that antipyretic drugs act by inhibiting the synthesis and release of this prostaglandin. As with all good theories, there are those who disagree, and only time will resolve this conflict.

REFERENCES

1. Bligh, J., and Milton, A. S. (1973): The thermoregulatory effects of prostaglandin E_1 when infused into a lateral cerebral ventricle of the Welsh mountain sheep at different ambient temperatures. *J. Physiol. (Lond.),* 229:30–31P.
2. Cammock, S., Dascombe, M. J., and Milton, A. S. (1976): Prostaglandins in thermoregulation. In: *Advances in Prostaglandin and Thromboxane Research, Vol. 1,* edited by B. Samuelsson and R. Paoletti, pp. 375–380. Raven Press, New York.
3. Cremades-Campos, A., and Milton, A. S. (1978): The effect on deep body temperature of the intraventricular injection of two prostaglandin endoperoxide analogues. *J. Physiol. (Lond.),* 282:38P.
4. Dey, P. K., Feldberg, W., Gupta, K. P., Milton, A. S., and Wendlandt, S. (1974): Further studies on the role of prostaglandin in fever. *J. Physiol. (Lond.),* 241:629–646.
5. Feldberg, W., Gupta, K. P., Milton, A. S., and Wendlandt, S. (1973): Effect of pyrogen and antipyretics on prostaglandin activity in cisternal C.S.F. of unanaesthetized cats. *J. Physiol. (Lond.),* 234:279–303.
6. Feldberg, W., and Milton, A. S. (1978): Prostaglandins and body temperature. In: *Handbook of Experimental Pharmacology, Vol. 50.1,* edited by J. R. Vane and S. H. Ferreira, pp. 615–656. Springer-Verlag, Berlin.
7. Harvey, C. A., and Milton, A. S. (1975): Endogenous pyrogen fever, prostaglandin release and prostaglandin synthetase inhibitors. *J. Physiol. (Lond.),* 250:18–20P.
8. Harvey, C. A., Milton, A. S., and Straughan, D. W. (1975): Prostaglandin E levels in cerebrospinal fluid of rabbits and the effects of bacterial pyrogen and antipyretic drugs. *J. Physiol. (Lond.),* 248:26–27P.
9. Milton, A. S. (1975): Morphine hyperthermia, prostaglandin synthetase inhibitors and naloxone. *J. Physiol. (Lond.),* 251:27–28P.
10. Milton, A. S. (1980): Prostaglandins in fever and mode of action of antipyretic agents. In: *Handbook of Experimental Pharmacology,* edited by A. S. Milton, chap. 12. Springer-Verlag, Berlin *(in press).*
11. Milton, A. S., Cremades-Campos, A., Sawhney, V. K., and Bichard, A. (1980): The effects of prostacyclin, 6-oxo-$PGF_{1\alpha}$ and two stable prostaglandin endoperoxide analogues on body temperature of cats and rabbits. In: *Thermoregulatory Mechanisms and their Therapeutic Implications,* edited by B. Cox, P. Lomax, A. S. Milton, and E. Schönbaum. S. Karger, Basel.
12. Milton, A. S., Smith, S., and Tomkins, K. B. (1977): Levels of prostaglandin F and E in cerebrospinal fluid of cats during pyrogen fever. *Br. J. Pharmacol.,* 59:447–448P.
13. Milton, A. S., and Wendlandt, S. (1968): The effect of 4-acetamidophenol in reducing fever produced by the intracerebral injection of 5-hydroxytryptamine and pyrogen in the conscious cat. *Br. J. Pharmacol.,* 34:215P.
14. Milton, A. S., and Wendlandt, S. (1970): A possible role for prostaglandin E_1 as a modulator for temperature regulation in the central nervous system of the cat. *J. Physiol., (Lond.),* 207:76–77P.
15. Milton, A. S., and Wendlandt, S. (1971): The effects of 4-acetamidophenol (paracetamol) on the temperature response of the conscious rat to the intracerebral injection of prostaglandin E_1, adrenaline and pyrogen. *J. Physiol. (Lond.),* 217:33–34P.
16. Milton, A. S., and Wendlandt, S. (1971): Effects on body temperature of prostaglandins of the A, E and F series on injection into the third ventricle of unanaesthetized cats and rabbits. *J. Physiol. (Lond.),* 218:325–336.

Fever, edited by James M. Lipton.
Raven Press, New York © 1980.

Prostaglandins and Fever in Rats

*Jacek A. Spławiński, **Zbigniew Górka, **Elżbieta Zacny, and
*Barbara Wojtaszek

*Department of Pharmacology, Copernicus Medical Academy; and **Institute of
Pharmacology, Polish Academy of Sciences, Cracow, Poland*

Over the last few years evidence has accumulated to the effect that endotoxin-induced fever is mediated by a metabolite of arachidonic acid (AA) (for references see Milton, *this volume*). The mechanism whereby this mediation occurs is still unknown.

NEUROCHEMISTRY OF ARACHIDONIC ACID AND ITS METABOLITES

Within mammalian tissues AA is enzymatically converted into the cyclic endoperoxides PGG_2 and PGH_2 (Fig. 1) (10). The cyclo-oxygenation of AA to PGG_2 is catalyzed by an aspirin-sensitive enzyme, and the PGG_2 peroxidase generates PGH_2 and a free hydroxy radical (15). The unstable PGH_2 may be reduced to $PGF_{2\alpha}$ or isomerized to PGE_2, PGD_2, thromboxane A_2 (TXA_2), or prostacyclin (PGI_2) (10,17,18). TXA_2 and PGI_2 are highly unstable in physiological media (18). PGE_2 and $PGF_{2\alpha}$ are relatively more stable provided that enzymes which degrade them (10) are not present. None of the products of AA metabolism are stored in tissue; they are formed within a cell on demand (10). Phospholipase A_2, the enzyme which splits the precursor AA from membrane phosphoglycerides, is believed to be the rate-regulating factor of AA metabolism (10). This means that whenever free AA is available for interaction with membrane-bound cyclo-oxygenase (3), the synthesis of PG, PGI_2 or TXA_2 occurs.

Is there any free precursor in brain cells? Brain ischemia in mice (2) and rats (4) was reported to increase the level of free AA, which in turn resulted in increased PG formation (24). Such an increase of free AA does not occur when rats are killed within 3 sec by a microwave beam (4). However, even with the latter technique substantial amounts of free fatty acids have been detected in the brain (4), and it could be calculated that there are approximately 100 ng of free AA in rat hypothalamus. It might well be that ischemia produced during the 3 sec of microwave treatment activated phospholipase A_2.

Yet other experiments indirectly suggest that there is a definite pool of free AA in the brains of normal animals. Five minutes after an intracerebral injection

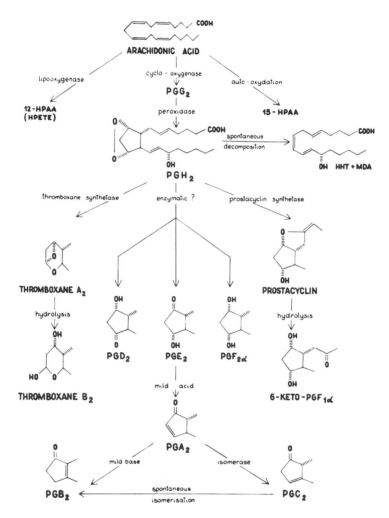

FIG. 1. Pathways of metabolism of arachidonic acid. Abbreviations: PG, prostaglandin; AA, arachidonic acid; MDA, malondialdehyde; HP, hydroperoxy; HHT, 12-hydroxy-5,8,10-heptadeca-trienoic acid; HPETE, 12-hydroperoxy-5,8,10,14-eicosatetraenoic acid ("12-HPAA").

of radiolabeled AA, 50% of the dose is incorporated into brain phospholipids; after 80 min, 2% of the injected dose is present in the free fatty acid fraction (34). If free AA is constantly available for membrane cyclo-oxygenation, it follows that constant metabolism of this acid takes place.

The route of AA metabolism is determined by the enzymatic equipment found in tissue, e.g., blood platelets cyclo-oxygenize AA primarily to TXA_2 (18), whereas in the aortic wall AA is converted mainly to PGI_2 (17). Recently, a great deal of attention has been paid to the lipoxygenase-mediated pathway of

AA metabolism (Fig. 1), a pathway present in the brain (24). AA is metabolized by lipoxygenase to unstable hydroperoxy-acids which break down to corresponding hydroxy acids [e.g., 12-hydroperoxy-5,8,10,14-eicosatetraenoic acid (HPETE)]. Brain ischemia in rats also leads to increased levels of HPETE (24). The significance of this pathway in fever is unknown. Sodium salicylate, an antipyretic drug comparable to aspirin, is a much weaker inhibitor of cyclo-oxygenase than aspirin (12). However, sodium salicylate appears to inhibit lipoxygenase (Seagall, *personal communication*). Bacteria have phospholipase activity (1), and the possibility exists that after entering the body they may release AA in the CNS thermoregulatory center as well as in other tissues. Also glia and neuronal cells of rabbit brain have been shown to contain phospholipase A_2 (33), and bacterial endotoxin or leukocyte pyrogens might stimulate this enzyme.

These facts provide a basis for investigating the effect of intracerebral injection of AA on body temperature of the rat. In these experiments we tried to simulate the chain of events according to the hypothesis (29) that bacterial endotoxins stimulate the release of AA, which in turn gives rise to PGE_2 formation. An additional reason for such investigation arises from research of Cranston et al. (7) and Laburn et al. (16) which suggests that in rabbits TXA_2, and not PGE_2, may mediate fever induced by pyrogens. In light of the facts presented above, it seems that the levels of TXA_2, as well as PGI_2 and PGs, are regulated *in vivo* by the availability of PGH_2, and therefore by the availability of AA.

ARACHIDONATE HYPERTHERMIA

AA sodium salt introduced into the brain ventricles of rats or into the anterior hypothalamic/preoptic nucleus (AH/PO) induced a rise in body temperature (29) accompanied by a rise in the skin temperature and a significant increase in CO_2 production (27). In contrast to the response to endotoxin (26), there was no correlation between the hyperthermic response to AA and the distance of the injected site from the AH/PO (27). The spontaneous generation of $PGF_{2\alpha}$ in homogenates of rat hypothalami is twice as great as the generation of PGE_2 (27). Also as in the case of AA, there is no correlation between the magnitude of the hyperthermic response to $PGF_{2\alpha}$ and the distance of the injected site from the AH/PO (27). The rise in body temperature following AA or $PGF_{2\alpha}$ was hyperthermia and not a regulated fever since the vegetative reactions in both cases were not integrated. Hyperthermia induced by AA but not by $PGF_{2\alpha}$ is attenuated by aspirin (29). Also, the $PGF_{2\alpha}/AA$ ratio of potency did not change over the relatively large distance in the brain, whereas the PGE_2/AA ratio of potency did change (Table 1). Furthermore, the mechanism by which PGE_2 increases body temperature of the rat is quite different from the mechanism and site of origination of AA-induced hyperthermia (see refs. 26 and 27). This evidence taken together suggests that the effect of exogenous AA is mediated mainly by $PGF_{2\alpha}$ and not by PGE_2.

TABLE 1. PGE_2 and $PGF_{2\alpha}$ to arachidonic acid ratios of potency in producing hyperthermia when injected into the rat brain

Localization	PGE_2 (0.02 μg)	RP^a	$PGF_{2\alpha}$ (1.0 μg)	RP	AA (10.0 μg)
AH/PO[b]	3.80 ±1.40[c]	500	2.33 ±0.75	10	1.07 ±0.47
Nucleus reticularis pontis caudalis	0.20[d]	—	1.20[e]	10	1.50[e]

[a] Approximate ratio of potency (to induce hyperthermia) as compared with AA.
[b] See text.
[c] Mean rate of esophageal temperature change (ΔT max./hr) ± SEM.
[d] Not significantly different from the control injection.
[e] Only two rats were used.

The possibility also exists that injected AA gives rise to hydroperoxy derivative formation partially mediated by cyclo-oxygenase (i.e., sensitive to aspirin). In fact, the magnitude of the hyperthermic response did not change when instead of freshly prepared AA sodium salt solution an auto-oxidized AA sodium salt solution (exposed to air for 4 days) was injected intraventricularly. The solutions of AA (100 μg dose in 10 μl) were equipotent; the rises in body temperature of 1.04 ± 0.26°C (fresh AA) and of 1.02 ± 0.12°C (auto-oxidized AA) were observed. The hydroperoxy derivatives of AA are lipoxygenase-mediated metabolites. Antagonism of the AA effect in cats by sodium salicylate (5) was observed.

It seems unlikely that exogenous AA follows the same pathway of metabolism as endogenous AA. The endogenous pool of substrate probably does not exceed 100 ng in the hypothalamus, yet enormous amounts of AA must be injected into the hypothalamus to produce hyperthermia. The threshold doses of AA required to cause hyperthermia in rats are 500 times greater than the threshold doses of PGE_2 and 50 times greater than threshold doses of $PGF_{2\alpha}$ (27). Furthermore, free hydroxy radicals formed from hydroperoxy acids are potent inhibitors of various enzymes including cyclo-oxygenase (9). It is therefore possible that with huge doses of AA, $PGF_{2\alpha}$ is formed nonenzymatically. This may explain why aspirin (29), as well as indomethacin (5), does not completely antagonize AA-induced hyperthermia. Finally, the sensitivity of the brain lipoxygenase to aspirin is as yet unknown.

TXA$_2$ AND PGI$_2$ FEVER IN RATS

The possibility that arachidonate hyperthermia in rats is medited by either TXA$_2$ or PGI$_2$ has been investigated. SC 19220, an antagonist of PGE_2 at its receptor on smooth muscle (28), inhibits the PGE_2-induced rise in body temperature of rabbits, but does not influence the response to either leukocyte pyrogen (7) or AA (16). The latter finding suggests that fever caused by pyrogens results from either the release of AA or the activation of cyclo-oxygenase and/or TXA_2 synthetase, providing that free precursor is available in the cell.

Our experiments do not support either possibility. The first possibility may be dismissed on the ground that, at least in rats, AA induces hyperthermia whereas endotoxin induces fever (26). The second possibility also seems unlikely since the study of AA conversion by hypothalamic homogenate has shown that TXA_2 is not the main metabolite formed and, in fact, only traces of TXA_2 could be detected in two out of eight experiments (27). In contrast to bovine aortic microsomes, microsomes from hypothalamic tissue do not convert PGH_2 to PGI_2 (27). Finally, if pyrogens were to produce fever by stimulation of cyclo-oxygenase (35), a rise of $PGF_{2\alpha}$ level in cerebrospinal fluid (CSF) would be expected. However, only the PGE_2 concentration of CSF increases during bacterial fever in rabbits (20). The participation of PGG_2 or PGH_2 in fever is unlikely because stable analogs of PGG_2 and PGH_2 do not induce a rise in the rat body temperature (13).

PGE_2 AND FEVER IN RATS

As far as the mechanism and site of origination of the body temperature change is concerned, among the AA metabolites, including AA itself, only PGE_2 fulfills the requirements for the role of mediator of endotoxin fever in rats. PGE_2, similar to endotoxin, induces a regulated rise in body temperature, probably representing fever (27). The central site of the fever-causing action of PGE_2, the AH/PO region, corresponds with the site responsible for endotoxin-induced fever (26,27).

The mechanism by which endotoxin increases the hypothalamic level of PGE_2 cannot be the release of AA for reasons already stated. Also as mentioned above, the lack of increase in PGF concentration in CSF during fever makes it unlikely that endotoxin stimulates cyclo-oxygenase. However, assuming that there is free AA within the hypothalamic cells, one may expect continuous synthesis of PGE_2. Endotoxin, therefore, may inhibit the breakdown of PGE_2 in hypothalamic tissue similar to the inhibition of PGE_1 degradation in lung and kidney homogenates obtained from endotoxemic rats (19). On the basis of preliminary findings, such a mechanism of endotoxin action in the rat hypothalamus was postulated (25).

Our indirect evidence further supports this notion. First, the inhibitor of 15-hydroxy PG dehydrogenase (PGDH), polyphloretin phosphate, when given i.p. in rats, significantly potentiates and prolongs endotoxin-induced fever as well as PGE_2-induced fever. Second, this inhibitor, when injected into the AH/PO, produces a dose-dependent rise in the rat body temperature, which is attenuated significantly by aspirin. Third, degradation of PGE_2 by the crude PGDH from rats with endotoxin fever is significantly slower than that of nonfebrile animals (30). The observed degradation of PGE_2 by control hypothalami obtained from nonfebrile rats is slow as compared with the degradation of PGE_1

by lung and kidney homogenates of rats (19). It is possible that type I PGDH (i.e., NAD dependent) is not very active in the hypothalamus (14). Nevertheless, other evidence suggests that PGDH may contribute to PGE_2 inactivation in the brain (32). Interestingly, degradation of PGE_2 by the crude NAD-dependent PGDH from the rat cerebral cortex does not occur (30).

These results indicate a possible mechanism by which endotoxins increase PGE_2 level in the hypothalamus. However, their relevance to the theory that PGE_2 mediates endotoxin fever in rats must wait until a causal relationship between endotoxin fever and endotoxin interaction with PGE_2 turnover in the hypothalamus is found. The results of Cranston et al. (7) indicate that the increased level of PGE_2 in cerebrospinal fluid during fever is a "side-effect" of pyrogen action.

ENDOTOXIN FEVER IN RATS

In sharp contrast to other species, *Escherichia coli* endotoxin injected intravenously produces a fall in body temperature of the rat, probably resulting from vasodilatation (31). Rats do not produce leukocyte pyrogen in response to i.v. endotoxin and in that respect differ from other animal species (31). However, injection of endotoxin into the AH produces a rise in the body temperature of the rat which probably represents fever (26). Interestingly, with repeated injections of endotoxin into the AH, the change in body temperature increases for some unknown reason (26).

The failure of i.v. endotoxin to induce fever probably results from its rapid detoxification. It has been demonstrated that a second i.v. injection of endotoxin given 48 hr after the first induces typical fever with a monophasic curve (31). This is due to the significant increase of availability of endotoxin because the level of circulating endotoxin after the second injection greatly increased (31).

PERIPHERIAL PGs AND RAT BODY TEMPERATURE

Of interest is the long-lasting (up to 90 min) hypothermia induced by PGE_2 or $PGF_{2\alpha}$ given intraperitoneally. These hypothermias are due neither to the cardiovascular effects of PGE_2 and $PGF_{2\alpha}$, which subside within 15 min, nor probably to PGE_2 and $PGF_{2\alpha}$ *per se,* as their metabolism in the body is very high (11). Both PGE_2 and $PGF_{2\alpha}$ given intravenously at doses of 1 to 10 mg/kg induce a rise in body temperature of the rat *(unpublished results)*. The fact that both PGE_2 and $PGF_{2\alpha}$ given i.p. induce hypothermia regardless of the ambient temperature and the changes in the tonus of skin vessels (Table 2) suggest that the hypothermic responses may be integrated by the CNS. After the brain was sectioned caudal to the hypothalamus, PGE_2 or $PGF_{2\alpha}$ given i.p. induced a rise in the rat body temperature which amounted to 1.93 ± 0.46°C and 2.20 ± 0.80°C ($N = 3$), respectively. It is known that in mice PG given i.p. produces nociceptive stimuli and the writhing reflex (6). Thus it is

TABLE 2. *Effect of ambient temperature (Ta) on hypothermia induced by i.p. administration of PGE$_2$ (0.3 mg/kg) and PGF$_{2\alpha}$ (3.0 mg/kg) in rats.*

Ta: Drug:	10 ± 1°C		22 ± 1°C		32 ± 1°C	
	PGE$_2$	PGF$_{2\alpha}$	PGE$_2$	PGF$_{2\alpha}$	PGE$_2$	PGF$_{2\alpha}$
T_e[a]	−2.06[d] ±0.17	−2.42 ±0.28	−1.72 ±0.21	−1.13 ±0.14	−1.20 ±0.18	−2.03 ±0.42
T_s[b]	−2.60 ±0.78	−3.40 ±0.62	1.13 ±0.62	1.08 ±0.20	ND	ND
N[c]	5	5	4	6	4	3

[a] Esophageal temperature.
[b] Skin temperature recorded at the base of the tail.
[c] Number of animals.
[d] Mean maximal changes ± SEM.

possible that PG given i.p. indirectly induces a hypothermic response. This indicates that whenever the central mechanism is investigated in rats or mice and PGs are included in the experimental protocol, PGs should not be administered intraperitoneally.

ENDOTOXIN AND ASPIRIN

In rats, in contrast to rabbits (21), salicylates induce hypothermia in nonfebrile animals (23). We have investigated the effect of aspirin (300 mg/kg, p.o.) on the body temperature of the rat at ambient temperatures of 22 and 10°C (Table 3). The results indicate that at a neutral ambient temperature aspirin promptly induces significant hypothermia, whereas the hypothermic effect of aspirin is much weaker at 10°C.

Recently we have studied the effect of endotoxin given either into the AH/

TABLE 3. *Effect of aspirin (300 mg/kg, p.o.) on esophageal temperature (T$_e$) of rats in cold and neutral ambient temperatures (T$_a$)*

T_a (°C)	Initial[a] T_e	Time (min) after aspirin administration					
		30	60	90	120	150	180
22	37.15 ±0.06[e]	−0.12[b,c]	−0.20	−0.32[d]	−0.42[c]	−0.35[c]	−0.38[c]
10	36.75 ±0.08	−0.08	−0.12	−0.14	−0.20[d]	−0.16	−0.11

[a] Mean of last three measurements after 2.5 hr exposure in the cold room.
[b] Mean change in T_e; (−) denotes the fall in T_e.
[c] $p < 0.01$ as compared with vehicle-treated animals.
[d] $p < 0.05$ as compared with vehicle-treated animals.
[e] Mean T_e ± SEM; eight animals in each group.

TABLE 4. *Effect of endotoxin (i.v.: 10.0 μg/rat, second injection; AH/PO[a]: 0.5 μg/rat, first injection) on the rat esophageal temperature (T_e) at various ambient temperatures (T_a)*

Ta (°C)	Route	N[b]	ΔT$_e$ max.[c]
22 ± 1	i.v.	5	1.20 ± 0.05[d]
10 ± 1	i.v.	7	0.18 ± 0.21
22 ± 1	AH/PO	6	0.97 ± 0.16[e]
10 ± 1	AH/PO	6	−0.05 ± 0.15

[a] See text.
[b] Number of animals.
[c] Mean maximal T_e as compared with initial T_e ± SEM.
[d] $p < 0.001$ as compared with saline-treated rats.
[e] $p < 0.05$ as compared with saline-treated rats.

PO or i.v. (two injections) on the body temperature of the rat in neutral and in cold environments. Endotoxin injected into the AH/PO or given i.v. at 22°C ambient temperature induced fever, whereas at 10°C no change in body temperature occurred (Table 4). PGE$_2$ given into the AH/PO still induced fever in the 10°C ambient temperature.

CAUSAL RELATIONSHIP AMONG ENDOTOXIN, PGs, AND FEVER

The indirect evidence cited in this chapter suggests that there is continuous synthesis and degradation of PGE$_2$ in the rat hypothalamus. It follows that PGE$_2$ in rats contributes to the thermoregulation of nonfebrile animals. It could be expected, then, that aspirin in such animals would lower the body temperature through inhibition of cyclo-oxygenase.

Indeed, such an effect of aspirin in rats was observed in the present experiments at the ambient temperature of 22°C. Therefore, the continuous generation in rats of PGE$_2$ or some other cyclo-oxygenase-mediated pyrogenic metabolite of AA constitutes a basis for endotoxin as well as aspirin activity at ambient temperature of 22°C. Endotoxin, through inhibition of breakdown of PGE$_2$ or of another AA metabolite, induces fever and aspirin through inhibition of cyclo-oxygenase-induced hypothermia. We have shown that the effect of endotoxin in rats is probably brought about through its action on the hypothalamus (30), and a similar site of hypothermic effect of aspirin may be proposed as sodium salicylate-induced hypothermia in rats is due to its influence on the thermoregulatory center (22). There is evidence that 300 μg of sodium salicylate microinjected into AH/PO of rats failed to change body temperature (11). However, there is only 27 μg of salicylate per gram of brain tissue after p.o. administration of 120 mg/kg (8).

Why is aspirin significantly less effective in a cold environment and why in such an environment does endotoxin lose its ability to produce fever in rats? On the other hand, PGE$_2$ evokes a febrile response in the cold as well as in 22°C environment. Our working hypothesis is that at the ambient temperature of 10°C, the continuous generation of PGE_2 in the rat hypothalamus is inhibited. In agreement with our working hypothesis is the finding that body temperature of rats transferred from 22°C environment to a cold room (10°C) fell significantly (by 0.40°C, $N = 12$, $p < 0.05$). Obviously, further studies are needed on causal relationships between the ability of endotoxin to produce fever and its interaction with PG system in the hypothalamus. Of special interest are the questions whether PGE_2 is continuously synthesized in the rat hypothalamus and whether in cold environment this synthesis is inhibited. If our working hypothesis is correct, the rate of PGE_2 synthesis in the rat hypothalamus would be under the control of sensory inputs.

ACKNOWLEDGMENTS

We are grateful to Prof. R. Gryglewski for his help in this study, to Prof. J. Lipton for his help in preparing the manuscript, and to Dr. J. Pike of Upjohn for providing us with samples of prostaglandins. This work was supported by NIH Special Foreign Currency Research Agreement No. 05–083–N.

REFERENCES

1. Audet, A., Nantel, G., and Proulx, P. (1974): Phospolipase A activity in growing *Escherichia coli* cells. *Biochim. Biophys. Acta,* 348:334–343.
2. Aveldano, M. I., and Bazan, N. G. (1975): Rapid production of diacylglycerols enriched in arachidonate and stearate during early brain ischemia. *J. Neurochem.,* 25:919–920.
3. Bito, L. Z. (1975): Are prostaglandins intracellular, transcellular or extracellular autacoids? *Prostaglandins,* 9:851–855.
4. Cenedella, R. J., Galli, C., and Paoletti, R. (1975): Brain free fatty acid levels in rats sacrificed by decapitation versus focused microwave irradiation. *Lipids,* 10:290–293.
5. Clark, W. G., and Cumby, H. R. (1976): Antagonism by antipyretics of the hyperthermic effect of a prostaglandin precursor, sodium arachidonate, in the cat. *J. Physiol. (Lond.),* 257:581–595.
6. Collier, H. O. J. (1971): Prostaglandins and aspirin. *Nature,* 232:17–19.
7. Cranston, W. I., Duff, G. W., Hellon, R. F., Mitchell, D., and Townsend, Y. (1976): Evidence that brain prostaglandin synthesis is not essential in fever. *J. Physiol. (Lond.),* 259:239–249.
8. Davison, C., Guy, J. L., Levitt, M., and Smith, P. K. (1961): The distribution of certain non-narcotic analgetic agents in the cns of several species. *J. Pharmacol. Exp. Ther.,* 134:176–183.
9. Egan, R. W., Paxton, J., and Kuehl, F. A., Jr. (1976): Mechanism for irreversible self-deactivation of prostaglandin synthetase. *J. Biol. Chem.,* 251:7329–7335.
10. Flower, R. J. (1978): Prostaglandins and related compounds. In: *Handbook of Experimental Pharmacology, Vol. 50.1,* edited by J. R. Vane and S. H. Ferreira, pp. 374–424. Springer-Verlag, Berlin.
11. Green, M. D., and Lomax, P. (1973): The effects of sodium salicylate on body temperature in the normothermic rat. *Proc. West. Pharmacol. Soc.,* 16:257–261.
12. Gryglewski, R. J. (1978): Screening and assessment of the potency of anti-inflammatory drugs in vitro. In: *Handbook of Experimental Pharmacology, Vol. 50.2,* edited by J. R. Vane and S. H. Ferreira, pp. 3–43. Springer-Verlag, Berlin.
13. Hawkins, M., and Lipton, J. M. (1977): Analogs of endoperoxide precursors of prostaglandins: Failure to affect body temperature when injected into primary and secondary central temperature controls. *Prostaglandins,* 13:209–218.
14. Kröner, E. E., and Peskar, B. A. (1976): On the metabolism of prostaglandins by rat brain homogenate. *Experientia,* 32:1114–1115.

15. Kuehl, F. A., Jr., Humes, J. L., Egan, R. W., Ham, E. A., Beveridge, G. C., and van Arman, C. G. (1977): Role of prostaglandin endoperoxide PGG_2 in inflammatory processes. *Nature,* 265:170–173.

16. Laburn, H., Mitchell, D., and Rosendorff, C. (1977): Effect of prostaglandin antagonism on sodium arachidonate fever in rabbits. *J. Physiol. (Lond.),* 267:559–570.

17. Moncada, S., Gryglewski, R., Bunting, S., and Vane, J. R. (1976): An enzyme isolated from arteries transforms prostaglandin endoperoxides to an unstable substance that inhibits platelet aggregation. *Nature,* 263:663–665.

18. Moncada, S., and Vane, J. R. (1978): Unstable metabolites of arachidonic acid and their role in haemostasis and thrombosis. *Br. Med. Bull.,* 34:129–135.

19. Nakano, J., and Prancan, A. V. (1973): Metabolic degradation of prostaglandin E_1 in the lung and kidney of rats in endotoxin shock. *Proc. Soc. Exp. Biol. Med.,* 144:506–508.

20. Philipp-Dormston, W. K., and Siegert, R. (1974): Prostaglandins of the E and F series in rabbit cerebrospinal fluid during fever induced by Newcastle disease virus, *E. coli*-endotoxin, or endogenous pyrogen. *Med. Microbiol. Immunol.,* 159:279–284.

21. Pittman, Q. J., Veale, W. L., and Cooper, K. E. (1976): Observations on the effect of salicylate in fever and the regulation of body temperature against cold. *Can. J. Physiol. Pharmacol.,* 54:101–106.

22. Polk, D. L., and Lipton, J. M. (1975): Effects of sodium salicylate, aminopyrine and chlorpromazine on behavioral temperature regulation. *Pharmacol. Biochem. Behav.,* 3:167–172.

23. Satinoff, E. (1972): Salicylate action on normal body temperature in rats. *Science,* 176:532–533.

24. Sautebin, L., Spagnuolo, C., Galli, C., and Galli, G. (1978): A mass fragmentographic procedure for the simultaneous determination of HETE and $PGF_{2\alpha}$ in the central nervous system. *Prostaglandins,* 16:985–988.

25. Spławiński, J. A. (1977): Mediation of hyperthermia by prostaglandin E_2: A new hypothesis. *Naunyn Schmiedebergs Arch. Pharmacol.,* 297:S95–S97.

26. Spławiński, J. A., Górka, Z., Zacny, E., and Kałuża, J. (1977): Fever produced in the rat by intracerebral *E. coli* endotoxin. *Pfluegers Arch.,* 368:117–123.

27. Spławiński, J. A., Górka, Z., Zacny, E., and Wojtaszek, B. (1978): Hyperthermic effects of arachidonic acid, prostaglandins E_2 and $F_{2\alpha}$ in rats. *Pfluegers Arch.,* 374:15–21.

28. Spławiński, J. A., Nies, A. S., Sweetman, B., and Oates, J. A. (1973): The effects of arachidonic acid, prostaglandin E_2 and prostaglandin F_2 on the longitudinal stomach strip of the rat. *J. Pharmacol. Exp. Ther.,* 187:501–510.

29. Spławiński, J. A., Reichenberg, K., Vetulani, J., Marchaj, J., and Kałuża, J. (1974): Hyperthermic effect of intraventricular injections of arachidonic acid and prostaglandin E_2 in the rat. *Pol. J. Pharmacol. Pharm.,* 26:101–107.

30. Spławiński, J. A., Wojtaszek, B., and Święs, J. (1979): Endotoxin fever in rats: Is it triggered by a decrease in breakdown of prostaglandin E_2? *Neuropharmacology,* 18:111–115.

31. Spławiński, J. A., Zacny, E., and Górka, Z. (1977): Fever in rats after intravenous *E. coli* endotoxin administration. *Pfluegers Arch.,* 368:125–128.

32. Tse, and Coceani, F. (1979): Does 15-hydroxy prostaglandin dehydrogenase contribute to prostaglandin inactivation in brain? *Prostaglandins,* 17:71–77.

33. Woelk, H., Goracci, G., Gaiti, A., and Porcellati, G. (1973): Phospholipase A_1 and A_2 activities of neuronal and glial cells of the rabbit brain. *Hoppe Seylers Z. Physiol. Chem.,* 354:729–736.

34. Yau, T. M., and Sun, G. Y. (1974): The metabolism of $(1-^{14}C)$ arachidonic acid in the neutral glycerides and phosphoglycerides of mouse brain. *J. Neurochem.,* 23:99–104.

35. Ziel, R., and Krupp, P. (1976): Influence of endogenous pyrogen on the cerebral prostaglandin-synthetase system. *Experientia,* 32:1451–1453.

Fever, edited by James M. Lipton.
Raven Press, New York © 1980.

Some Tests of the Prostaglandin Hypothesis of Fever

*R. F. Hellon, **W. I. Cranston, **Y. Townsend, *D. Mitchell,
*N. J. Dawson, and **G. W. Duff

*National Institute for Medical Research; and **Department of Medicine, St. Thomas'
Hospital Medical School, London, England

Within the last 9 years, a hypothesis has emerged to explain the central action of endogenous pyrogens and the means by which antipyretic drugs act. The hypothesis has been summarized recently by two of its originators (7). Endogenous pyrogens stimulate the production of arachidonic acid from the phospholipids metabolized through the pathways shown in Fig. 1. Prostaglandin synthetase (cyclo-oxygenase) catalyzes the formation of the endoperoxides PGG_2 and PGH_2. These in turn give rise to prostacyclin (PGI_2), thromboxane A_2, or PGE_2. This last prostaglandin causes a condition similar to a pyrogen fever if it is injected into the cerebral ventricles or directly into the anterior hypothalamus. During a pyrogen fever there is a sharp rise in the concentration of PGE_2 in cerebrospinal fluid. The nonsteroidal antipyretic drugs, such as indomethacin and salicylate, are known to inhibit brain prostaglandin synthetase (1,12). When antipyretic drugs are given to an animal with pyrogen fever, there is a reduction in the CSF concentration of PGE_2 at the same time as the fever is diminished. In essence, this is the prostaglandin hypothesis of fever. But when the hypothesis is subjected to critical testing, its validity becomes doubtful.

If the prostaglandin hypothesis is correct, it should not be possible to give a pyrogen to an animal and cause fever without there being, at the same time, a rise in the amount of PGE in the CSF. We infused endogenous pyrogen continuously into rabbits to produce a steady state submaximal fever (5). There was the predicted rise in the PGE content of CSF collected from the cisterna magna. In similar experiments rabbits were given an additional infusion of sodium salicylate (9 μmole/min after an initial priming dose of 1.5 mmole). As illustrated in Fig. 2, rectal temperature rose with the same latency and rate to a level which was not significantly different from that reached by the rabbits not receiving salicylate. In contrast, the levels of PGE did not increase and were not significantly different from those in the controls. The least inference which can be drawn from these results is that the elevation of prostaglandin levels in cisternal CSF cannot be used as an argument that PGE is an essential mediator of pyrogen fever. By the same token, it can no longer be argued

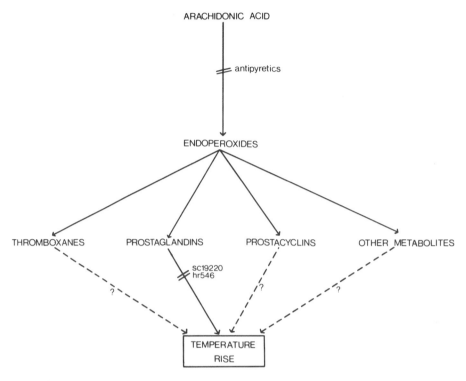

FIG. 1. Metabolic pathways of the degradation products of arachidonic acid.

that the depression of the appearance of PGE in cisternal CSF by antipyretic drugs is evidence that these act by inhibiting prostaglandin synthesis.

More compelling evidence against the PG hypothesis has come from experiments in which prostaglandin antagonists were used (4). Two antagonists, SC 19220 and HR 546, were first shown to be effective in blocking the temperature rise in rabbits to PGE_2 injected into the cerebral ventricles (Fig. 3A). When similar temperature rises were caused by the intraventricular injection of endogenous pyrogen, the antagonists were without effect (Fig. 3B). Clearly, in these experiments the central prostaglandin receptors had been effectively blocked and yet the pyrogen fever was unaffected. The brain prostaglandin which is synthesized in pyrogen fever does not appear to be an essential factor in the genesis of the fever.

The possibility that fever might depend on metabolites of arachidonic acid other than PGE is raised by the work of Laburn et al. (10). They found that arachidonic acid, the precursor of prostaglandin (see Fig. 1), produced a hyperthermia which was not changed by the presence of the two prostaglandin antagonists SC 19220 and HR 546. The other possible pyrogenic metabolites would be the thromboxanes, endoperoxides, or prostacyclin. These metabolites are

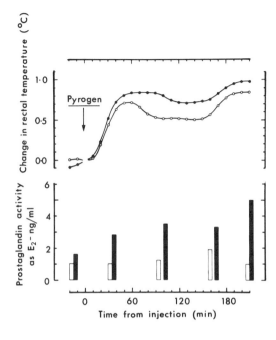

FIG. 2. Changes in rectal temperature and PGE concentration in CSF in two groups of rabbits. One group (*closed symbols*, N = 8) received a bolus and then continuous infusion of endogenous pyrogen. The other group (*open symbols*, N = 8) received in addition a bolus and continuous infusion of sodium salicylate starting 60 min before time 0. (Adapted from Cranston et al., ref. 5.)

unstable in tissue, having half-lives of, at most, only a few minutes. Attempts to use stable analogs of the metabolites to produce a fever-like condition have given equivocal results (6). There is additional evidence which does not support the role of prostaglandin synthesis in pyrogen fever. If developing rats are fed a diet free of essential fatty acids, the mature animals are markedly deficient in prostaglandin precursors. Nevertheless, the deficient rats show the same fever-like response as normals when injected with activated yeast (8).

If fever does not depend on the production of metabolites of arachidonic acid, then the idea that antipyretic drugs act by inhibiting the enzyme prostaglandin synthetase cannot be correct. The antipyretic drugs could act in quite different systems as has been shown recently in the case of indomethacin. This drug is known to inhibit protein kinase at a concentration of only one-hundredth of that needed to inhibit prostaglandin synthetase (9).

There has been a separate approach to the question of the mediators of fever, and this concerns the process of protein synthesis. It has been known for some time that the fever in conditions such as Hodgkin's disease can be reduced by giving the patient a protein synthesis inhibitor, cycloheximide (13). The explanation offered was that cycloheximide was inhibiting the synthesis of endogenous pyrogen by the leukocytes and the cells of the reticuloendothelial system. This explanation was shown to be invalid by Siegert et al. (11). When three different exogenous pyrogens were used to produce fever in rabbits, cycloheximide was effective in preventing those fevers. Endogenous pyrogen fever was also blocked. The implication of these results is that cycloheximide was acting not on the

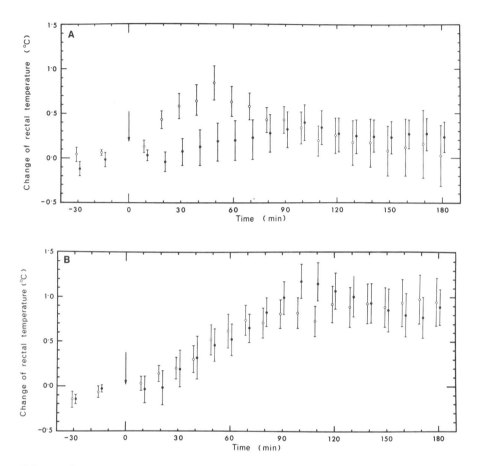

FIG. 3. **A:** Changes in rectal temperature for two groups of rabbits given intraventricular injections of 2.5 nmole PGE₂ (*open circles, N = 9*) or PGE₂ plus SC 19220 (*solid circles, N = 10*) at the *arrow*. **B:** Similar experiments with endogenous pyrogen (*open circles, N = 6*) or endogenous pyrogen plus SC 19220 (*solid circles, N = 6*). (From Cranston et al., ref. 4, with permission.)

production of endogenous pyrogen, but by interfering with the action of endogenous pyrogen on its target tissue, the anterior hypothalamus. If this is the case, and if arachidonic acid metabolites are not essential mediators of fever, it should be possible to block a fever caused by endogenous pyrogen but not a fever due to arachidonic acid.

We (2) gave groups of rabbits equipotent intraventricular injections of 245 nmole arachidonic acid or endogenous pyrogen. When these two treatments were preceded by intravenous cycloheximide (14 to 18 µmole/kg) given 100 min earlier, the fever following endogenous pyrogen was significantly attenuated (Fig. 4). In contrast, the hyperthermic effect of arachidonic acid was unaffected by pretreatment with cycloheximide. Since it is known that cycloheximide does

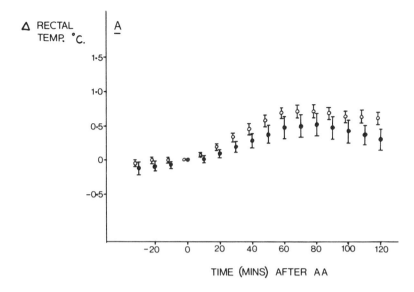

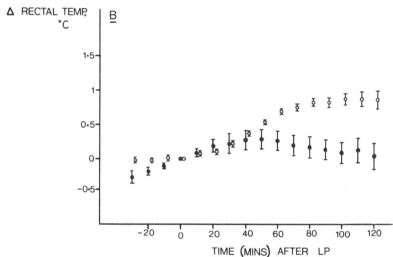

FIG. 4. A: Changes in rectal temperature for two groups of rabbits given an intraventricular injection of 245 nmole arachidonic acid (*open circles*, N = 9) or arachidonic acid preceded by intravenous cycloheximide given 100 min before time 0 (*solid circles*, N = 9). B: Similar experiments using endogenous pyrogen alone (*open circles*, N = 9) or endogenous pyrogen preceded by cycloheximide (*solid circles*, N = 9).

not prevent the production of PGE in pyrogen fever (11), these results suggested that it was unlikely that any metabolite of arachidonic acid was responsible for the production of fever. Subsequently we have found that cycloheximide in the same dose can block the hyperthermic action of PGE₂. This made it difficult to interpret the apparent lack of inhibition of the hyperthermic effect of arachidonic acid by cycloheximide; for this reason, these experiments have been repeated. The latest evidence suggests that cycloheximide may indeed attenuate the temperature rise caused by arachidonic acid. If this is the case, the possibility exists that an arachidonic acid metabolite may be a mediator of pyrogen-induced fever, although it is unlikely that PGE_2 is the essential agent, for the reasons mentioned above.

Cycloheximide does not affect central thermoregulatory mechanisms, because the central temperature responses to intravenous infusion of cold Hartmann's solution (3) are unaffected by its administration.

The mechanism whereby cycloheximide decreases temperature responses to endogenous pyrogen and arachidonic acid is not known. We have recently found that cycloheximide given in this way inhibits the uptake of radioactive leucine into hypothalamic protein; whether this is the mechanism responsible for its antipyretic action or whether it has some entirely different pharmacological action remains to be established.

The evidence reviewed in this chapter shows that although PGE is undoubtedly synthesized by brain tissue during fever, it does not appear to be essential for the febrile process. The new evidence suggests that endogenous pyrogen may act through some process involving protein synthesis.

REFERENCES

1. Collier, H. O. J. (1971): Prostaglandins and aspirin. *Nature,* 232:17–19.
2. Cranston, W. I., Dawson, N. J., Hellon, R. F., and Townsend, Y. (1978): Contrasting actions of cycloheximide on fever caused by arachidonic acid and by pyrogen. *J. Physiol.,* 285:35P.
3. Cranston, W. I., Duff, G. W., Hellon, R. F., and Mitchell, D. (1976): Thermoregulation in rabbits during fever. *J. Physiol.,* 257:767–777.
4. Cranston, W. I., Duff, G. W., Hellon, R. F., Mitchell, D., and Townsend, Y. (1976): Evidence that brain prostaglandin synthesis is not essential in fever. *J. Physiol.,* 259:239–249.
5. Cranston, W. I., Hellon, R. F., and Mitchell, D. (1975): A dissociation between fever and prostaglandin concentration in cerebrospinal fluid. *J. Physiol.,* 253:583–592.
6. Cremades-Campos, A., and Milton, A. S. (1978): The effect on deep body temperature of the intraventricular injections of two prostaglandin endoperoxide analogues. *J. Physiol.,* 282:38P.
7. Feldberg, W., and Milton, A. S. (1978): Prostaglandins and body temperature. In: *Handbook of Experimental Pharmacology, Vol. 50.1,* edited by G. V. R. Born, A. Farah, H. Herken, and A. D. Welch, pp. 617–656. Springer-Verlag, Berlin.
8. Frens, J., van Miert, A. S. J. P. A. M., and van Duin, C. Th.M. (1978): Prostaglandins are not essential in experimental fever of rats. *Br. J. Pharmacol.,* 64:439P.
9. Kantor, H. S., and Hampton, M. (1978): Indomethacin in submicromolar concentrations inhibits cyclic AMP-dependent protein kinase. *Nature,* 276:841–842.
10. Laburn, H., Mitchell, D., and Rosendorff, C. (1977): Effects of prostaglandin antagonism on sodium arachidonate fever in rabbits. *J. Physiol.,* 267:559–570.
11. Siegert, R., Philipp-Dormston, W. K., Radsak, K., and Menzel, H. (1976): Mechanism of fever induction in rabbits. *Infect. Immun.,* 14:1130–1137.
12. Vane, J. R. (1971): Inhibition of prostaglandin synthesis as a mechanism of action for aspirin-like drugs. *Nature [New Biol.],* 231:232–235.
13. Young, C. W., and Dowling, M. D. (1975): Antipyretic effect of cycloheximide, an inhibitor of protein synthesis, in patients with Hodgkin's disease or other malignant neoplasms. *Cancer Res.,* 35:1218–1224.

Fever, edited by James M. Lipton.
Raven Press, New York © 1980.

Studies of Fever Associated with Cerebral Trauma and Intracranial Hemorrhage in Experimental Animals

Thomas A. Rudy

School of Pharmacy, University of Wisconsin, Madison, Wisconsin 53706

As discussed elsewhere in this volume, it is thought that the vast majority of fevers are caused by an action of a blood-borne endogenous pyrogen on certain neural systems within the rostral hypothalamus. There is excellent, but not unequivocal, evidence that prostaglandins released by endogenous pyrogen are the ultimate mediators of this action. Regardless of whether the effect of the pyrogen on the hypothalamus is direct or mediated through prostaglandins, the functional consequence is that the thermoregulatory "set-point" is elevated so that body temperature is regulated at a higher than normal level. Antipyretics, probably by inhibiting prostaglandin biosynthesis, antagonize the effect of endogenous pyrogen, permitting body temperature to again be regulated at the normal level.

Some "fevers," however, are atypical in that they are mediated by mechanisms not involving blood-borne endogenous pyrogen. Examples are heatstroke, malignant hyperpyrexia, and the hyperthermia associated with thyrotoxicosis. "Fevers" of this sort are additionally atypical in that they do not respond to antipyretics and because, in contrast to the situation during ordinary fever, the elevated core temperature is not defended. As these unregulated hyperthermias possess none of the characteristics of ordinary, pyrogen-mediated fevers, it would seem inappropriate to employ the term "fever" in describing them.

The primary subject of this chapter is yet another kind of hyperpyrexic condition—that which appears in association with cerebral trauma or intracranial hemorrhage. As indicated by the extensive clinical literature dealing with this subject (20,21), moderate to severe hyperthermia following cerebral injury and/or intracranial bleeding is not uncommon. Hyperthermia has been observed in association with cerebral trauma or intracranial hemorrhage resulting from penetrating and nonpenetrating cranial injury, various neurosurgical procedures, rapid expansion of intracranial tumors, embolic cerebral infarction, hypertensive intraparenchymal hemorrhage, ruptured intracranial aneurysms, cerebral venous sinus thrombosis, cerebral anoxia, and invasive diseases.

Many of the hyperthermic episodes which arise after cerebral insult are ordinary fevers caused by concomitant intracranial or systemic infection. However, many instances of posttraumatic or posthemorrhagic hyperthermia cannot be accounted for by concomitant sepsis and are therefore believed to be mediated by mechanisms not involving circulating endogenous pyrogen. A survey of the clinical and experimental literature dealing with these so-called neurogenic or central hyperthermias or fevers revealed that they are usually attributed to injury of the thermoregulatory pathways and/or to the pyrogenic effects of blood which has extravasated into the ventricular or subarachnoid cerebrospinal fluid.

DIRECT OR SECONDARY INJURY TO THE THERMOREGULATORY PATHWAYS

Physical damage to the central neural pathways which subserve thermoregulation is frequently cited as a cause of neurogenic hyperthermia. Injury to the thermoregulatory pathways could arise through acute mechanical disruption caused by a penetrating injury, centrifugal forces, or high-pressure intracranial bleeding, or it could be a secondary consequence of vasospasm, hypoxia, and edema or mechanical displacement by an expanding intracranial hematoma. Damage could also arise through expansion of an intracranial tumor or through invasive disease.

Although hyperthermia has been observed in association with injury to any of several areas of the brain and even with lesions of the upper cervical cord, an unequivocal cause–effect relationship has been established for only one area— the rostral hypothalamic/preoptic region. In several animal species intentional injury of this area produces hyperthermia, and major temperature increases have been observed in man after hypothalamic trauma caused by head injury, neurosurgical procedures, and various disease states (21).

If we accept the contention that injury to the rostral hypothalamus can produce neurogenic hyperthermia, we then encounter the problem of explaining how such an injury results in an elevation of body temperature. Speculations regarding the mechanism of action have, with rare exception, attributed the hyperthermia to a failure or disorganization of thermoregulation characterized by autonomous hyperactivity of the centers controlling heat production and/ or by a crippling of the heat dissipation mechanisms. Obviously, a temperature increase brought about by unbridled thermogenesis in combination with impaired thermolysis would not be regulated and thus would be more akin to malignant hyperpyrexia and the other unregulated hyperthermic conditions than to ordinary fever. Indeed, in several reviews dealing with thermoregulatory disorders, it has been stated or implied that neurogenic hyperthermias are unregulated (9,17,18).

The impairment of heat dissipation mentioned by several authors (2,8,22,24) was apparently thought to be a consequence of the loss or temporary disablement of the centers or pathways responsible for the activation of heat loss mechanisms. The persistent thermogenesis has most frequently been attributed to the release of heat gain centers from a tonic inhibition normally emanating from the injured region or to an ill-defined "irritating" or "inflammatory" effect of the lesion on heat gain pathways situated in the surviving perilesional tissue (2,4,5,8,14, 24,27). A somewhat different view was espoused by Barbour and Wing (7) and by Kornblum (15). They proposed that tissue injury caused fever through the release of chemical "toxins." Barbour and Wing suggested that the neurotoxins consisted of the "decomposition products" of killed cells, and Kornblum spoke of "toxins liberated from sudden and extensive destruction of brain tissue" and of "an alteration in the metabolism of brain cells, giving rise to toxic products." Kornblum believed that all fevers were mediated by "toxins," and therefore that the fever associated with cerebral trauma did not differ in its mechanism from other fevers encountered clinically. Barbour and Wing wrote in 1913, Kornblum in 1925.

We now know, some 50 years later, that injury to brain tissue does alter cellular metabolism, with the result that prostaglandins are rapidly synthesized and released (28,29). Prostaglandins of the E series are highly pyrogenic when introduced directly into the rostral hypothalamic/preoptic region or injected intracerebroventricularly (12). Thus, it seems reasonable to suppose that the hyperthermia associated with hypothalamic trauma might be mediated by prostaglandins released from injured tissue. However, fevers produced by the intracranial injection of prostaglandins, like ordinary fevers, are known to be regulated (13,16,25,26). Therefore, any neurogenic fever mediated by prostaglandins should also be regulated. This, of course, is contrary to the prevailing notions about the functional characteristics of neurogenic hyperthermia.

The idea that prostaglandins may mediate neurogenic hyperthermia is also in conflict with statements that the hyperpyrexias associated with cerebral trauma are resistant to antipyretic therapy (3,18); all antipyretics are prostaglandin synthesis inhibitors and thus should attenuate any fever mediated by prostaglandins. However, it should be pointed out that these claims of resistance to antipyretics appear to be based on clinical impression for, to my knowledge, no study evaluating the effect of antipyretics in neurogenic hyperthermia has been published.

Because the hypothesis that neurogenic hyperthermia associated with hypothalamic trauma might be prostaglandin-mediated seemed reasonable and since the arguments against the idea appeared to be based on speculation and/or anecdotal information, it was thought worthwhile to evaluate the hypothesis under controlled conditions. This required that a reliable and simple method be developed which would produce neurogenic hyperthermias of a relatively uniform magnitude in laboratory animals. In this regard, we found that "old is good," and our present technique is nothing more than a slightly updated version of the classic *Wärmestich* (heat puncture) technique first employed by Aronsohn and Sachs (5) in 1885. In our studies, neurogenic hyperthermia was elicited in unanesthetized rats by lowering a sterile stainless steel stylet through a chronically implanted guide tube situated above the rostral hypothalamic/

preoptic region on one side. Pressing the stylet down to the base of the brain produces instantaneous unilateral destruction of the rostral hypothalamus and the preoptic region. Details of the method have been reported elsewhere (21). At an ambient temperature of 24°C, this procedure evoked, with greater than 90% reliability, an increase in core temperature of about 2°C which began almost immediately after puncture, reached peak amplitude within 1 to 1.5 hr, and lasted for 8 to 16 hr. None of the problems commonly associated with bilateral rostral hypothalamic lesions, such as persistent hyperactivity, pulmonary edema, or a high incidence of rapid deaths, were encountered.

Using this model of neurogenic hyperthermia, we examined the ability of the prostaglandin synthesis inhibitor indomethacin to prevent or reverse the temperature rise. Experiments were carried out using four groups of 12 rats each. One group received no treatment prior to the production of lesions. The second and third groups received, respectively, 5 and 15 mg/kg of indomethacin i.p. 1 hr before lesions were made. The fourth group was pretreated with the vehicle for indomethacin (60% DMSO–40% normal saline). As reported elsewhere (21), the low dose of indomethacin significantly attenuated the hyperthermia and the high dose nearly abolished it. The indomethacin vehicle had no significant effect on fever magnitude. The ability of indomethacin to reverse an established neurogenic hyperthermia was examined in eight rats. An i.p. injection of 10 to 15 mg/kg of indomethacin during the plateau stage of hyperthermia produced prompt defervescence in every animal tested.

These findings are evidence that at least one form of neurogenic hyperthermia—that produced by unilateral rostral hypothalamic trauma—is mediated by prostaglandins released in association with acute tissue injury. Presumably, the released prostaglandins caused hyperthermia by acting on surviving ipsilateral and contralateral rostral hypothalamic/preoptic tissue. The source of the prostaglandins is not known, but we presume it to be the traumatized hypothalamic tissue. Since platelet aggregation is accompanied by the release of prostaglandins (10,23), blood extravasated into the injured region is another possible source. However, we found no obvious correlation between the degree of local hemorrhage and fever magnitude.

To test further the hypothesis that prostaglandins mediate the neurogenic hyperthermia produced by hypothalamic trauma and to examine the validity of the belief that neurogenic hyperthermias are unregulated, we studied the characteristics of the hyperthermia elicited in rats by a unilateral puncture of the rostral hypothalamic/preoptic region. Two general approaches were used. In the first, groups of 5 to 10 rats were lesioned at five different ambient temperatures: 10, 15, 26, 32, and 36°C. The effect of ambient temperature on the size of the fever expressed in two different ways is summarized in Figs. 1 and 2. The rats kept in the hot environment (36°C) were hyperthermic prior to lesioning and experienced only a small additional increase in core temperature after hypothalamic puncture. The rats in the other four groups all experienced large hyperthermias after lesioning. The maximum increase in core temperature and

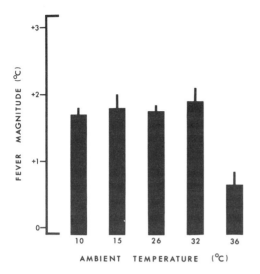

FIG. 1. Effect of ambient temperature on the magnitude of neurogenic hyperthermia. *Ordinate,* maximum increase in colonic temperature occurring within 3 hr after lesioning. *Bars,* mean, and *vertical lines,* SEM, for groups of rats subjected to unilateral hypothalamic puncture at the ambient temperatures shown on the abscissa. Number of animals per group: 5 for 10 and 36°C and 10 for the other ambient temperatures.

the areas under the fever curves did not differ significantly among these four groups. The failure of cold ambient conditions to inhibit the temperature increase and of hot ambient conditions to augment it suggests that the hyperthermia is a regulated one. The diminution in fever magnitude in the rats which were hyperthermic prior to lesioning (the 36°C group) is also consistent with this conclusion.

In the second approach, four rats kept at 26°C were subjected to acute thermal stress during the plateau phase of neurogenic hyperthermia. Body temperature was increased or decreased by means of a water-perfused polyethylene coil implanted in the peritoneal cavity of each rat. In addition to colonic temperature,

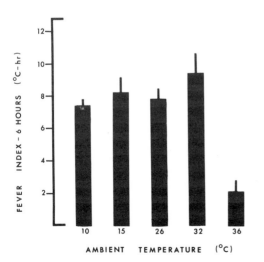

FIG. 2. Effect of ambient temperature on the magnitude of neurogenic hyperthermia. *Ordinate,* area in °C-hr between the colonic temperature curve and the extrapolated baseline temperature for the first 6 hr after unilateral hypothalamic puncture. Other features as in Fig. 1.

thigh muscle electromyographic activity and tail skin temperature were monitored throughout the experimental sessions. The EMG activity served as an
index of shivering thermogenesis. Tail thermal conductivity, an index of thermoregulatory vasomotor tone, was computed from the tail skin, core, and ambient temperature data.

The results for three rats are illustrated in Fig. 3. Note the log scale for
tail thermal conductivity and the fact that this index takes into account the
passive changes in tail skin temperature caused by the experimentally induced
changes in core temperature. The figure shows that (a) the evolution of hyperthermia following hypothalamic puncture was a consequence of a coordinated activation of thermogenic and heat retentive mechanisms; (b) core temperature perturbations introduced during the plateau phase were quickly corrected, with core
temperature returning to the level of hyperthermia existing prior to perturbation;
and (c) the defense against the correction of these perturbations were both
coordinated and active.

Our conclusion, based on both the experiments carried out at various ambient
temperatures and the perturbation studies, is that the neurogenic hyperthermia
produced by unilateral puncture of the rostral hypothalamic/preoptic region
is a well-coordinated, tightly defended temperature change. Neurogenic hyperthermia of this type thus has functional characteristics similar to fevers caused
by prostaglandins, a finding which provides indirect confirmation of our previous
conclusion that the effect is prostaglandin mediated.

In summary, the conclusions that can be drawn from our studies are (a)
that the hyperthermia is mediated by prostaglandins released from the damaged
tissue and/or from blood extravasated into the lesioned region, and (b) that
the elevated core temperature existing during the neurogenic hyperthermia is
a regulated temperature rise functionally equivalent to an elevated set-point.
Thus, at least for neurogenic hyperthermias associated with unilateral injury
in the vicinity of the rostral hypothalamus, it can be said that hypothesized
mechanisms of action based on loss of function, disinhibition, and/or nonspecific
irritation or inflammation are not applicable. It can also be inferred from our
conclusions that the notion that neurogenic hyperthermias are unregulated is
invalid, at least with respect to the type of central fever modeled by our technique.
Furthermore, our results provide no support for claims that neurogenic hyperthermias are resistant to antipyretics. Finally, I would like to point out the
considerable similarity of ordinary fever and neurogenic hyperthermia evoked
by unilateral hypothalamic trauma. Both are probably mediated by prostaglandins, in both the temperature increase is regulated, and both respond to antipyretics. Thus, this type of neurogenic fever differs from ordinary fever only with
respect to its initiation by trauma rather than by circulating endogenous pyrogen.

It must be stressed that the preceding inferences may not be applicable to
neurogenic hyperthermias associated with bilateral rostral hypothalamic damage
or to hyperthermias associated with trauma to other portions of the central
nervous system. It may well be that other "pyrexias of nervous origin" are

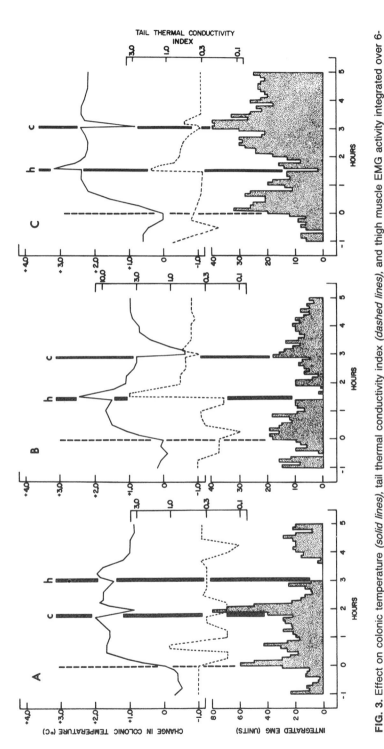

FIG. 3. Effect on colonic temperature *(solid lines)*, tail thermal conductivity index *(dashed lines)*, and thigh muscle EMG activity integrated over 6-min periods *(stippled histograms)* of unilateral puncture of the rostral hypothalamus and of forced deviations in core temperature during the plateau stage of hyperthermia. Panels A, B, and C represent data from individual rats. *Heavy vertical dashed lines* indicate the time of puncture injury. *Solid vertical bars* indicate periods of internal heating (h) and cooling (c). Heating = perfusion of the implanted coil (see text) with 50°C water.

Cooling = perfusion of the coil with 15°C water. Tail thermal conductivity = $\dfrac{T_{tail} - T_{ambient}}{T_{colonic} - T_{tail}} \times 10$. Note that the ordinate for tail thermal conductivity is logarithmic.

mediated by entirely different mechanisms and have different functional characteristics. On the other hand, it should be recognized that the ability to synthesize and release prostaglandins following injury is a characteristic which is not unique to rostral hypothalamic tissue. The unique characteristic of hypothalamic trauma is that the traumatized region which serves as the prostaglandin source is in close proximity to the tissue which mediates the hyperthermic effect of the released prostaglandins. Thus, major tissue injury at sites distant from the hypothalamus could conceivably cause fever by a mechanism analogous to that operative in hypothalamic trauma. All that is required is that the released prostaglandins reach the rostral hypothalamic/preoptic region (by diffusion through tissue or by transport in the cerebrospinal fluid or cerebral circulation) and that the hypothalamofugal pathways necessary for effecting the hyperthermic response be intact.

PYROGENIC EFFECTS OF BLOOD IN THE CEREBROSPINAL FLUID

The second general mechanism thought to be involved in the genesis of some instances of central fever relates to the presence of extravasated blood in the cerebrospinal fluid. Hyperpyrexia has been observed in association with both subarachnoid and intraventricular hemorrhage (20). Instances of posthemorrhagic fever which cannot be accounted for by sepsis or hypothalamic injury have frequently been attributed to an aseptic meningeal irritation produced by the presence of blood within the subarachnoid spaces (20). Blood reaching the subarachnoid spaces does provoke a delayed meningeal inflammatory reaction, and it is certainly possible that phagocytes involved in this response may secrete leukocytic pyrogen and/or prostaglandins which might eventually reach the rostral hypothalamus. Fever associated with subarachnoid bleeding which is not accompanied by major tissue damage or intraventricular hemorrhage is usually of moderate intensity, delayed in onset, and accompanied by nuchal rigidity and other signs of meningeal inflammation (6,11). These characteristics are compatible with a mechanism of fever genesis based on the proinflammatory effects of blood in the subarachnoid space.

Intraventricular hemorrhage, on the other hand, can evoke an intense, fulminating hyperpyrexia which sometimes begins almost immediately after the hemorrhage (20). This suggests that an entirely different mechanism may be responsible for the hyperpyrexia associated with intraventricular bleeding. Intraventricular hemorrhage is a catastropic event which is frequently associated with extensive cerebral injury. Thus large amounts of prostaglandins may be released into the ventricular CSF. Since the prostaglandin-sensitive structures lie just beneath the ependyma of the walls of the ventral portion of the third ventricle, the released prostaglandins would have ready access to a site of action, and intense hyperthermia might result. According to this purely speculative explanation, blood *per se* plays no active role in the genesis of hyperthermia consequent to intraventricular hemorrhage. Rawlins and Cranston (19), however, have postulated an active role for blood in the mediation of the hyperthermia. They suggested that blood contains or releases a pyrogenic substance which diffuses through the ventricular walls to a hypothalamic site of action.

To examine the possibility that some factor contained in or released by blood may contribute to the hyperthermia of intraventricular hemorrhage, we have carried out studies in unanesthetized cats (20). In these experiments, we observed the effect on body temperature of intraventricular injections of 500 µl of fresh autogenous unanticoagulated blood. The blood was drawn from a foreleg or jugular vein using aseptic technique and immediately injected into the dorsal or ventral third ventricle through a chronically implanted guide tube. The guide tube tips were located in the ventricular space, and the blood was injected slowly (over 2 min). The goal was to ensure filling of the ventral third ventricle while simultaneously keeping tissue trauma to an absolute minimum. The cats were killed 4 hr after injection and the brains examined immediately to ascertain the distribution of the injected blood.

In 7 of the 15 cats, the injections were aberrant in that the blood did not reach the ventral third ventricle, but instead entered the lateral dorsal third or fourth ventricles and/or the subarachnoid spaces. This was indeed fortunate, for it allowed us to observe the effect of intraventricular and subarachnoid bleeding in a situation in which the blood did not reach the postulated site of action. None of these cats became febrile within 4 hr. In the remaining cats, the blood had reached the ventral aspect of the third ventricle; the distribution of clotted blood in the other ventricles and in the basilar subarachnoid spaces varied from cat to cat. Seven out of eight of these cats developed a fever within 4 hr. The afebrile cat was found to have a blood clot which was limited to the posterior half of the ventral third ventricle. Examination of a matrix of the blood distributions in the 15 cats revealed that only one distribution locus was consistently correlated with the development of a short-latency fever. This locus was the ventral portion of the third ventricle; in particular, its rostral aspect. In other experiments *(unpublished)* in which the blood was injected into a lateral ventricle, similar results were obtained. If the blood clotted in the lateral ventricle before it could pass through the intraventricular foramen, no fever was seen. In animals which experienced fever, a string of clotted blood could be traced from the lateral ventricle through the foramen and into the front part of the ventral third ventricle.

These findings provide evidence that blood freshly extravasated into the ventricular cerebrospinal fluid can cause a short-latency hyperthermia by a mechanism which does not involve concomitant tissue destruction. Furthermore, they indicate that a rapidly appearing fever is produced only if the blood has access to the rostral portion of the ventral third ventricle within whose walls are situated structures capable of mediating the pyrogenic action of prostaglandins. Even massive quantities of clotted blood in the other ventricles or in the subarachnoid spaces were totally without effect in the short term, and bleeding into these spaces therefore cannot be responsible for a fever which appears soon after an intracranial hemorrhage. However, our investigations did not provide any basis for the notion that intraventricular bleeding causes fulminating hyperpyrexia through a direct action of blood. The blood-induced fevers we observed were relatively small (mean maximum amplitude, 1.4°C) and developed gradually over a period of 3 to 4 hr. Extreme hyperpyrexia associated with intraventricular hemorrhage may be a consequence of the joint pyrexic effects of blood and of direct tissue trauma or of some other factor associated with *in vivo* ventricular bleeding which was not mimicked by our model.

ACKNOWLEDGMENTS

This work was supported by United States Office of Naval Research Contract N00014–75–C–0939.

REFERENCES

1. Ackerman, D., and Rudy, T. A. (1977): The effect of ambient temperature on the hyperthermia evoked by acute mechanical damage to the hypothalamus. *Neurosci. Abstr.,* 3:393.
2. Alpers, B. J. (1936): Hyperthermia due to lesions in the hypothalamus. *Arch. Neurol. Psychiatry,* 35:30–42.
3. Anderson, E., and Haymaker, W. (1962): Disorders of the hypothalamus and pituitary gland. In: *Clinical Neurology, Vol. 3, 2nd Ed.,* edited by A. B. Baker, pp. 1338–1405. Hoeber-Harper, New York.
4. Andersson, B., Gale, C. C., Hokfelt, B., and Larsson, B. (1965): Acute and chronic effects of preoptic lesions. *Acta Physiol. Scand.,* 65:45–60.
5. Aronsohn, E., and Sachs, J. (1885): Die Beziehungen des Gehirns zur Körperwärme und zum Fieber. *Pfluegers Arch.,* 37:232–301.
6. Bannister, R. (1973): *Brain's Clinical Neurology, 4th Ed.,* pp. 227–231. Oxford University Press, London.
7. Barbour, H. G., and Wing, E. S. (1913): The direct application of drugs to the temperature centers. *J. Pharmacol. Exp. Ther.,* 5:105–147.
8. Clark, G., Magoun, H. W., and Ranson, S. W. (1939): Hypothalamic regulation of body temperature. *J. Neurophysiol.,* 2:61–80.
9. Cranston, W. I. (1959): Fever—Pathogenesis and circulatory changes. *Circulation,* 20:1133–1142.
10. Ferreira, S. H., Ubatuba, F. B., and Vance, J. R. (1976): Platelets, acute inflammation and inflammatory mediators. *Agents Actions,* 6:313–319.
11. Gurdjian, E. S., and Thomas, L. M. (1975): Traumatic intracranial hemorrhage. In: *Brock's Injuries of the Brain and Spinal Cord,* edited by E. H. Feiring, pp. 203–282. Springer, New York.
12. Hellon, R. F. (1975): Monoamines, pyrogens and cations: Their actions on central control of body temperature. *Pharmacol. Rev.,* 26:289–321.
13. Hori, T., and Harada, Y. (1974): The effects of ambient and hypothalamic temperatures on the hyperthermic responses to prostaglandins E_1 and E_2. *Pfluegers Arch.,* 350:123–134.
14. Keller, A. D., and McClaskey, E. B. (1964): Localization, by the brain slicing method, of the level or levels of the cephalic brainstem upon which effective heat dissipation is dependent. *Am. J. Phys. Med.,* 43:181–213.
15. Kornblum, K. (1925): A clinical and experimental study of hyperthermia. *Arch. Neurol. Psychiatry,* 13:754–766.
16. Lin, M. T. (1978): Effects of intravenous and intraventricular prostaglandin E_1 on thermoregulatory responses in rabbits. *J. Pharmacol. Exp. Ther.,* 204:39–45.
17. Minard, D., and Copman, L. (1963): Elevation of body temperature in disease. In: *Temperature,*

Its Measurement and Control in Science and Industry, Vol. 3, edited by C. M. Herzfeld, pp. 253–273. Reinhold, New York.

18. Petersdorf, R. G. (1977): Disturbances of heat regulation. In: *Harrison's Principles of Internal Medicine, 8th Ed.,* edited by G. W. Thorn, R. D. Adams, E. Braunwald, K. J. Isselbacker, and R. G. Petersdorf, pp. 53–59. McGraw-Hill, New York.
19. Rawlins, M. D., and Cranston, W. I. (1973): Clinical studies on the pathogenesis of fever. In: *The Pharmacology of Thermoregulation,* edited by E. Schonbaum and P. Lomax, pp. 264–277. S. Karger, Basel.
20. Rudy, T. A., Westergaard, J. L., and Yaksh, T. L. (1978): Hyperthermia produced by simulated intraventricular hemorrhage in the cat. *Exp. Neurol.,* 58:296–310.
21. Rudy, T. A., Williams, J. W., and Yaksh, T. L. (1977): Antagonism by indomethacin of neurogenic hyperthermia produced by unilateral puncture of the anterior hypothalamic/preoptic region. *J. Physiol.,* 272:721–736.
22. Schmeling, W. T., and Hosko, M. J. (1976): Hypothermia induced by Δ^9-tetrahydrocannabinol in rats with electrolytic lesions of preoptic region. *Pharmacol. Biochem. Behav.,* 5:79–83.
23. Smith, J. B., Ingerman, C., Kocsis, J. J., and Silver, M. J. (1973): Formation of prostaglandins during the aggregation of human blood platelets. *J. Clin. Invest.,* 52:965–969.
24. Squires, R. D., and Jacobson, F. H. (1968): Chronic deficits of temperature regulation produced in cats by preoptic lesions. *Am. J. Physiol.,* 214:549–560.
25. Stitt, J. T. (1973): Prostaglandin E_1 fever induced in rabbits. *J. Physiol.,* 232:163–179.
26. Veale, W. L., and Whishaw, I. Q. (1976): Body temperature responses at different ambient temperatures following injections of prostaglandin E_1 and noradrenaline into the brain. *Pharmacol. Biochem. Behav.,* 4:143–150.
27. White, W. H. (1890): The effect upon the bodily temperature of lesions of the corpus striatum and optic thalamus. *J. Physiol.,* 11:1–24.
28. Wolfe, L. S., and Mamer, O. A. (1975): Measurement of prostaglandin $F_{2\alpha}$ levels in human cerebrospinal fluid in normal and pathological conditions. *Prostaglandins,* 9:183–192.
29. Wolfe, L. S., Pappius, H. M., and Marion, J. (1976): The biosynthesis of prostaglandins by brain tissue *in vitro.* In: *Advances in Prostaglandin and Thromboxane Research, Vol. 1,* edited by B. Samuelsson and R. Paoletti, pp. 345–355. Raven Press, New York.

Fever, edited by James M. Lipton.
Raven Press, New York © 1980.

Ontogenetic Development of Fever Mechanisms

Clark M. Blatteis

Department of Physiology and Biophysics, University of Tennessee Center for the Health Sciences, Memphis, Tennessee 38163

It is a common clinical observation that fever, the hallmark of infection in children and adults, is rarely high and often absent in infected neonates (12,14). Although no systematic studies have been conducted to determine why human neonates do not readily develop fever, a number of laboratory animal studies have established that the principal affector [viz., endogenous (leukocytic) pyrogen (LP) production] and effector (viz., autonomic and behavioral thermoregulatory abilities) subsystems needed for fever production are present and functional from birth. By elimination, therefore, a deficiency in the central transduction of the affector component into the appropriate, coordinated thermoeffector response, i.e., fever, is implicated. Blatteis and Smith (6) recently presented evidence that the low reactivity of neonatal guinea pigs to pyrogen may be due to a relative insensitivity of the primary hypothalamic site that is responsive to LP in later life, i.e., from 8 days after birth. The purpose of this chapter is to review the work leading up to this conclusion and to speculate on the mechanism(s) of the pyrogenic insensitivity of this hypothalamic region in neonates.

DEVELOPMENT OF FEBRILE RESPONSIVENESS

The postnatal development of febrile responsiveness has been investigated in detail in lambs (26–29) and guinea pigs (3–6,19,32–37) and less completely in rabbits and kittens (19,31,33,35,37). It was demonstrated that the pyrogenic response to intravenous endotoxin in doses that consistently caused fever in adult animals did not develop in lambs under 4 days (26,27) and in guinea pigs under 8 days of age (3,4), although some degree of pyrogenic reactivity was present from birth in both species. However, the conclusion that the pyrogenic reaction of neonates is reduced is not justified without evidence that the thermoeffector mechanisms that normally underlie it also are unresponsive to the effect of pyrogens. Such evidence was provided by Blatteis (3), who showed that endotoxin did not elicit in newborn guinea pigs the expected heat conservation and heat production responses at both cool (Fig. 1) and neutral temperatures. By contrast, these neonates showed prompt and typical responses to cold, which evokes the same pattern of thermoeffector activity as do pyrogens (3,8). Insufficient thermoeffector capability therefore could not account for the apparently

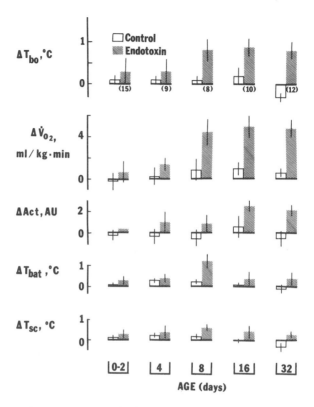

FIG. 1. Thermoregulatory responses of guinea pigs exposed to 23°C ambient temperature at various ages after saline *(open bars)* or endotoxin *(hatched bars)* injections. Values are means (± SE), expressed as the differences between the maximum values obtained following the injection of saline or endotoxin (2.0 μg/kg *Salmonella enteritidis* i.v.) and the mean of consecutive readings made over a 20-min period beginning at 40 min after the onset of treatment. The numbers in parentheses under the hatched bars represent the *N* of each endotoxin-treated group; the *N-s* of the respective saline-treated animals were 17, 10, 8, 11, and 9. T_{bo}, body (colonic) temperature; $\dot{V}_{O_2}$, rate of O_2 consumption; Act, visible shivering activity; T_{bat}, subcutaneous temperature over the interscapular brown fat pad; T_{sc}, subcutaneous temperature over the sacrospinalis muscle. (From Blatteis, ref. 3, with permission.)

deficient pyrogenic sensitivity of neonatal guinea pigs. Hence, the absence of fevers during the first 8 days of life represented a true inability of these animals to respond in the expected thermoregulatory manner to an endotoxic challenge. After 8 days of age, pyrogenic responses were evoked regularly. Endotoxin-induced thermogenesis occurred principally in brown adipose tissue; it gradually shifted from nonshivering to shivering means during the first month of life (Fig. 1), in conformity with well-established observations in newborn guinea pigs exposed to a cool environment (9).

Why, then, is the apparently functional thermoregulatory machinery of the neonate reactive to one, but not another, type of stimulation from birth? Several possibilities might account for this effect.

PRESENSITIZATION TO ENDOTOXIN

Pittman et al. (26,27) have suggested that prior immunological sensitization to endotoxin may be necessary before fever can occur for the first time because 4- and 60-hr-old lambs which received an initial intravenous injection of endotoxin did not develop fever, whereas 60-hr-old animals challenged for the second time did so. Thus, a reduced ability of leukocytes from animals at this age to form LP might be inferred. The injected endotoxin might be cleared disproportionately rapidly, thereby exposing the leukocytes too briefly to too little endotoxin, or the leukocytes might themselves be unable to recognize the endotoxin or to synthesize LP even though stimulated. However, fetal lambs given endotoxin *in utero* also did not consistently develop fever 60-hr postnatally (12), whereas guinea pigs (Fig. 1) responded with fever to the first challenge of a standard dose of endotoxin, provided they were older than 8 days (3) (although the possibility could not be excluded in the latter animals that they had become sensitized through inhaled or ingested endotoxin contaminants in the days before the tests). On the other hand, the number of animals reactive to endotoxin could be increased from birth by increasing the dose of pyrogen injected. Febrile rises in response to high doses of endotoxin similarly were demonstrated in new born guinea pigs, rabbits, and kittens by Székely (33,35) and Székely and Szelényi (37). Furthermore, an increasing number of animals became responsive to endotoxin as they aged and matured (5,23,27). Sensitization to endotoxin, therefore, probably is not a prerequisite for fever production in all species.

ONTOGENY OF ENDOGENOUS PYROGEN PRODUCTION

If the ability of leukocytes to form LP after endotoxin challenge were reduced in neonates as compared with adults, the hypothalamic "set-point" either would not be displaced or would be displaced little by the action of the injected pyrogen; therefore, little or no fever would be evoked. This could account for the low febrile responsiveness of neonates. This possibility, however, was refuted by the following results (5). Leukocytes from neonates incubated with a standard amount of endotoxin (25×10^6 WBC/8 μg of *Salmonella enteritidis* endotoxin) yielded sufficient LP to produce fever in guinea pigs provided that they were older than 8 days and that the LP was administered in doses commensurate with their body weight (adults, Fig. 2; neonates, Fig. 3, *top*). There was no evidence that more endotoxin was required during the early postnatal period to generate LP. However, when LP was injected at 10 times the dose that would be expected to be effective based on body weight, febrile responses could be evoked in guinea pigs younger than 8 days (Fig. 3, *bottom*). Similarly, LP

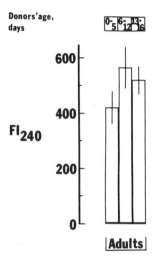

FIG. 2. Mean (± SE) fever indices (°C·min) of adult guinea pigs that received 1.0 ml LP i.v. produced by incubating 8 μg of *Salmonella enteritidis* endotoxin per 25 × 10⁶ leukocytes from 0- to 5-, 6- to 12-, and 13- to 16-day-old guinea pigs. (From Blatteis, ref. 5, with permission.) sion.)

derived from adult donors produced fever in newborn recipients when administered in large, but not in small, doses. Thus the reduced pyrogenic reactivity of neonatal guinea pigs could not be ascribed to an incapacity of their leukocytes to produce sufficient LP. To the contrary, this substance clearly was generated in adequate febrigenic quantities from birth. Indeed, it may even be formed

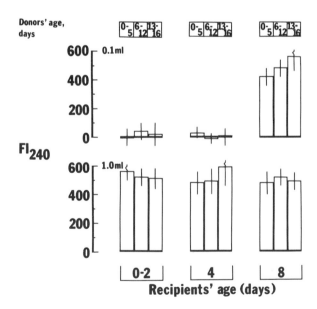

FIG. 3. Mean (± SE) fever indices (°C·min) of 0- to 2-, 4-, and 8-day-old guinea pigs that received 0.1 *(upper bars)* and 1.0 ml *(lower bars)* LP i.v. produced by incubating 8 μg of *Salmonella enteritidis* endotoxin per 25 × 10⁶ leukocytes from 0- to 5-, 6- to 12-, and 13- to 16-day-old guinea pigs. (From Blatteis, ref. 5, with permission.)

prenatally since leukocytes from the cord blood of infants born after 33 to 36 weeks of gestation released LP when stimulated by phagocytosis (16). Hence it is apparent that, although the potential for pyrogenesis was present from birth, more of the pyrogenic endogenous mediator was required early in life than after a few days in order to activate fever production.

HYPOTHALAMIC INSENSITIVITY TO LP

Blatteis (5) concluded that an insensitivity of hypothalamic fever-producing mechanisms to low levels of LP might account for the pyrogenic refractoriness of neonates. This possibility was investigated by comparing the pyrogenic responsiveness of adult and newborn guinea pigs to localized hypothalamic microinjections of LP (6). The primary site of LP sensitivity in guinea pigs was found to be the preoptic region (PO). Injections of LP into this locus produced rapidly developing, brief, monophasic fevers, whereas injections into circumjacent sites evoked smaller fevers with longer latencies. Interestingly, equal volumes (1.0 μl bilaterally) of various dilutions of stock LP (e.g., 1:2, 1:4) injected into the PO of adult guinea pigs induced fevers as rapidly, high, and protracted as did the undiluted stock; sterile saline had no effect. However, appropriate dose-response relations were obtained when different volumes of stock LP (e.g., 0.25, 0.50, and 1.00 μl) were microinjected into the PO region; again, equal volumes of apyrogenic saline were without effect. These findings suggested that the minimal dose of LP capable of triggering a febrile response in guinea pigs could be rather small. By inference, therefore, the occurrence of fever appeared to depend not so much on whether a sufficient dose of LP was administered as on whether an adequate (threshold?) population of LP-sensitive cells was stimulated. Thus the intensity of a febrile response may be related to the size of the drop of LP injected, its diffusion rate, and the brain area that it suffused, i.e., to the number of sensitive cells that it activated simultaneously.

Although febrile responses to 0.25 μl injections of LP could be evoked, it should be noted that the 0- to 5-day-old guinea pigs which developed fever after this dose were few in number (Fig. 4, *top left*) and larger in weight (Table 1) than the average (95 ± 3 g); "small-for-age" neonates became hypothermic. However, the number of reactive animals could be increased by doubling the dose of LP at any age (Fig. 4, *bottom*). Also, with age, an increasing number of guinea pigs became capable of developing fever after both doses (Fig. 4), analogously to the results obtained when endotoxin or LP was injected intravenously in lambs (27) or in guinea pigs (5). Clearly, individual animals grew and matured at different rates. Indeed, as noted above, those guinea pigs which were, at birth, already sensitive to the lower volume of LP were large for their age. On the presumption that they were more mature than their smaller counterparts, the occurrence of fever in the former may reflect their greater development. Thus, if the number of LP-sensitive cells stimulated simultaneously were a critical factor in fever production, it may be that the lack of febrile responsiveness in

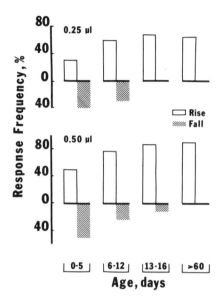

FIG. 4. Percent frequency distribution of guinea pigs 0–5, 6–12, 13–16, and > 60 days of age that reacted with either a rise *(open bars)* or a fall *(hatched bars)* to 0.25 *(upper bars)* and 0.50 *(lower bars)* μl of intrapreoptic LP produced by incubating 8 μg of *Salmonella enteritidis* endotoxin per 25 × 10⁶ leukocytes from adult guinea pigs. (From Blatteis and Smith, ref. 6, with permission.)

the smaller guinea pigs was due to an insufficient number of such receptive cells or to a low sensitivity of these cells to the action of LP. The density of functional cells per unit volume of PO tissue might be expected to be greater in a mature than in a maturing animal (1); consequently, in the latter, it might be necessary to perfuse a larger volume of tissue in order to stimulate an equivalent number of functional units. This interpretation would explain why the large-for-age neonates (at birth) were able to develop a fever in response to the smaller volume of LP. It also would explain why the instances of fever could be increased by increasing the volume of LP injected.

These results suggested, therefore, that the postnatal emergence of febrile responsiveness may depend on the development of the central LP-receptive mechanism. This maturational process would seem to be complete in lambs within 10 days (23), in guinea pigs within 13 to 16 days (3,6), and in rabbits within

TABLE 1. *Body weight and ages of guinea pigs that reacted with either a rise (Pos) or a fall (Neg) in body temperature ($\Delta T_{re} > 0.5°C$) to two doses of leukocytic pyrogen (LP) injected into the PO region*

	Age (days)					
	0–5		6–12		13–16	
LP doses (μl)	Pos	Neg	Pos	Neg	Pos	Neg
0.25	107 ± 3[a]	84 ± 3	114 ± 24	119 ± 11	161 ± 7	—
0.50	78 ± 7	95 ± 8	97 ± 3	105 ± 2	156 ± 16	144 ± 24

[a] g, mean ± SE.

14 days (31) after birth. In summary, the reduced febrile responsiveness of neonates may be due to insufficient development of the intrapreoptic fever-activating mechanism, resulting in the impediment of the central transduction of the affector component (LP) into the expected thermoeffector response (fever).

POSSIBLE CAUSES OF THE APPARENT HYPOTHALAMIC INSENSITIVITY OF NEONATES TO LP

The immaturity of the hypothalamic febrigenic system could be biochemical and/or morphological in nature. Thus, (a) owing to neuronal or chemical immaturity of the relevant cells in the PO, the excitation caused by LP might be inadequate to produce fever; or alternatively, (b) LP might adequately sensitize hypothalamic neurons, but again, owing to neuronal or chemical immaturity, the generated signals might not be processed or might be processed incompletely for transmission to the thermoregulatory effectors.

NEUROCHEMICAL IMMATURITY

Despite the development of a number of neurophysiological models, the precise neuronal pathways by which LP-induced activity in the PO influences the effector system remain obscure. Various putative neurotransmitter substances have been implicated as mediators in the febrile response, e.g., prostaglandins of the E series, biogenic amines (norepinephrine, serotonin), acetylcholine, cyclic AMP, and brain peptide(s). Several of these putative intermediates are at immature levels during the first days of postnatal life in most species. Nevertheless, newborn animals respond to their central application in the appropriate thermoregulatory manner (29,33,39,40). Although their function in fever production is equivocal, their deficiency conceivably could result in noncompletion or reduction of the expected febrile response.

Pittman et al. (28,29) investigated this possibility by microinjecting PGE_1 into the lateral ventricles (i.c.v.) of lambs 4 to 16 hr old and both PGE_1 and PGE_2 into 44 sites within the hypothalamus of lambs 50 to 70 hr old. In both tests, the animals failed to develop fevers consistently, although they responded in the expected manner to intrapreoptic injections of norepinephrine and serotonin. Intrapreoptic PGE_2 also had no consistent effect on the temperatures of 0- to 5-day-old guinea pigs (C. M. Blatteis, *unpublished observations*). On the other hand, Székely and Komáromi (36) found that i.c.v. PGE_1 caused fever in 0- to 3-day-old guinea pigs, and concluded that this compound contributed to the febrile response to endotoxin. Székely (34,35) also postulated a role for serotonin in fever because pretreatment with p-chlorophenylalanine (PCPA) moderated a fall between two rising phases after i.c.v. *Eschericia coli* endotoxin in newborn guinea pigs; indomethacin prevented the first rise and the otherwise consequent fall, but not the second rise. Serotonin i.c.v. produced an initial temperature rise in neonatal kittens, but a fall in newborn guinea pigs. In both species, a temperature rise which could be prevented by indomethacin pretreatment followed these initial effects (33). In kittens, the single febrile rise after i.c.v. endotoxin was attenuated by PCPA (35). On the other hand, the hypothalamic levels of both norepinephrine and serotonin were not changed after i.c.v. endotoxin alone in newborn guinea pigs and kittens (19). Thus, although it is possible that before complete maturation of its neurochemical systems an organism might go through a period during which certain functions that depend on neurochemical maturity would appear inoperative, it cannot be assumed from the results available that low levels of these substances at birth account for the low pyrogenic sensitivity of neonates. Indeed, evidence has been adduced that fever can occur without the central involvement of any of these compounds (21).

MORPHOLOGICAL IMMATURITY

Cell development continues for some time after birth in the brains of most species (1). Although specific data on the PO are lacking, it has been demonstrated for other phylogenetically old brain areas that long-axoned cells are mature at birth, whereas the dendrites of many short-axoned interneurons and of neuroglia cells (which may exert a modulatory influence on neurons) develop and make synaptic contact with the long-axoned cells postnatally (1). If these dendrites were essential to LP sensitivity and if they were formed late in the PO, their delayed appearance might account for the deficient pyrogenic responsiveness of neonates. In this context, DNA (17), several enzymes (18), and amino acids (15) do not attain adult levels in the hypothalami of animals until several days after birth. Since most of these components are necessary for the functional integrity of that area, it may be that their relative deficiency at birth also accounts for the reduction or the absence of the expected febrile response.

ENDOGENOUS ANTIPYRESIS

Kasting et al. (22) found that fever caused by endotoxin or LP was suppressed in pregnant ewes from 2 to 4 days prepartum until several hours postpartum. The febrile rises induced by endotoxin in term rabbits also were reduced (24). An endogenous antipyretic elaborated by either the pregnant female or its fetus and probably acting after LP has been formed could therefore also account for the lack of febrile responsiveness of certain neonates. This possibility is discussed in greater detail elsewhere in this volume.

NEUROPHYSIOLOGICAL MODELS OF FEVER PRODUCTION

The results described in the preceding paragraphs lend themselves to several interpretations. Three of these interpretations based on the neuronal model of the central integrative parts of the temperature control system of guinea pigs developed by Brück (7) are summarized in Fig. 5. It should be remembered that, in contrast to the unresponsiveness of most neonates to pyrogens, thermoregulatory ability is fully functional from birth in most animals (8). This difference implies that those neurons which relay afferent temperature signals to thermoeffectors may be spatially and functionally distinct from those which are sensitive to LP. This view conflicts with the prevalent concept, based on electrophysiological evidence, of an action of LP on the thermal sensitivity of neurons within the preoptic/anterior hypothalamus (PO/AH) (Fig. 5A) (20). However, since both thermosensory and thermointegrative functions within the PO/AH are developed at birth, it seems improbable that they would be reactive to temperature and to neurotransmitters but not to endogenous pyrogen. Hence the upward shift of the thermoregulatory "set-point" conceivably may be due to an action of LP on other neurons which are specific LP-receptive units (Fig. 5B and C). At birth, the majority of these may be chemically immature or not yet connected synaptically to the integrative structures, as suggested above.

In apparent conflict with this notion, however, is the report by Satinoff et

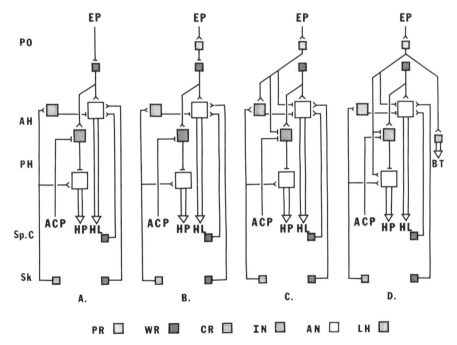

FIG. 5. Four models of neuronal pathways by which EP-induced activity in the PO may influence thermoeffector systems. The possible effects of EP are superimposed on the model of thermoregulation in guinea pigs proposed by Brück (7). For explanation, see text. PO, preoptic area; AH, anterior hypothalamus; PH, posterior hypothalamus; Sp.C, spinal cord; Sk, skin; EP, endogenous (leukocytic) pyrogen; ACP, ascending catecholaminergic pathways; HP, heat production effectors; HL, heat loss effectors; BT, behavioral thermoregulatory effectors; PR, pyrogen receptors; WR, warm receptors; CR, cold receptors; IN, inhibitory (inter)neurons; AN, activating neurons; LH, lateral hypothalamus. (Modified from ref. 7, with permission.)

al. (31) and Kleitman and Satinoff *(this volume)* that neonatal rabbits, although unable to develop a fever autonomically in response to an intraperitoneal injection of exogenous pyrogen, nevertheless did so behaviorally by selecting a higher ambient temperature in a thermal gradient chamber. These workers suggested that the efferent networks subserving behavioral thermoeffectors are functional from birth, whereas those controlling autonomic responses mature somewhat later. However, the observation in several species that both these thermoeffector modes are present from birth (10) argues against the possibility of a differential maturation rate of these two networks. Alternatively, two separate pathways may project from the proposed LP-sensitive sites (Fig. 5D); one, which may be immature at birth, to autonomic integrators and another, which may be functional at birth, to behavioral integrators. This would imply that these integrative structures may be separate and independent, a concept for which there is increasing support (11,30). From a related point of view, another possibility may be that LP acts at more than one brain site to drive the full complement of fever-producing mechanisms, i.e., sensors which activate behavioral responses may be reactive to LP from birth whereas those which initiate autonomic responses may not be reactive until several days later. Several workers (2,13,25,38) have postulated the existence of subsidiary sites of LP action; these are presumed to become revealed when the primary site is nonfunctional, as may be the case in neonates.

CONCLUSIONS

On the basis of the results reviewed in this chapter, it is suggested that the reduced pyrogenic responsiveness of newborn animals may be due to morphological and/or biochemical immaturity of LP-sensitive neurons within the PO. Since thermoregulatory capability is present from birth in these animals, the site within the PO where LP acts may not be the same as those where local hypothalamic temperature is sensed or where the signals from these sensors are integrated.

ACKNOWLEDGMENTS

The research reported herein was supported by Public Health Service Grants AI-09957 and AI-13244.

REFERENCES

1. Altman, J. (1970): Postnatal neurogenesis and the problem of neural plasticity. In: *Developmental Neurobiology,* edited by W. A. Himwich, pp. 197–237. Charles C Thomas, Springfield, Ill.
2. Andersson, B., Gale, C. C., Hökfelt, B., and Larsson, B. (1965): Acute and chronic effects of preoptic lesions. *Acta Physiol. Scand.,* 65:45–60.
3. Blatteis, C. M. (1975): Postnatal development of pyrogenic sensitivity in guinea pigs. *J. Appl. Physiol.,* 39:251–257.
4. Blatteis, C. M. (1976): Effect of propranolol on endotoxin-induced pyrogenesis in newborn and adult guinea pigs. *J. Appl. Physiol.,* 40:35–39.

5. Blatteis, C. M. (1977): Comparison of endotoxin and leukocytic pyrogen pyrogenicity in newborn guinea pigs. *J. Appl. Physiol.*, 42:355–361.
6. Blatteis, C. M., and Smith, K. A. (1979): Hypothalamic sensitivity to leukocytic pyrogen of adult and newborn guinea-pigs. *J. Physiol. (Lond.) (in press).*
7. Brück, K. (1976): Cold adaptation in man. In: *Regulation of Depressed Metabolism and Thermogenesis,* edited by L. Janský and X. J. Musacchia, pp. 42–63. Charles C Thomas, Springfield, Ill.
8. Brück, K. (1978): Heat production and temperature regulation. In: *Perinatal Physiology,* edited by U. Stave, pp. 455–498. Plenum Press, New York.
9. Brück, K., and Wünnenberg, B. (1965): Über die Modi der Thermogenese beim neugeborenen Warmblüter. *Pfluegers Arch.,* 282:362–375.
10. Cabanac, M. (1974): Thermoregulatory behavior. In: *Environmental Physiology, Vol. 1,* edited by D. Robertshaw, pp. 231–269. Butterworths, London.
11. Cabanac, M. (1975): Temperature regulation. *Annu. Rev. Physiol.,* 37:415–439.
12. Cooper, K. E., Veale, W. L., Kasting, N., and Pittman, Q. J. (1979): Ontogeny of fever. *Fed. Proc.,* 38:35–38.
13. Cooper, K. E., Veale, W. L., and Pittman, Q. J. (1976): The pathogenesis of fever. In: *Brain Dysfunction in Infantile Febrile Convulsions, Vol. 2,* edited by M. A. B. Brazier and F. Coceani, pp. 107–115. Raven Press, New York.
14. Craig, W. S. (1963): The early detection of pyrexia in the newborn. *Arch. Dis. Child.,* 38:29–39.
15. Davis, J. M., Himwich, W. A., and Agrawal, H. C. (1968): Free amino acids of newborn and adult guinea pig brain. *Dev. Psychobiol.,* 1:24–29.
16. Dinarello, I. A., and Wolff, S. M. (1978): Pathogenesis of fever in man. *N. Engl. J. Med.,* 298:607–612.
17. Dobbing, J., and Sands, J. (1970): Growth and development of the brain and spinal cord of the guinea pig. *Brain Res.,* 17:115–123.
18. Flexner, L. B. (1955): Enzymatic and functional patterns of the developing mammalian brain. In: *Biochemistry of the Developing Nervous System,* edited by H. Waelsch, pp. 281–300. Academic Press, New York.
19. Hahn, Z., and Székely, M. (1979): Hypothalamic monoamine contents in endotoxin fever of new-born guinea pigs and kittens. *Neurosci. Lett.,* 11:279–282.
20. Hammel, H. (1965): Neurons and temperature regulation. In: *Physiological Controls and Regulations,* edited by W. S. Yamamoto and J. R. Brobeck, pp. 71–97. W. B. Saunders, Philadelphia.
21. Hellon, R. F. (1975): Monoamines, pyrogens, and cations: Their action in central control of body temperature. *Pharmacol. Rev.,* 26:289–321.
22. Kasting, N. W., Veale, W. L., and Cooper, K. E. (1978): Suppression of fever at term of pregnancy. *Nature,* 271:245–246.
23. Kasting, N. W., Veale, W. L., and Cooper, K. E. (1979): Development of fever in the newborn lamb. *Am. J. Physiol.,* 236:R184–R187.
24. Kullander, S. (1978): Fever and parturition: An experimental study in rabbits. *Acta Obstet. Gynecol. Scand.,* 66:77–85.
25. Lipton, J. M., and Trzcinka, G. P. (1976): Persistence of febrile responses to pyrogens after POAH lesion in squirrel monkey. *Am. J. Physiol.,* 231:1638–1648.
26. Pittman, Q. J., Cooper, K. E., Veale, W. L., and Van Petten, F. R. (1973): Fever in newborn lambs. *Can. J. Physiol. Pharmacol.,* 51:868–872.
27. Pittman, Q. J., Cooper, K. E., Veale, W. L., and Van Petten, F. R. (1974): Observations on the development of the febrile response to pyrogens in sheep. *Clin. Sci. Mol. Med.,* 46:591–602.
28. Pittman, Q. J., Veale, W. L., and Cooper, K. E. (1975): Temperature responses of lambs after centrally injected prostaglandins and pyrogens. *Am. J. Physiol.,* 228:1034–1038.
29. Pittman, Q. J., Veale, W. L., and Cooper, K. E. (1977): Effect of prostaglandin, pyrogen and noradrenaline, injected into the hypothalamus, on thermoregulation in newborn lambs. *Brain Res.,* 128:473–483.
30. Satinoff, E. (1974): Neural integration of thermoregulatory responses. In: *Limbic and Autonomic Nervous Systems Research,* edited by L. V. DiCara, pp. 41–80. Plenum Press, New York.
31. Satinoff, E., McEwen, G. N., Jr., and Williams, B. A. (1976): Behavioral fever in newborn rabbits. *Science,* 193:1139–1140.

32. Székely, M. (1978): Biphasic endotoxin fever in the newborn rabbit. *Acta Physiol. Acad. Sci. Hung.,* 51:389–392.
33. Székely, M. (1978): 5-Hydroxytryptamine-induced changes in body temperature of newborn kittens and guinea-pigs and the effect of indomethacin thereon. *Experientia,* 34:58–59.
34. Székely, M. (1978): Endotoxin fever in the newborn guinea-pig and the modulating effects of indomethacin and *p*-chlorophenylalanine. *J. Physiol. (Lond.)* 281:467–476.
35. Székely, M. (1978): Endotoxin fever in para-chlorophenylalanine (PCPA) treated newborn guinea pigs and kittens. *Life Sci.,* 22:1585–1588.
36. Székely, M., and Komáromi, I. (1978): Endotoxin and prostaglandin fever of newborn guinea pigs at different ambient temperatures. *Acta Physiol. Acad. Scient. Hung.,* 51:293–298.
37. Székely, M., and Szelényi, Z. (1977): The effect of *E. coli* endotoxin on body temperature in the newborn rabbit, cat, guinea pig and rat. *Acta Physiol. Acad. Sci. Hung.,* 50:293–298.
38. Veale, W. L., and Cooper, K. E. (1975): Comparison of sites of action of prostaglandin E and leukocyte pyrogen in brain. In: *Temperature Regulation and Drug Action,* edited by P. Lomax, E. Schönbaum, and J. Jacob, pp. 218–226. S. Karger, Basel.
39. Zeisberger, E., and Brück, K. (1971): Comparison of the effects of local hypothalamic acetylcholine and RF-heating on non-shivering thermogenesis in the guinea pig. *Int. J. Biometeorol.,* 15:305–308.
40. Zeisberger, E., and Brück, K. (1971): Central effects of noradrenaline on the control of body temperature in the guinea pig. *Pfluegers Arch.,* 322:152–166.

Fever, edited by James M. Lipton.
Raven Press, New York © 1980.

Models of Endogenous Antipyresis

N. W. Kasting, W. L. Veale, and K. E. Cooper

*Division of Medical Physiology, Faculty of Medicine, University of Calgary,
Calgary, Alberta T2N 1N4, Canada*

The experiments which have provided evidence for an endogenous antipyretic within the brain of the sheep originally arose out of inquires into the development of the fever mechanism in the newborn animal. It is well known that the human infant can suffer severe infection without becoming febrile (6,13,15,26,36). One explanation for reduced fever capacity in the newborn concerns a learned immunological process, a function of the immune system occurring shortly after birth (11). Our initial studies were with lambs since the young of this species are born with a mature thermoregulatory system—they vasoconstrict in the cold and vasodilate in the heat; they change respiratory heat loss in relation to environmental temperature and body temperature; and they are able to shiver and maintain stable, normal body temperatures in response to severe cold exposure. Furthermore, the lamb is born with a good insulating coat which becomes effective as soon as it is dry after delivery (2,32).

Initial experiments (32) were performed using lambs 4 hr old that were given i.v. injections of bacterial endotoxin derived from *Salmonella abortus equi.* The dose (0.3 µg) chosen produced a fever of approximately 1°C in adult sheep. All of the lambs that received this initial dose of endotoxin 4 hr after birth remained afebrile. Nor did another group of lambs given the same dose of endotoxin 60 hr after delivery develop fever. A third group of lambs given a dose of endotoxin 4 hr after delivery, and a second dose 60 hr postdelivery became febrile, with the fevers being of similar characteristics to those observed in the adult animal.

These observations suggested that the newborn animal was unable to produce fever and that the process of having a fever in response to i.v. endotoxin represented a priming or triggering of some mechanism by the first exposure to the bacterial products. The fact that the animal, once primed with a small dose of endotoxin, could experience fever at 60 hr suggests that, after the priming dose, the efferent systems mediating fever were mature and one could not explain the nonsensitized animal's failure to respond at 60 hr by a lack of maturity of mechanisms in the central nervous system. The concept that an initial priming of some unknown mechanism is important in the genesis of fever in the newborn receives support from experiments by Podoprigora (33) in which it was demonstrated that newborn germ-free mini-pigs and germ-free mice did not develop fever in response to endotoxin for several weeks after birth. Further studies showed that exposure of the fetus *in utero* to endotoxin did not achieve the priming necessary to enable a second dose of endotoxin given 60 hr after delivery to cause fever unless the initial dose of endotoxin was given to the fetus shortly before delivery (32).

However, at about the same time it was demonstrated that large doses of endotoxin could induce fever before 60 hr of age in the guinea pig (7). There was also evidence that large doses of endotoxin could induce a monophasic fever in the newborn rabbit but that the ability to get a biphasic fever in response to endotoxin occurred later in development in that species (38).

Further experiments on the lamb (23) have demonstrated that 30.0 μg *S. abortus equi* endotoxin administered i.v. does not produce fever 5 hr after delivery, but does produce fever when given 32 to 60 hr after delivery, even if the animal has not been previously primed with endotoxin. At 5 hr after birth there is, if anything, a modest fall in body temperature in response to this large dose of endotoxin, although the animals do not appear to be in "endotoxin shock." Furthermore, the response of lambs to sheep endogenous pyrogen was similar to the response produced by endotoxin, namely, a small fall in temperature when the substance was administered intravenously 5 hr after delivery and a brisk fever when the substance was given for the first time at 32 or 60 hr after delivery. It was tempting to postulate not only that a priming mechanism is necessary for the animal to respond to a small dose of endotoxin after delivery, but also that a large dose of endotoxin drives the heat production and heat conservation mechanisms without initial priming, although the latter effect becomes apparent only between 5 and 32 hr after delivery. The refractoriness of the lamb to endotoxin given 5 hr after delivery, even the large dose, remained a puzzle. One possible explanation was that there could be some substance in the blood or within the CNS which acted as an antipyretic in the newborn lamb. Such a substance might be one of the many hormones whose levels change rapidly at about the time of delivery. If such a substance were present in the newborn lamb, it might also occur in the ewe at around the time of parturition.

Another model of endogenous antipyresis was sought and evidence was obtained that an endogenous substance, produced under abnormal circumstances, suppresses fever in the rabbit. While we were observing febrile responses of near-term rabbits, some animals were observed to develop only small fevers (Fig. 1). These rabbits did not subsequently give birth, and when they were killed and their uteri examined, they were found to be resorbing the fetuses. Several rabbits were subsequently induced to resorb their fetuses artificially by administering diethylstilbestrol s.c. on the 18th day of gestation. These rabbits resorbed their fetuses, but had normal febrile responses. However, when the horns of the uteri of these rabbits were examined, the resorbing fetuses were markedly different in appearance, texture, and color from the naturally resorbing fetuses. This evidence suggests that naturally resorbing fetuses in the rabbit

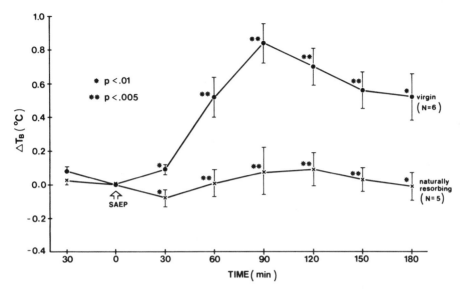

FIG. 1. The change in body temperature in response to 0.1 μg *Salmonella abortus equi* endo-toxin (BP) of virgin rabbits and females resorbing their fetuses.

may lead to the elaboration of a natural antipyretic, which we were unable to reproduce in the artificial resorption model.

The sheep was, therefore, utilized in further studies of this antipyretic phenomenon and, consequently, the ability of the ewe to develop fever close to the expected date of delivery was studied. Several attempts were made to see if previous exposure of the pregnant ewe to bacterial pyrogen could alter the afebrile period in the newborn lamb. It was found that such an exposure of the ewe does not alter the afebrile period of the lamb. A more interesting observation was made, however, namely, that several ewes, especially those near parturition, did not respond to i.v. bacterial pyrogen with fevers of a normal magnitude. In subsequent studies it was found that, beginning about 4 days before term, ewes progressively lost their ability to respond to bacterial pyrogen with fever. This afebrile condition lasted until parturition and for at least 5 hr postpartum. The response of postparturient ewes at 32 hr was normal. In order to determine at which step in the sequence of events leading to fever such an inhibition might occur, endogenous pyrogen (EP) was administered i.v. The EP-induced fevers in near-term ewes were observed to be greatly diminished in comparison to control animals. Because the EP fever was also diminished, it was likely that the inhibition occurred after the synthesis and release of EP and probably, therefore, within the preoptic/anterior hypothalamic region of the brain in which EP is thought to exert its pyrogenic effects. None of the ewes responded to bacterial pyrogen or EP with a fever of normal magnitude during this period

(21,22). Thus at 5 hr after birth neither ewe nor lamb can produce a fever to bacterial pyrogen or EP, whereas this ability returns (or begins) by 32 hr postpartum (Fig. 2). The coincidental occurrence of this afebrile period in ewe and lamb suggested a similar mechanism and the most consistent explanation seemed to be that some agent, common to or shared by both ewe and fetus, increased near term and acted in the central nervous system to prevent a febrile response to pyrogens.

The search for a possible agent with which to attribute this decreased ability to produce fever required that we assume that the plasma levels of this substance parallel the period of time during which fevers were suppressed. The literature was examined for reports of hormonal fluctuations in the sheep near term. The criteria which were selected for this search were that the concentration of the substance in the blood should (a) increase in the blood of both ewe and fetus, (b) increase about 4 days before term and reach the highest levels at term, and (c) return to normal by 32 hr postpartum.

The hormone which best met the criteria before delivery was arginine vasopressin (AVP). Alexander et al. (1) reported that plasma levels of AVP (as measured by bioassay) in both ewe and fetus started to rise about 4 days after delivery. AVP reached higher concentrations in fetal plasma than maternal plasma, but in both animals it appeared to be above that required for maximum antidiuresis. It was also reported that AVP did not cross the placenta; therefore, the increased AVP levels must be due to increased secretion by both maternal and fetal brains. Other hormones, such as steroids with known antipyretic activity, which were

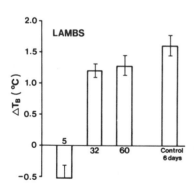

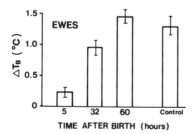

FIG. 2. The change in body temperature in response to 30.0 μg *Salmonella abortus equi* endotoxin (BP) of lambs and ewes at 5, 32, and 60 hr after birth.

initially considered the most likely for such a role, did not fit the criteria as well as AVP.

AVP was considered a putative agent for a role as an endogenous antipyretic in the sheep by virtue of its apparent correlations with the period of decreased ability to produce fevers. There is other evidence that AVP could also be involved in thermoregulation. It was shown that AVP (Pitressin®) caused hypothermia in rats whether administered i.v., i.c., or i.p. (30; *personal observations*). Pigs exposed to high ambient temperatures showed no increases in plasma vasopressin until an ambient temperature of 45°C, at which point the heat load could not be balanced and the body temperatures of the pigs rose. After body temperatures had risen about 1°C, a sudden increase in vasopressin occurred in the plasma and continued until heating was stopped. Vasopressin levels fell before body temperature decreased. The heat-induced increase in vasopressin levels could be abolished by cooling thermodes in the preoptic hypothalamic region of the brain. This evidence suggests that AVP is released when hypothalamic temperatures reach levels not encountered under normal circumstances (16). In another study, in which heating thermodes were implanted in the preoptic hypothalamus and ventrolateral septum of dogs, it was reported that heating these areas increased AVP levels in the blood (37). These reports reached no conclusions about AVP involvement in thermoregulation, nor did they arrive at any definite physiological role for AVP in these circumstances aside from that of a generalized water conservation effect based on antidiuresis.

Since AVP was considered to be the best candidate for an endogenous antipyretic in our experiments, it was decided to determine if AVP perfused in discrete sites of the brain had any effect on febrile responses to i.v. bacterial pyrogen and particularly when the AVP was given into the preoptic/anterior hypothalamic nuclei which have been traditionally recognized as the site of action of pyrogens (5,9,19,34,41).

Guide cannulae were stereotaxically implanted above the hypothalamus and surrounding brain areas in nonpregnant female sheep. This technique allows perfusion of discrete brain tissue sites in conscious unstressed animals (28). The push–pull perfusion technique was utilized to introduce AVP into the brain and to allow collection of perfusates. Iso-osmotic sucrose was chosen as the vehicle for perfusion since, of all vehicles tested, it alone had no effect on body temperature. Perfusions (40 μl/min) began at the same time as i.v. bacterial pyrogen injections, and body temperature was measured using a thermistor placed in the vagina.

Perfusions in the septal area with vehicle and AVP (4.0 μg/ml) resulted in significantly decreased fevers in four sheep, whereas fevers during perfusion with vehicle alone were not significantly different from those of nonoperated controls. Perfusions with vehicle and AVP had no effect on normal body temperature, which indicates that antipyretic activity was not due to a nonspecific hypothermic effect (20).

Push–pull perfusions have an estimated exchange of up to about 10% with tissue extracellular fluid, 90% of the perfusate returning directly into the withdrawal cannula (40). The best estimate of AVP exchanged with the tissue would be a maximum of 6.4 μg over a period of 200 min. On a molar basis, this is considerably less than that required for antipyresis by cortisol or salicylate injected directly into the brain of rabbits (8,14,39).

Perfusions with AVP in the posterior hypothalamus, lateral hypothalamus, fornix, anterior hypothalamus, preoptic hypothalamus, ventral surface of septal area, and rostrum of corpus callosum had no effect on the febrile response.

AVP was infused i.v. to determine if circulating AVP could affect fever responses. Infusions of 0.24, 2.4, or 24 μg of AVP over 200 min were designed to cover the estimated amount of AVP administered during central perfusion experiments (6.4 μg). These infusions were carried out during i.v. bacterial pyrogen fevers, but fevers were unaffected at any dose (10). Several sheep were infused with 150 μg AVP/200 min and achieved plasma levels of 1,000 pg/ml, well in excess of levels seen in physiological states. Fevers in these sheep were similar to fevers in control animals. Experiments designed to alter neurohypophyseal function and release of AVP, such as intracarotid infusion of hypertonic saline, i.v. infusion of ethanol, and mild dehydration, had no significant effects on fevers in sheep. The tentative conclusion was made that if AVP has a physiological antipyretic role in the CNS, it appears to be unrelated to normal neurohypophyseal function, and, in addition, fevers could not be altered by high blood levels of AVP.

The mechanism of action of AVP as an endogenous antipyretic remains obscure. However, it is interesting that antipyretic drugs have antidiuretic actions in the kidney by increasing water resorption in distal tubules (29,35), and PGE, a substance often implicated in the brain mechanism of fever, has been shown to antagonize AVP action in the kidney (3,4,17,18,31).

It is appropriate to ask the purpose of such a period of decreased ability to produce fever. Since fever has been suggested to be beneficial to the host organism (12,24,25), the lack of fever in the near-term sheep would seem paradoxical. Therefore, fever in this circumstance would appear to be more detrimental to the survival of the ewe and/or the lamb than the consequence of infectious processes unmodified by fever. Such a detrimental effect may involve lung surfactant, the secretory mechanism of which matures in the last few days of intrauterine life and which has been demonstrated to exert a significantly more decreased pressure at 41°C than at 37°C (27). Thus fever in the last few days of pregnancy or in the newborn could adversely affect the surfactant function; consequently, respiratory distress might result with greatly reduced chances of survival of the lamb. Another possible survival value may lie in the observation that the lamb must be able to stand and suckle within 1 or 2 hr of birth or the mother will ignore it. Thus the formation of a newborn–maternal bond depends on a lamb and ewe which are mobile and responsive soon after birth. These responses would likely be absent if either the ewe or lamb were affected by the symptoms of infection, especially fever.

ACKNOWLEDGMENTS

This research was supported by the Medical Research Council of Canada. N. W. K. is a predoctoral student of the MRC. Dr. G. Moore kindly supplied the AVP.

REFERENCES

1. Alexander, D. P., Bashore, R. A, Britton, H. G., and Forsling, M. A. (1974): Maternal and fetal arginine vasopressin in the chronically catheterized sheep. *Biol. Neonate,* 25:242–248.
2. Alexander, G. (1975): Body temperature control in mammalian young. *Br. Med. Bull.,* 31:62–68.
3. Anderson, R. J., Berl, T., McDonald, K. M., and Schrier, R. W. (1975): Evidence for an *in vivo* antagonism between vasopressin and prostaglandin in the mammalian kidney. *J. Clin. Invest.,* 56:420–426.
4. Beck, N. P., Kanecko, T., Zor, U., Field, J. B., and Davis, B. B. (1971): Effects of vasopressin and prostaglandin E_1 on the adenyl cyclase–cyclic $3',5'$-adenosine monophosphate system of the renal medulla of the rat. *J. Clin. Invest.,* 50:2461–2465.
5. Bennett, I. L., Jr., Petersdorf, R. G., and Keene, W. R. (1975): Pathogenesis of fever: Evidence for direct cerebral action of bacterial endotoxin. *Trans. Assoc. Am. Physicians,* 70:64–72.
6. Bergstrom, T., Larson, H., Lincolm, K., and Winberg, J. (1972): Studies of urinary tract infections in infancy and childhood. Eighty consecutive patients with neonatal infection. *J. Pediatr.,* 80:858–866.
7. Blatteis, C. M. (1977): Comparison of endotoxin and leukocytic pyrogen pyrogenicity in newborn guinea pigs. *J. Appl. Physiol.,* 42:355–361.
8. Chowers, I., Conforti, N., and Feldman, S. (1968): Local effect of cortisol in the preoptic area on temperature regulation. *Am. J. Physiol.,* 214:538–542.
9. Cooper, K. E., Cranston, W. I., and Honour, A. J. (1967): Observations on the site and mode of action of pyrogens in the rabbit brain. *J. Physiol.,* 191:325–337.
10. Cooper, K. E., Kasting, N. W., Lederis, K., and Veale, W. L. (1979): Evidence supporting a role for endogenous vasopressin in natural suppression of fever in the sheep. *J. Physiol. (Lond.) (in press).*
11. Cooper, K. E., Veale, W. L., Kasting, N., and Pittman, Q. J. (1979): Ontogeny of fever. *Fed. Proc.,* 38:35–38.
12. Covert, J. B., and Reynolds, W. W. (1977): Survival value of fever in fish. *Nature,* 267:43–45.
13. Craig, W. S. (1963): The early detection of pyrexia in the newborn. *Arch. Dis. Child.,* 38:29–39.
14. Cranston, W. I., and Rawlins, M. D. (1972): Effects of intracerebral microinjection of sodium salicylate on temperature regulation in the rabbit. *J. Physiol.,* 222:257–266.
15. Epstein, H. C., Hochwald, A., and Ashe, R. (1951): Salmonella infections of the newborn infant. *J. Pediatr.,* 38:723–731.
16. Forsling, M. L., Ingram, D. M., and Stanier, M. W. (1976): Effects of various ambient temperatures and of heating and cooling the hypothalamus and cervical spinal cord on antidiuretic hormone secretion and urinary osmolality in pigs. *J. Physiol.,* 257:673–686.
17. Grantham, J. J., and Orloff, J. (1968): Effect of prostaglandin E_1 on the permeability in response of the isolated collecting tubule to vasopressin, $3',5'$-monophosphate, and theophylline. *J. Clin. Invest.,* 47:1154–1161.
18. Hall, W. J., and Martin, J. D. G. (1974): Effect of calcium and vasopressin on the response of frog skin to PGE_1. *J. Physiol.,* 240:595–608.
19. Jackson, D. L. (1967): A hypothalamic region responsive to localized injections of pyrogens. *J. Neurophysiol.,* 30:586–602.
20. Kasting, N. W., Cooper, K. E., and Veale, W. L. (1979): Antipyresis following perfusion of brain sites with vasopressin. *Experientia,* 35:208–209.
21. Kasting, N. W., Veale, W. L., and Cooper, K. E. (1978): Suppression of fever at term of pregnancy. *Nature,* 271:245–246.

22. Kasting, N. W., Veale, W. L., and Cooper, K. E. (1978): Evidence for a centrally active endogenous antipyretic near parturition in the sheep. In: *Current Studies of Hypothalamic Function, 1978. Part II. Metabolism and Behavior,* edited by K. Lederis and W. L. Veale, pp. 63–71. S. Karger, Basel.

23. Kasting, N. W., Veale, W. L., and Cooper, K. E. (1979): Development of fever in the newborn lamb. *Am. J. Physiol.,* 236:R184–R187.

24. Kluger, M. J., and Vaughn, L. K. (1978): Fever and survival in rabbits infected with *Pasteurella multocida. J. Physiol. (Lond.),* 282:243–251.

25. Kluger, M. J., Ringler, D. H., and Anver, M. R. (1975): Fever and survival. *Science,* 188:166–168.

26. Marzetti, G., Laurenti, F., Caro, M. D., Conca, L., and Orzalesi, M. (1973): *Salmonella munchen* infections in newborns and small infants. *Clin. Pediatr.,* 12:93–97.

27. Meban, C. (1978): Influence of pH and temperature on behavior of surfactant from human neonatal lungs. *Biol. Neonate,* 33:106–111.

28. Myers, R. D. (1970): An improved push–pull cannula system for perfusing an isolated region of the brain. *Physiol. Behav.,* 5:243–246.

29. Nusynowitz, M. L., and Forsham, P. H. (1966): The antidiuretic action of acetaminophen. *Am. J. Med. Sci.,* 252:429–435.

30. Okuno, A., Yamamoto, M., and Itoh, S. (1965): Lowering of the body temperature induced by vasopressin. *Jpn. J. Physiol.,* 15:378–387.

31. Parisi, M., and Piccinni, Z. F. (1972): Aspirin potentiates the hydrosmotic effect of antidiuretic hormone in toad urinary bladder. *Biochim. Biophys. Acta,* 279:209–212.

32. Pittman, Q. J., Cooper, K. E., Veale, W. L., and Van Petten, G. R. (1974): Observations on the development of the febrile response to pyrogens in sheep. *Clin. Sci. Mol. Med.,* 46:591–602.

33. Podoprigora, G. I. (1978): Body temperature and response to pyrogen in germ-free and ordinary animals. *Bull. Exp. Biol. Med. (USSR).,* 85:272–273.

34. Sheth, U. K., and Borison, H. L. (1960): Central pyrogenic action of *Salmonella typhosa* lipopolysaccharide injected into the lateral cerebral ventricle in cats. *J. Pharmacol. Exp. Ther.,* 130:411–417.

35. Silverstein, M. E., Feldman, R. C., Henderson, L. W., and Engelman, K. (1975): Acute effects of indomethacin (Indo) and aspirin (ASA) on human renal function. *Clin. Res.,* 23:374A.

36. Smith, R. T., Platou, E. S., and Good, R. A. (1956): Septicemia of the newborn. *Pediatrics,* 17:549–575.

37. Szczepanska-Sadowska, E. (1974): Plasma ADH increase and thirst suppression elicited by preoptic heating in the dog. *Am. J. Physiol.,* 226:155–161.

38. Székely, M., and Szelényi, Z. (1977): The effect of *E. coli* endotoxin on body temperature in the newborn rabbit, cat, guinea pig and rat. *Acta Physiol. Acad. Sci, Hung.,* 50:293–298.

39. Vaughn, L. K., Veale, W. L., and Cooper, K. E. (1979): Sensitivity of hypothalamic sites to salicylate and prostaglandin. *Can. J. Physiol. Pharmacol.,* 57:118–123.

40. Veale, W. L. (1971): Behavioral and physiological changes caused by the regional alteration of sodium and calcium ions in the hypothalamus of the unanesthetized cat. Ph.D. thesis, Purdue University, Lafayette, Ind.

41. Villablanca, J., and Myers, R. D. (1965): Fever produced by microinjection of typhoid vaccine into hypothalamus of cats. *Am. J. Physiol.,* 208:703–707.

Fever, edited by James M. Lipton.
Raven Press, New York © 1980.

Fever in Normal and Maternally Neglected Newborn Rabbits

Naomi Kleitman and Evelyn Satinoff

Departments of Psychology and Physiology and Biophysics, University of Illinois at Urbana-Champaign, Champaign, Illinois 61820

Although fever is the most common sign of infection in adults, in infected newborn babies it is often low grade or absent (32), and body temperature may even be below normal (17). In fact, when a human newborn does develop high fever, it generally indicates a serious, life-threatening illness (24). In cases of less severe superficial infections, only about half the infants develop any fever at all (16). The same effects have been found in controlled studies on newborns of other species. For instance, doses of pyrogen that cause fever in adult guinea pigs, rabbits, and sheep do not lead to rises in body temperature in newborns of these species (5,15) or to any increase in oxygen consumption (5,27). However, if the dose of pyrogen is well above the dose that causes fever in adults, then newborn rabbits and guinea pigs do develop fevers (6,34, 35).

These results are somewhat unexpected because we know that from birth all of these species, as well as others, increase metabolic rate in the cold [rabbits (18,27); guinea pigs (10); humans (8); lambs (1); mice (20,33); rats (14)]. Why, then, do they not become febrile except when given very high doses of pyrogen or in cases of very severe infection?

In a previous paper, Satinoff et al. (26) confirmed that newborn rabbits do not become febrile when they are injected with a dose of pyrogen that causes fever in older animals. However, when the pups were given an opportunity to select their preferred position in a thermally graded alleyway, they chose much warmer positions than did controls injected with saline, and their body temperature rose to febrile levels. Thus the drive towards fever was present in these newborn rabbits, but was only expressed behaviorally.

These results imply that somewhere in the central nervous system of newborn rabbits there is a separation between the neural networks controlling behavioral and reflexive responses to pyrogen. This hypothesis is strengthened by results showing that adult rats with large preoptic lesions cannot regulate their body temperatures reflexively in a cold environment (30), but they can maintain near-normal body temperatures if given the opportunity to press a bar to turn on a heat lamp (13,28). Similarly, such rats will die of hyperthermia in a hot environment, but not if they can turn the heat lamp off and a cooling fan on

(23). Rats with small lesions in the lateral hypothalamus have the opposite defect: they can thermoregulate reflexively in the cold, but they do not perform behavioral acts to obtain heat (29,36).[1]

In the present paper we show that doses of pyrogen large enough to produce a fever reflexively in newborn rabbits produce a behavioral fever that is much higher still. Thus behavioral measures are much more sensitive than autonomic measures as an indication of infection in newborn rabbits. In addition, we show that malnourished, hypothermic rabbit pups that do not develop fevers autonomically, even at doses of pyrogen that produce such fevers in normals, select extremely high temperatures in a thermal gradient and develop fevers behaviorally. We will present the data to support these statements and then discuss some of their implications both for a model of brain function during fever and as an animal model for the human situation.

RESPONSES TO PYROGEN IN NORMAL RABBIT PUPS

In the present experiments we injected 1- to 3-day-old New Zealand white rabbits intraperitoneally with pyrogen (Piromen®; 50, 500, and 5,000 μg/kg). Pups were housed individually in an incubator kept at 33°C for 30 min to 2½ hr before and 2 hr after injection. They were then placed in a thermal gradient, an aluminum alley 75 cm long with a temperature range of 19 to 55°C. The pups were placed in a position corresponding to a floor temperature of 30°C. Their position in the gradient was recorded each minute until they remained at one place for 5 consecutive minutes, up to a maximum of 30 min. This was the first behavioral measure: the selected temperature at which the pups first stayed for at least 5 min. All pups were left in the gradient for 30 min. Then they were removed, their rectal temperatures were recorded, and they were returned to the incubator for another 2 hr. This was the second measure of the efficacy of the pups' behavior: rectal temperature after 30 min in the gradient. All pyrogen-injected groups were compared to littermate controls injected with an equivalent volume of saline vehicle (2 ml/kg) and tested concurrently.

Figure 1 shows the mean data from the pups injected with pyrogen (50 μg/kg). Both groups had higher mean rectal temperatures after 2 hr in the incubator, but at this dose there was no significant difference between body temperature of experimental and control pups. However, the pups injected with pyromen selected significantly warmer gradient positions than did the pups injected with saline (mean difference, 1.6°C, $p < 0.02$), and after 30 min in the gradient their rectal temperatures averaged 39.2 ± 0.3°C compared with 38.3 ± 0.2°C for the controls. Thus, had we looked only at rectal temperature

---

[1] Actually, the concept of two separate neural systems, one for behavior and one for reflexes, is an oversimplification (see ref. 25 for a more detailed analysis of the central control of thermoregulation). However, since in this chapter we are discussing only two responses—movement in a gradient and changes in metabolic rate—it is sufficient for our purposes.

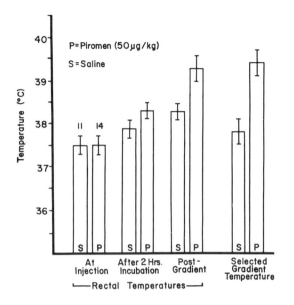

FIG. 1. Mean of rectal temperatures (T_R) of 1– to 3-day-old normal rabbit pups at time of injection with saline or pyrogen (50 μg/kg); maximum T_R recorded during 2 hr at ambient temperature of 33°C; T_R after 30 min in thermal gradient alley; and temperature at which pups settled in gradient for 5 min. Numbers over bars are number of pups in each group; bars at ± 1 SEM.

changes in the incubator after pyrogen, we would have concluded that the dose was too low to elicit fever in these newborn rabbits. Only when the rabbits were given the opportunity for behavioral temperature selection did we see that they developed fever and therefore were sensitive to the effects of the drug.

In Fig. 2 we see the effects of 500 μg/kg pyrogen, 10 times the previous

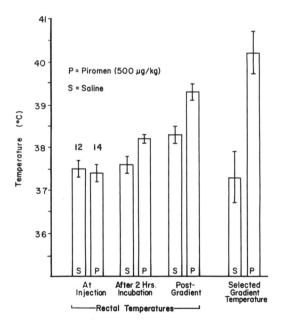

FIG. 2. Dose of pyrogen 500 μg/kg. See Fig. 1.

dose. After 2 hr in the incubator, the pups' rectal temperatures rose an average of 0.8°C over the controls. Satinoff et al. (26) observed a smaller (0.5°C) difference in temperature between their groups. In that study with 11 pups, the difference was not significant. In the present experiment there was less variance within the groups, perhaps because the pups were preincubated for at least 30 min, and the difference is statistically significant ($p < 0.01$). Newborn rabbit pups' body temperatures are labile, and individual and litter differences can be marked. The 0.8°C difference observed in this experiment represents febrile responses (that is, increases at or above the highest increase seen in controls) in only 64% of the pyrogen-injected pups. Nonetheless, as in the Satinoff et al. (26) experiment, our pyrogen-injected pups selected substantially higher gradient temperatures than controls, thereby raising their body temperature further. The pyrogen-injected pups chose a gradient position that was higher by 2.6°C. After 30 min their rectal temperatures averaged 39.4 ± 0.2°C, significantly higher than the mean of 38.4 ± 0.2°C of the saline controls ($p < 0.01$) and also significantly higher than their pregradient body temperature of 38.3 ± 0.1°C ($p < 0.001$).

Figure 3 demonstrates that pyrogen (5,000 μg/kg) caused a mean rise of 1.4 ± 0.2°C in the experimental pups' temperature compared with 0.2 ± 0.1°C for the saline group. These pups chose the highest gradient position—42.4 ± 0.6°

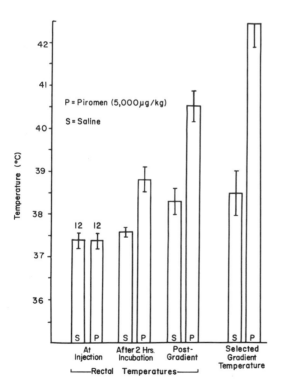

FIG. 3. Dose of pyrogen 5,000 μg/kg. See Fig. 1.

versus $38.5 \pm 0.5°C$ for controls, thereby raising their body temperature $2.1 \pm 0.6°C$ further. Table 1 summarizes these data. When the pups were placed back in the incubator after 30 min in the gradient, their temperatures quickly fell to pregradient levels.

In summary, we found separate dose-response curves for the development of fever autonomically and behaviorally. Rectal temperatures rose higher in the incubator with increasing doses of pyrogen. However, they rose even higher after the pups had been in the gradient. Even at the lowest dose of pyrogen, at which many animals showed no reflexive fever, behavioral fever was clear.

One possible explanation for these results is that the central threshold for activating reflexive responses to pyrogen is higher than the threshold for behavioral responses. Behavior will therefore be the first and, if the dose is low enough, possibly the only response to a pyrogen injection. Not only the activating thresholds were different, however. The fact that behavioral fevers were always higher than reflexive fevers implies that the controller equations for these individual responses were different as well. A second intriguing possibility is that there are two central integrators, one activating responses to cold, the other activating responses to pyrogen, and these two integrators receive input from two different sets of thermosensitive units. The units whose activity eventually leads to behavioral changes may be more mature and thus more sensitive to the effects of pyrogen on their firing rates. Of course, these two possibilities are not mutually exclusive. There may be different afferent inputs for cold and for pyrogens as well as different sensitivities of the pathways controlling various responses.

One could argue that it is simply easier to increase body temperature in a thermal gradient and that, in fact, infant rabbits cannot do so reflexively. However, the dose-response curves argue against this. The pups given pyrogen (5,000 $\mu g/kg$) were able to raise their body temperatures in the incubator by a mean of 1.2°C relative to saline-injected controls. This was higher than the increase seen in pups given pyrogen (50 $\mu g/kg$) after 30 min in the gradient, whereas during incubation body temperature rose only 0.4°C in the latter group. Thus the pups given the low dose of pyrogen had the autonomic capacity to raise their body temperatures but they did not do so.

In summary, infant rabbits can increase their body temperatures by autonomic means if the dose of pyrogen is sufficiently high. They then increase it even

TABLE 1. *Comparison of pyrogen-injected and saline-injected pups: mean differences in selected temperatures and in changes in rectal temperature (ΔT_R)*

Pyrogen ($\mu g/kg$)	Difference in selected temp. (°C)	ΔT_R during 2 hr at 33°C (°C)	ΔT_R from injection to postgradient (°C)
50	1.6	0.4	0.8
500	2.6	0.8	1.1
5,000	3.9	1.2	2.5

further by temperature selection. Even at doses of pyrogen that do not cause changes in body temperature in the incubator, the animals become febrile in the behavioral situation. All infants seek heat when they are below their thermoneutral zone. These data imply a separation in the central nervous system between behavioral and autonomic mechanisms of heat production in response to a cold environment and in response to pyrogen injection.

RESPONSES TO PYROGEN IN MATERNALLY NEGLECTED RABBIT PUPS

In normal pups there was a certain amount of variability in responses to pyrogen. Some pups did not develop a fever even after 5,000 μg/kg pyrogen, whereas others did at 50 μg/kg. However, 75% of the pups had elevated body temperatures after 5,000 μg/kg, whereas only 36% showed elevations at 50 μg/kg. Furthermore, 22% of pups injected with saline raised their body temperatures to febrile levels either in the incubator or in the gradient. This variability of responses to pyrogen that we saw at all doses is reminiscent of the situation in human newborns. In any group of infected infants, some develop fevers and some do not (16,17,24,32). Prematurity, low birth weight, malnutrition, and other stresses affect heat production in newborns (9,11,31) and could be important factors in the development of febrile responses.

Several times during our testing of normal pups we noted that some rabbit mothers did not build proper nests or feed their young. As a result, these pups had low body temperature, did not gain or even lost weight, and rarely survived longer than 3 days. We separated these neglected litters from the normal litters and tested their responses to pyrogen (5,000 μg/kg), the dose at which almost all normal pups developed fevers in the incubator. They were tested in the manner described above, and Fig. 4 shows the results with these animals. In this figure we have included the body temperatures of the animals when they were removed from the nests. They were an average of 3°C lower than temperatures of pups from normal litters. Body weights averaged 48 g ($N = 23$) compared with 64 g ($N = 75$) for normal pups. The pups were incubated for several hours after removal from the nest, but their body temperatures still did not reach normal levels. Two hours after injection, again at the incubation temperature of 33°C, body temperature had not changed significantly in either group, indicating that the neglected pups were unable to develop a fever autonomically. However, when they were placed in the thermally graded alley, pups injected with pyrogen chose the highest positions of any group—42.8 ± 0.2°C—and at the end of 30 min their body temperatures were elevated 0.9°C over the saline controls. Thus, although the pyrogen did not induce metabolic heat production in these neglected pups, it did induce behavioral heat-seeking at higher than normal levels, just as it does in normal pups injected with pyrogen.

In summary, pups from litters that are not cared for do not develop fever reflexively even at a dose of pyrogen high enough to produce fever in almost

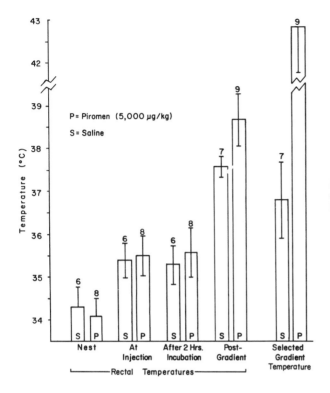

FIG. 4. For neglected pups, dose of pyrogen 5,000 μg/kg. See Fig. 1.

all normal pups. Nevertheless, these pups do show a strong behavioral response to the pyrogen and choose the warmest positions in the thermal gradient of any group.

Even after 4 to 5 hr incubation at 33°C, the mean body temperature of the neglected pups was 35.5°C. Normal saline-injected pups usually had body temperatures over 37°C. This could mean that 33°C was below thermoneutrality for the neglected pups and they could not increase their metabolic rate due to the effects of starvation on brown fat (12), or it could mean that a low body temperature is an adaptation to conserve calories. Although we have not yet measured the metabolic rates of these neglected pups in the cold, results of others suggest that oxygen consumption would not be raised. Normal rabbit pups increase their metabolic rate in the cold (21,27), but starved ones do not (18,22). The same is true for malnourished rats up to the age of 16 days (2,4,19) and human infants up to 16 months (7). This is probably not due to an inability to increase internal heat production in the cold, that is, to an inadequate substrate mobilization, but rather is an active neural process designed to conserve energy. Bignall et al. (3) have shown that the oxygen consumption of starved, intact rats declines in the cold, whereas starved decerebrate rat pups maintain near maximal oxygen consumption levels in both cold and thermoneutral environments. The lack of internal heat production to a high dose of pyrogen in our neglected rabbit pups may similarly be an energy conserving response.

In conclusion, since behavioral heat-seeking in response to pyrogen in our neglected pups is even more pronounced than in normal pups, we feel that behavioral measures, rather than the presence or absence of metabolically induced elevations of body temperature, may be the most sensitive indicator of infection in all newborns and especially in small premature or malnourished infants.

ACKNOWLEDGMENTS

The work described in this chapter was supported in part by Grant #BNS77-03151 from NSF, Contract #N00014-77-C-0465 from the Office of Naval Research, and a University of Illinois Biomed Research Grant awarded to Evelyn Satinoff and an NSF Pre-doctoral Fellowship awarded to Naomi Kleitman. We thank Dr. Philip Teitelbaum for his helpful comments on the manuscript and Travenol Laboratories for generously supplying us with Piromen.

REFERENCES

1. Alexander, G. (1961): Temperature regulation in the newborn lamb. III. Effect of environmental temperature on metabolic rate, body temperatures, and respiratory quotient. *Aust. J. Agric. Res.,* 12:1152–1174.
2. Bignall, K. E., Heggeness, F. W., and Palmer, J. E. (1974): Effects of acute starvation on cold induced thermogenesis in the preweanling rat. *Am. J. Physiol.,* 227:1088–1093.
3. Bignall, K. E., Heggeness, F. W., and Palmer, J. E. (1975): Effect of neonatal decerebration on thermogenesis during starvation and cold exposure in the rat. *Exp. Neurol.,* 49:174–188.
4. Blackmore, D. W. (1972): The effects of limited, moderate and lengthy daily separation from the mother during the early postnatal period of the rat on concurrent and subsequent growth, and on concurrent oxygen consumption at, as well as below, thermal neutrality. *Biol. Neonate,* 21:268–281.
5. Blatteis, C. M. (1975): Postnatal development of pyrogenic sensitivity in guinea pigs. *J. Appl. Physiol.,* 39:251–257.
6. Blatteis, C. M. (1977): Comparison of endotoxin and leukocytic pyrogen pyrogenicity in newborn guinea pigs. *J. Appl. Physiol.,* 42:355–361.
7. Brooke, O. G., Harris, M., and Salvosa, C. B. (1973): The response of malnourished babies to cold. *J. Physiol.,* 223:75–91.
8. Brück, K. (1961): Temperature regulation in the newborn infant. *Biol. Neonate,* 3:65–119.
9. Brück, K., Parmelee, A. H., Jr., and Brück, M. (1962): Neutral temperature range and range of "thermal comfort" in premature infants. *Biol. Neonate,* 4:32–51.
10. Brück, K., and Wünnenberg, B. (1965): Blockade der chemischen Thermogenese und Auslosüng von Muskelgitten durch Adrenolytica und Ganglienblockade beim neugeborenen Meerschweinchen. *Pfluegers Arch.,* 282:376–389.
11. Buetow, K. C., and Klein, S. W. (1964): Effect of maintenance of "normal" skin temperature on survival of infants of low birth weight. *Pediatrics,* 34:163–170.
12. Cardasis, C. A., and Sinclair, J. C. (1972): The effects of ambient temperature on the fasted newborn rabbit. I. Survival time, weight loss, body temperature and oxygen consumption. *Biol. Neonate,* 21:330–346.
13. Carlisle, H. J. (1969): Effect of preoptic and anterior hypothalamic lesions on behavioral thermoregulation in the cold. *J. Comp. Physiol. Psychol.,* 69:391–402.
14. Conklin, P., and Heggeness, F. W. (1971): Maturation of temperature homeostasis in the rat. *Am. J. Physiol.,* 220:333–336.

15. Cooper, K. E., Pittman, Q. J., and Veale, W. L. (1975): Observations on the development of the "fever" mechanism in the fetus and the newborn. In: *Temperature Regulation and Drug Action,* edited by P. Lomax, E. Schönbaum, and J. Jacob, pp. 43–50. S. Karger, Basel.
16. Craig, W. S. (1963): The early detection of pyrexia in the newborn. *Arch. Dis. Child.,* 38:29–39.
17. Epstein, H. C., Hochwald, A., and Ashe, R. (1951): Salmonella infections of the newborn infant. *J. Pediatr.,* 38:723–731.
18. Hardman, M. J., Hey, E. N., and Hull, D. (1969): The effect of prolonged cold exposure on heat production in newborn rabbits. *J. Physiol.,* 205:39–50.
19. Heim, T., and Szelényi, Z. (1965): Temperature regulation in rats semistarved since birth. *Acta Physiol. Acad. Sci. Hung.,* 27:247–255.
20. Hill, R. W. (1976): The ontogeny of homeothermy in neonatal *Peromyscus leucopus. Physiol. Zool.,* 49:292–306.
21. Hull, D. (1965): Oxygen consumption and body temperature of newborn rabbits and kittens exposed to cold. *J. Physiol.,* 177:192–202.
22. Hull, D., and Segall, M. M. (1965): Heat production in the newborn rabbit and the fat content of the brown adipose tissue. *J. Physiol.,* 181:468–477.
23. Lipton, J. M. (1968): Effects of preoptic lesions on heat-escape responding and colonic temperature in the rat. *Physiol. Behav.,* 3:165–169.
24. McCarthy, P. L., and Dolan, T. F. (1976): The serious implications of high fever in infants during their first three months. *Clin. Pediatr.,* 15:794–796.
25. Satinoff, E. (1978): Neural organization and evolution of thermal regulation in mammals. *Science,* 201:16–22.
26. Satinoff, E., McEwen, G. N., Jr., and Williams, B. A. (1976): Behavioral fever in newborn rabbits. *Science,* 193:1139–1140.
27. Satinoff, E., McEwen, G. N., Jr., and Williams, B. A. (1976): Behavioral and physiological responses to pyrogen in newborn rabbits. *Neurosci. Abstr.,* 2:226.
28. Satinoff, E., and Rutstein, J. (1970): Behavioral thermoregulation in rats with anterior hypothalamic lesions. *J. Comp. Physiol. Psychol.,* 71:77–82.
29. Satinoff, E., and Shan, Y. Y. (1971): Loss of behavioral thermoregulation after lateral hypothalamic lesions in rats. *J. Comp. Physiol. Psychol.,* 77:302–312.
30. Satinoff, E., Valentino, D., and Teitelbaum, P. (1976): Thermoregulatory cold-defense deficits in rats with preoptic/anterior hypothalamic lesions. *Brain Res. Bull.,* 1:553–565.
31. Scopes, J. W., and Ahmed, I. (1966): Range of critical temperatures in sick and premature newborn babies. *Arch. Dis. Child.,* 41:417–419.
32. Smith, R. T., Platou, E. S., and Good, R. A. (1956): Septicemia of the newborn: Current status of the problem. *Pediatrics,* 17:549–575.
33. Stanier, M. W. (1975): Effect of body weight, ambient temperature and huddling on oxygen consumption and body temperature of young mice. *Comp. Biochem. Physiol.,* 51A:79–82.
34. Székely, M. (1978): Biphasic endotoxin fever in the newborn rabbit. *Acta Physiol. Acad. Sci. Hung.,* 51:389–392.
35. Székely, M., and Szelényi, Z. (1977): The effects of *E. coli* endotoxin on body temperature in the newborn rabbit, cat, guinea pig and rat. *Acta Physiol. Acad. Sci. Hung.,* 50:293–298.
36. Van Zoeren, J. G., and Stricker, E. M. (1977): Effects of preoptic, lateral hypothalamic, or dopamine-depleting lesions on behavioral thermoregulation in rats exposed to the cold. *J. Comp. Physiol. Psychol.,* 91:989–999.

Fever, edited by James M. Lipton.
Raven Press, New York © 1980.

Behaviorally Mediated Fever in Aquatic Ectotherms

*William Wallace Reynolds, *Martha Elizabeth Casterlin, and
**Jerry B. Covert

*Department of Biology, Pennsylvania State University, Wilkes-Barre, Pennsylvania 18708;
and **Department of Biology, Pennsylvania State University, Hazleton, Pennsylvania 18201*

Aquatic ectotherms (23,24) are excellent subjects for thermoregulatory studies. Although they are able to heat and cool at different rates following a sudden ambient temperature change (21), under steady state conditions their core body temperatures differ little from ambient water temperatures (29), particularly in animals weighing less than 1 kg. Thermoregulatory responses of aquatic ectotherms are, therefore, largely behavioral (23,24,29,30).

Behavioral thermoregulation in aquatic ectotherms involves selection of appropriate water temperatures (24,30). Because radiation and evaporation are not effective routes of thermal exchange in water, postural orientations utilized by some terrestrial ectotherms (23) are ineffective. Each species exhibits a characteristic "final thermal preferendum" (24,30) which is species specific and unaffected by previous thermal history of the individual.

Many ectotherms are capable of precise behavioral thermoregulation when presented with a suitable choice of environmental temperatures, as in a conventional laboratory gradient trough (30) or an electronic shuttlebox (20,29). An Ichthyotron-type shuttlebox (20) is particularly convenient for experimental studies because it allows the animal to actually control water temperatures, and therefore body temperatures, by means of normal unconditioned locomotor movements.

Aquatic ectotherms are also convenient for studies involving experimental manipulation of the animals' body temperatures, which the experimenter can easily control by adjusting the water temperature as desired (9). Baseline data on normothermic final temperature preferenda, upper and lower lethal temperatures, and optima for various physiological processes are available in the literature for many species (30).

Aquatic lower vertebrates (lampreys, sharks, bony fishes, and amphibian larvae) are useful for investigations of the evolutionary history of CNS thermoregulatory control mechanisms which have culminated in homeoendothermy in the higher vertebrates (birds and mammals). Aquatic invertebrates, such as arthropods, provide further evolutionary perspective on thermoregulatory mechanisms (5,6).

---

* Present address: Center for Life Sciences, University of New England, Biddeford, Maine 04005

FEVER IN AQUATIC ECTOTHERMS

A number of aquatic ectotherm species, both lower vertebrates and invertebrates, have been found to exhibit "behavioral fever" (25), manifested as an increase in preferred temperature above the species-specific normothermic final preferendum (24,30), when injected with various pyrogens (4–6,9,16,22,25–28). Similar responses have been observed in terrestrial ectotherms (1,12,13,16,31). Mammals also exhibit a behavioral component among their febrile mechanisms (8,11,19,31), which develops earlier in ontogeny in some mammal species (31) than do the physiological thermoregulatory mechanisms. Behavioral fever, and behavioral thermoregulation generally, apparently precede physiological thermoregulation and fever ontogenetically and phylogenetically, suggesting that physiological mechanisms such as fine control of blood flow and metabolic rate and evaporative cooling have been added on to more ancient behavioral mechanisms for controlling body temperature.

It is our purpose to review existing data on behavioral fever in aquatic ectotherms, including both previously published results and more recent unpublished data for lower vertebrates and invertebrates. Kluger (12) has recently reviewed studies of fever in terrestrial ectothermic vertebrates (reptiles and adult anuran amphibians). Numerous other publications (e.g., 8,10,11,14,19,31,32) have dealt with mammalian fever.

Febrile responses are elicited in mammals by bacterial pyrogens (14,31) or endotoxins, which induce the release of endogenous leukocytic pyrogen (14). Behavioral fever is induced in lizards (13), neonatal mammals (31), and adult

TABLE 1. *Summary of aquatic ectotherm species found to exhibit behavioral fever, and pyrogenic agents used*

Species	Pyrogen
Amphibians	
Rana pipiens tadpoles	*Aeromonas hydrophila* (killed)
Rana catesbeiana tadpoles	*Aeromonas hydrophila* (killed)
Fishes	
Lepomis macrochirus	*Aeromonas hydrophila* (killed)
Lepomis macrochirus	*Escherichia coli* endotoxin
Lepomis macrochirus	*Staphylococcus aureus* (killed)
Micropterus salmoides	*Aeromonas hydrophila* (killed)
Carassius auratus	*Aeromonas hydrophila* (live)
Carassius auratus	*Escherichia coli* endotoxin
Decapod crustaceans	
Cambarus bartoni	*Aeromonas hydrophila* (killed)
Cambarus bartoni	Prostaglandin E_1
Penaeus duorarum	Prostaglandin E_1
Homarus americanus	Prostaglandin E_1
Chelicerate arthropods	
Limulus polyphemus	Prostaglandin E_1

frogs (16) by injecting them with live or killed bacteria or with bacterial extracts. Induction of behavioral fever by bacterial pyrogens has been observed in three bony fish species (Table 1): the bluegill sunfish *Lepomis macrochirus* (22,25–27), the largemouth bass *Micropterus salmoides* (25,27), and the goldfish *Carassius auratus* (9,27,28). Both Gram-positive *(Staphylococcus aureus)* and Gram-negative *(Aeromonas hydrophila)* bacteria induce fever when injected i.p. into fishes (9,22,25–28). Both live (9) and killed (22,25–28) bacteria are pyrogenic to fish when injected i.p. in doses of 1 to 4×10^9 cells. Lyophilized *E. coli* lipopolysaccharide endotoxin (28) is also pyrogenic to fish. Killed *A. hydrophila* is pyrogenic to two species of anuran amphibian tadpoles, *Rana pipiens* and *R. catesbeiana* (4,27), and to the freshwater decapod crustacean (Arthropoda) *Cambarus bartoni* (5). Nagai and Iriki (17) have reported an autonomic response of goldfish to bacterial pyrogen. However, endotoxin injected into the bass *M. salmoides* in a homogeneous thermal environment causes no increase in either oxygen consumption or core temperature (W. W. Reynolds and M. E. Casterlin, *unpublished data*), indicating that fever in fishes is mediated entirely by behavior.

PHARMACOLOGY OF FEVER IN AQUATIC ECTOTHERMS

Clark and Lipton (8) observed that "agents which alter the set-point for physiological thermoregulatory activity [in mammals] produce a complementary shift in the behavioural set-point as well." Polk and Lipton (19) further observed that "to characterize drug actions on thermoregulatory processes it is necessary to know whether compounds which alter body temperature also cause changes in thermoregulatory motivation." These observations are particularly relevant to comparisons of thermoregulatory and febrile responses of endotherms and ectotherms. If various drugs which affect thermoregulation or induce fever in mammals also do so in ectotherms, this may have profound implications for understanding the central mechanisms controlling thermoregulation in various taxa.

Prostaglandins of the E series, such as PGE_1, are known to induce fever in mammals (10,11,32), and are hypothesized to play an integral role in mediating fever (32). Antipyretics such as salicylate and acetaminophen are thought to reduce fever by blocking PGE synthesis (10,11,22,32). PGE induces behavioral as well as physiological fever in mammals (11). PGE_1 is known to exert a direct excitatory effect on neurons (7), whereas prostaglandin-blocking antipyretics such as sodium salicylate influence central thermoregulatory mechanisms (19) without acting directly on thermosensitive neurons (14). Prostaglandins are known to be synthesized by lower vertebrates (2,3,7) and invertebrates (3, 15,18). Does PGE_1 induce fever in these ectotherms?

PGE_1 has been found to induce fever in the frog *R. esculenta* (16), in the crayfish *Cambarus bartoni* (6), in the marine decapod crustaceans *Penaeus duorarum* and *Homarus americanus* (Table 1; M. E. Casterlin and W. W. Reynolds, *unpublished data*), and in the primitive chelicerate arthropod *Limulus polyphe-*

mus (Table 1; M. E. Casterlin and W. W. Reynolds, *unpublished data*), as well as in terrestrial scorpions (M. Cabanac, *personal communication*). The antipyretic acetaminophen prevents bacterial fever in *C. bartoni* (M. E. Casterlin and W. W. Reynolds, *unpublished data*). Although a great deal of further experimentation is necessary to firmly establish the precise mechanisms involved in thermoregulatory responses of arthropods, and of the role of prostaglandins in thermoregulatory mechanisms of vertebrates and invertebrates, the observation that PGE_1 induces fever in animals as taxonomically diverse as mammals, frogs, and arthropods, and the finding that acetaminophen is antipyretic in mammals (10), fishes (22), and arthropods (M. E. Casterlin and W. W. Reynolds, *unpublished data*), suggest commonalities among thermoregulatory mechanisms of animals which promise to open new avenues of investigation that may lead to better understanding of thermoregulatory neuropharmacology.

SURVIVAL VALUE OF FEVER

Covert and Reynolds (9) found that fever has adaptive value in goldfish, improving survival from a bacterial infection (Fig. 1) with live *A. hydrophila*. This parallels similar findings with lizards (1,12,13). Apparently, bacterial growth is limited by reduced iron availability at febrile temperatures (13), and blood flow is enhanced by elevated febrile temperatures (21), which speeds the movement of leukocytes to the site of infection (1). Serum copper is also elevated during fever (M. J. Kluger, *personal communication*), and copper is known to be toxic to prokaryotes such as bacteria, perhaps acting synergistically with elevated temperatures. Similar mechanisms may operate in invertebrates, which suggests further avenues for experimentation.

There is great significance in the fact that animals as diverse as mammals,

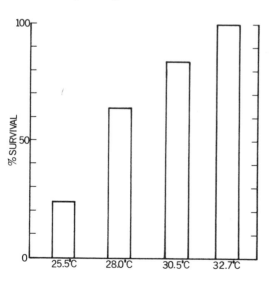

FIG. 1. Comparative survival after 72 hr of goldfish injected (i.p.) with live pathogenic *Aeromonas hydrophila* and held in aquaria at hypothermic (25.5°C, N = 25), normothermic (28.0°C; N = 25), or hyperthermic (30.5°C; N = 25) temperatures, or thermoregulating behaviorally at febrile (32.7°C; N = 10) temperature in an electronic shuttlebox (20). (Data from Covert and Reynolds, ref. 9.)

fishes, and arthropods respond to infection with fever. This implies that fever evolved hundreds of millions of years ago in very primitive animals, or that it evolved independently in more than one evolutionary lineage. Whichever is the case, it is reasonable to infer that fever has profound adaptive value in enhancing survival after infection.

ACKNOWLEDGMENTS

We are grateful for financial support from PSU Grants SAF–74–071, SAF–77–113, and SAF–78–050, and NSF Grant PCM 78–05691, to W.W.R. We also thank Dr. James Lipton for inviting us to contribute to this volume and for arranging for travel funds which permitted us to attend the symposium.

REFERENCES

1. Bernheim, H. A., Bodel, P. T., Askenase, P. W., and Atkins, E. (1978): Effects of fever on host defense mechanisms after infection in the lizard *Dipsosaurus dorsalis. Br. J. Exp. Pathol.,* 59:76–84.
2. Bishai, I., and Coceani, F. (1976): Presence of 15-hydroxy prostaglandin dehydrogenase, prostaglandin-Δ^{13}-reductase and prostaglandin E-9-keto (α)-reductase in the frog spinal cord. *J. Neurochem.,* 26:1167–1174.
3. Bito, L. Z. (1972): Comparative study of concentrative prostaglandin accumulation by various tissues of mammals and marine vertebrates and invertebrates. *Comp. Biochem. Physiol.,* 43A:65–82.
4. Casterlin, M. E., and Reynolds, W. W. (1977): Behavioural fever in anuran amphibian larvae. *Life Sci.,* 20:593–596.
5. Casterlin, M. E., and Reynolds, W. W. (1977): Behavioral fever in crayfish. *Hydrobiologia,* 56:99–101.
6. Casterlin, M. E., and Reynolds, W. W. (1978): Prostaglandin E_1 fever in the crayfish *Cambarus bartoni. Pharmacol. Biochem. Behav.,* 9:593–595.
7. Caulford, P. G., and Coceani, F. (1977): Microiontophoresis of 5-hydroxytryptamine, epinephrine, and prostaglandin E_1 on spinal neurons in the frog. *Can. J. Physiol. Pharmacol.,* 55:293–300.
8. Clark, W. G., and Lipton, J. M. (1974): Complementary lowering of the behavioural and physiological thermoregulatory set-points by tetrodotoxin and saxitoxin in the cat. *J. Physiol.,* 238:181–191.
9. Covert, J. B., and Reynolds, W. W. (1977): Survival value of fever in fish. *Nature,* 267:43–45.
10. Crawford, I. L., Kennedy, J. I., Lipton, J. M., and Ojeda, S. R. (1979): Effects of central administration of probenecid on fevers produced by leukocytic pyrogen and PGE_2 in the rabbit. *J. Physiol.,* 287:519–533.
11. Crawshaw, L. I., and Stitt, J. T. (1975): Behavioural and autonomic induction of prostaglandin E_1 fever in squirrel monkeys. *J. Physiol.,* 244:197–206.
12. Kluger, M. J. (1979): Fever in ectotherms: Evolutionary implications. *Am. Zool.,* 19:295–304.
13. Kluger, M. J., and Rothenburg, B. A. (1979): Fever and reduced iron: Their interaction as a host defense response to bacterial infection. *Science,* 203:374–376.
14. Lipton, J. M., and Kennedy, J. I. (1979): Central thermosensitivity during fever produced by intra-PO/AH and intravenous injections of pyrogen. *Brain Res. Bull.,* 4:23–34.
15. Morse, D. E., Kayne, M., Tidyman, M., and Anderson, S. (1978): Capacity for biosynthesis of prostaglandin-related compounds: Distribution and properties of the rate-limiting enzyme in hydrocorals, gorgonians, and other coelenterates of the Caribbean and Pacific. *Biol. Bull.,* 154:440–452.
16. Myhre, K., Cabanac, M., and Myhre, G. (1977): Fever and behavioural temperature regulation in the frog *Rana esculenta. Acta Physiol. Scand.,* 101:219–229.

17. Nagai, M., and Iriki, M. (1978): Autonomic response of the fish to pyrogen. *Experientia,* 34:1177–1178.
18. Ogata, H., Normura, T., and Hata, M. (1978): Prostaglandin biosynthesis in the tissue homogenates of marine animals. *Bull. Jpn. Soc. Sci. Fish.,* 44:1367–1370.
19. Polk, D. L., and Lipton, J. M. (1975): Effects of sodium salicylate, aminopyrine and chlorpromazine on behavioral temperature regulation. *Pharmacol. Biochem. Behav.,* 3:167–172.
20. Reynolds, W. W. (1977): Fish orientation behavior: An electronic device for studying simultaneous responses to two variables. *J. Fish. Res. Board Can.,* 34:300–304.
21. Reynolds, W. W. (1977): Thermal equilibration rates in relation to heartbeat and ventilatory frequencies in largemouth blackbass, *Micropterus salmoides. Comp. Biochem. Physiol.,* 56A:195–201.
22. Reynolds, W. W. (1977): Fever and antipyresis in the bluegill sunfish, *Lepomis macrochirus. Comp. Biochem. Physiol.,* 57C:165–167.
23. Reynolds, W. W. (1979): Perspective and introduction to the symposium: Thermoregulation in ectotherms. *Am. Zool.,* 19:193–194.
24. Reynolds, W.W., and Casterlin, M. E. (1979): Behavioral thermoregulation and the "final preferendum" paradigm. *Am. Zool.,* 19:211–224.
25. Reynolds, W. W., Casterlin, M. E., and Covert, J. B. (1976): Behavioural fever in teleost fishes. *Nature,* 259:41–42.
26. Reynolds, W.W., Casterlin, M. E., and Covert, J.B. (1978): Febrile responses of bluegill *(Lepomis macrochirus)* to bacterial pyrogens. *J. Thermal Biol.,* 3:129–130.
27. Reynolds, W. W., and Covert, J. B. (1977): Behavioral fever in aquatic ectothermic vertebrates. In: *Drugs, Biogenic Amines and Body Temperature,* edited by K. E. Cooper, P. Lomax, and E. Schönbaum, pp. 108–110. S. Karger, Basel.
28. Reynolds, W. W., Covert, J. B., and Casterlin, M. E. (1978): Febrile responses of goldfish *Carassius auratus* to *Aeromonas hydrophila* and to *Escherichia coli* endotoxin. *J. Fish Dis.,* 1:271–273.
29. Reynolds, W. W., McCauley, R. W., Casterlin, M. E., and Crawshaw, L. I. (1976): Body temperatures of behaviorally thermoregulating largemouth blackbass *(Micropterus salmoides). Comp. Biochem. Physiol.,* 54A:461–463.
30. Richards, F. P., Reynolds, W. W., McCauley, R. W., Crawshaw, L. I., Coutant, C. C., and Gift, J. J. (1977): Temperature preference studies in environmental impact assessments: An overview with procedural recommendations. *J. Fish. Res. Board Can.,* 34:728–761.
31. Satinoff, E., McEwen, G. N., Jr., and Williams, B. A. (1976): Behavioral fever in newborn rabbits. *Science,* 193:1139–1140.
32. Veale, W. L., Cooper, K. E., and Pittman, Q. J. (1977): Role of prostaglandins in fever and temperature regulation. In: *The Prostaglandins, Vol. 3,* edited by P. W. Ramwell, pp. 145–167. Plenum Press, New York.

Fever, edited by James M. Lipton.
Raven Press, New York © 1980.

Extreme Pyrexia in Man

Harvey B. Simon

*Infectious Disease Unit and Department of Medicine, Massachusetts General Hospital
and Harvard Medical School, Boston, Massachusetts 02115*

Ever since antiquity fever has been recognized as a cardinal manifestation of disease. Clinically accurate temperature measurements have been performed for about 100 years, and during this time many careful observations of the febrile response to infectious and noninfectious diseases have been devoted to the diagnostic evaluation of febrile illnesses; hence "fever of unknown origin" has become a classic exercise in differential diagnosis. Over the past 30 years, however, great strides have been made in the understanding of the pathogenesis of fever; the elegant studies presented in this volume provide a stimulating review of what is now known about the origins of fever.

The early clinical studies of fever devoted substantial effort to categorizing fever "patterns." Attempts were made to classify illnesses into those producing intermittent, remittent, sustained, or relapsing fevers, and the natural history of clinical recovery was divided into defervescence by lysis or by crisis. At the present time such terminology is of little practical use, for in most patients antipyretics alter the pattern of fever, antibiotics or other treatments alter the course of the underlying disease, and obviously much more accurate diagnostic information is available. Although the use of fever patterns in diagnosis is obsolete, some of the early observations of high fever have continued to influence current beliefs about the significance of extreme pyrexia in man. The classic studies of Wünderlich in 1868 provided the basis for the doctrine that temperatures in excess of 41.1°C (106°F) are rare (10). Moreover, it is believed that a hypothalamic "set-point" prevents body temperature from rising above 41°C in man (1,10). As a result, although infection is surely the most common cause of clinical fever, extreme pyrexia in man has been regarded as a manifestation of thermoregulatory failure rather than of infection or other inflammatory states.

My plan in this consideration of extreme pyrexia in man is first to review briefly the clinical aspects of normal thermoregulatory control mechanisms. Next, I will consider the differentiation between pyrexia due to thermoregulatory failure and fever due to infection and other inflammatory states; although these causes of fever can be distinguished on the basis of physiologic measurements, clinical differentiation is not possible on the basis of the magnitude of the temperature elevation alone. I will then review some of the specific syndromes of thermoregulatory failure which can produce dramatic examples of extreme pyrexia.

Finally, I will evaluate some of the consequences of extreme pyrexia and discuss the physiologic management of patients with high fever.

THERMOREGULATORY MECHANISMS: CLINICAL CONSIDERATIONS

Although other contributors to this volume have explored the neuropharmacology of thermoregulation in detail, I would like to review the clinical aspects of thermal economy in order to provide a framework for the consideration of extreme pyrexia.

Within the limits of the diurnal cycle, body temperature is closely regulated by homeostatic mechanisms; like other warm-blooded animals, man maintains a nearly constant core temperature over a wide range of environmental temperatures. Body temperature is the product of a balance between heat production and heat loss. Heat production is the result of all metabolic processes. At rest, liver, heart, and skeletal muscle account for the bulk of heat production, whereas the much greater thermal by-product of exercise is due to increased muscular activity. Even at rest the amount of heat produced is considerable, amounting to 1 cal/kg body weight/hr. Thus if no heat were lost, body temperature would rise about 1°C/hr. Heat is dissipated at the body surfaces, with the skin accounting for about 90% of the heat loss and the lungs contributing most of the remainder.

In man, only heat loss by radiation and evaporation are under significant homeostatic control. Surface temperature can be varied over a tremendous range, largely by alterations in cutaneous blood flow. Hence the amount of heat lost to the environment by radiation can be controlled by neural alteration of cutaneous blood flow. But as the environmental temperature approaches body temperature, heat cannot be dissipated by radiation or convection. Heat loss by evaporation is then the dominant factor. Even at rest without obvious sweating, heat loss by the evaporation of insensible perspiration accounts for 25% of the basal heat loss. In response to thermal stress, the rate of sweat production can increase enormously, up to 1.1 liters/hr, which, if entirely evaporated, would dissipate 900 Cal. Obviously the ability to dissipate heat by evaporation depends on the ambient humidity.

Looking at the other side of the coin, heat can be conserved by cutaneous vasoconstriction and cessation of sweating. Increased heat production depends primarily on skeletal muscle, either in the form of an imperceptible increase in muscle tension or by overt shivering. Shivering is under the control of the somatic nervous system, but this function is unconscious and automatic.

The preoptic nucleus of the anterior hypothalamus functions as a thermostat. In response to surface cooling and/or to declining core temperature (the temperature of blood perfusing the hypothalamus), the thermoregulatory center can drive cutaneous vasoconstriction, an autonomic response, and reduce the rate of heat lost to the environment. When more drastic cold stress occurs, the somatic nervous system is brought into play to generate heat via shivering. On the other hand, rising core temperature is the main stimulus to heat dissipation. Again, the autonomic nervous system is crucial to thermocontrol as it mediates heat loss through cutaneous vasodilatation and sweating.

The anterior hypothalamus, then, functions both as a thermal sensor and as a thermal control center. In a sense, it uses the rest of the body to maintain its own temperature. Accordingly, core temperature is much more constant than surface temperature—and is much more important to measure accurately. For clinical purposes, rectal temperature is used as an accurate approximation of "core" temperature. Oral temperature measurements are acceptable but they are generally slightly lower than rectal values and they are more variable. For precise physiologic measurements, tympanic membrane temperature is most accurate.

Thermoregulatory control mechanisms are ordinarily extremely effective in maintaining body temperature within the normal range. In fact, most clinical fever is due not to a failure of thermoregulation, but to an upward resetting of the hypothalamic set-point. In these situations, infection or other inflammatory states stimulate the production and release of endogenous pyrogen by phagocytic leukocytes (9). Endogenous pyrogen (EP) is carried in the systemic circulation to the central nervous system. The preoptic nucleus of the anterior hypothalamus responds to EP by raising its thermal set-point. Thermal control mechanisms are then brought into play so that body temperature is regulated around this new higher setting.

The clinical signs and symptoms of fever can be readily understood on the basis of these physiologic control mechanisms. Some patients with fever are completely asymptomatic. More common is a sensation of warmth or flushing, usually with malaise and fatigue. Myalgias are common and may be severe. These are probably best explained by the fact that in order to raise body temperature to its new set-point, the hypothalamus, via somatic efferents, increases muscle tone and this may be painful. These same factors account for one of the most dramatic manifestations of fever, the shaking chill or rigor. It is taught that rigor is a manifestation of bacteremia, but in fact any stimulus which raises the hypothalamic set-point rapidly may produce a rigor. Patients experiencing a rigor exhibit uncontrolled violent shaking and trembling and characteristically heap themselves with blankets even as their temperatures are rapidly rising. This phenomenon also has a physiologic basis. Despite the high central or core temperature, these patients subjectively feel cold because surface temperature is reduced. In order to generate fever in response to hypothalamic stimuli, cutaneous vasoconstriction occurs, skin temperature falls, and cold receptors in the skin sense the reduction in local temperature. Quite the reverse occurs during defervescence—body temperature falls in response to cutaneous vasodilatation, and drenching sweats typically terminate an episode of fever.

ETIOLOGIES OF EXTREME PYREXIA: INFECTIONS VERSUS THERMOREGULATORY FAILURE

In can be readily appreciated that patients with fever due to infection and other inflammatory states have intact thermoregulatory control mechanisms—in fact, they develop fever precisely because these mechanisms raise body temperature to the hypothalamic set-point which has been elevated by the action of endogenous pyrogen. It has been demonstrated that patients with clinical fever of this type are able to utilize homeostatic mechanisms to defend the elevated set-point against environmental stress (25). Hence physical cooling with alcohol sponging, hypothermic mattresses, or ice is likely to provoke further vasoconstriction and shivering. In contrast, aspirin or acetaminophen act on central thermoregulatory mechanisms, either as competitive antagonists of endogenous pyrogen or as inhibitors of PGE synthesis. As a result aspirin and acetaminophen lower the elevated set-point and thus stimulate vasodilatation, sweating, and cooling.

Hyperthermia due to thermoregulatory failure is quite different physiologically (25). In these circumstances, elevated body temperature results from a new excess of heat production relative to heat dissipation. Such an imbalance may result from increased heat production, defective heat dissipation, hypothalamic dysfunction, or a combination of these factors. Because the primary problem in these patients is defective thermoregulation, physical cooling would be expected to be more effective than antipyretic drugs. Table 1 outlines some of these thermoregulatory disorders.

From a physiologic viewpoint, one can differentiate elevated body temperature due to infection or inflammation from that caused by thermoregulatory failure, and thermal physiologists define the former as "fever" and the latter as "hyperthermia." As noted previously, extreme elevations of body temperature are generally attributed to defective thermoregulation (1,10,25). A standard text (14) states that "Hyperthermia—temperatures in excess of 41.1°C (106°F)—is rarely

TABLE 1. *Failures of thermoregulation*

Increased heat production	Exercise hyperthermia
	Thyrotoxicosis
	Pheochromocytoma
	Malignant hyperthermia of anesthesia
Decreased heat dissipation	Heat stroke
	Drug toxicity (atropine)
	Autonomic dysfunction
	Dehydration
	Occlusive dressings
Hypothalamic disorders	Infections (granulomas, encephalitis, etc.)
	Tumor, trauma, vascular insults
	Drugs (phenothiazines)

caused by infection." But can the clinician rely on the height of his patient's fever to distinguish between infection and thermoregulatory failure?

In an attempt to elucidate the causes of extreme pyrexia in man, 28 patients with temperatures in excess of 41.1°C (106°F) were studied (23). All were hospitalized at the Massachusetts General Hospital between 1970 and 1975. The group contained 23 males and 5 females, ranging in age from 6 to 74 (mean, 39) years. All had documented rectal temperatures between 41.4 and 42.2°C (106 to 108°F) with a mean of 41.4°C (106.6°F). In 39% infection was the sole identifiable cause of fever, whereas thermoregulatory failure was the sole etiology in only 18%. Both infection and thermoregulatory defects could be implicated in 32% of these patients, and in a final 10% no diagnosis could be firmly established.

In total, 71% of these 28 patients with extreme pyrexia had active infections at the time of diagnosis. In the great majority the infections were severe, including 12 patients with bacteremia; 3 with pyelonephritis; 2 with pneumonia; and 1 each with mediastinitis, malaria, viral encephalitis, and miliary tuberculosis. Gram-negative bacilli were the etiologic agents in 80% of these infections.

Potential thermoregulatory defects were present in 50% of these patients with extreme pyrexia, but severe infection was also present in 9 of these 14 patients. Impaired heat dissipation was the most common problem: three patients had heatstroke, four had burns requiring extensive occlusive dressings, and three had neurologic diseases leading to significant autonomic dysfunction which might impair cutaneous vasodilatation or sweating. Although cases of extreme pyrexia were seen throughout the year, elevated ambient temperatures may have contributed to fever by impeding heat loss in some patients, since 64% of these cases occurred in the three summer months. In three patients with intracranial hemorrhage and one with encephalitis, hypothalamic dysfunction seemed likely, but "central" fever was not proved in any of these individuals. No cases of extreme pyrexia due to excessive heat production were recognized; however, cases of extreme pyrexia due to thyroid storm and malignant hyperthermia of anesthesia have been encountered since this study.

Children are generally considered to be more thermolabile than adults. In one study (26) of 108 children with temperatures exceeding 40°C (104°F), only 2 had fevers above 41.1°C (106°F). However, in a large study of febrile children seen in the Yale–New Haven Hospital emergency ward (18), 100 children with temperatures in excess of 41.1°C (106°F) were identified. Of these patients, 56% were under 2 years of age and only 14% were older than 5 years. Although thermoregulatory defects were not specifically sought in this group, 63% were found to have infections, 37% had no clear diagnosis, and primary heat control defects were not recognized. The infections in these children with extreme pyrexia were serious and included bacterial meningitis, bacteremia, pneumonia, and otitis media.

Although these studies may be biased because only patients at urban university hospitals were included, it seems clear that extreme pyrexia in both children and adults results more often from infection than from defective thermoregulation. Although the true incidence of extreme pyrexia cannot be calculated, it is not a rare problem in current clinical practice. The height of the temperature does not allow differentiation of the "fever" of infection from the "hyperthermia" of defective thermoregulation, and these distinctions seem better suited to physiologic study than to the bedside practice.

THERMOREGULATORY DEFECTS: SELECTED SYNDROMES

If thermoregulatory defects are uncommon causes of fever, they are important nonetheless, both because of the dramatic fever which results and because urgent therapy is required in these high mortality situations. Table 1 classifies these syndromes according to the underlying homeostatic defect; although these are complex problems with mixed or incompletely defined physiologic bases in many instances, this simplified scheme may prove useful for clinical discussion.

Increased Heat Production

Malignant hyperthermia of anesthesia (2) is one of the most dramatic causes of fever in man. Although the syndrome was not described until 1962, over 600 cases have been reported. Estimates of the frequency of malignant hyperthermia have varied widely, but 1 occurrence in 14,000 instances of general anesthesia is a reasonable figure.

In the typical patient, administration of a muscle relaxant such as succinylcholine results in muscular rigidity. After subsequent administration of an anesthetic via inhalation there is an abrupt rise in body temperature, which may occur immediately or after a delay of several hours. Body temperature can rise with extreme rapidity and often exceeds 41.4°C (106°F); temperatures above 45°C (113°F) have been documented. About two-thirds of the patients exhibit marked muscular rigidity. Other clinical features present in most cases include tachypnea, cyanosis, hypotension, and ventricular arrhythmias. Laboratory findings include hypoxia, hypercarbia, and acidosis. Hyperkalemia occurs early and is usually severe. Other abnormalities which are recognized later include elevated muscle enzyme levels, myoglobinuria and acute renal failure, and disseminated intravascular coagulation.

The primary disorder in malignant hyperthermia of anesthesia is in skeletal muscle (3). Although details of the pathogenesis of this syndrome are still under study, it is known that a genetically determined defect in muscle metabolism permits anesthetic agents to produce abnormally high myoplasmic calcium concentrations. Elevated muscle calcium levels in turn produce increased muscle contraction, increased catabolism of muscle glycogen, and uncoupling of oxidative phosphorylation. The net result is increased heat production. As a secondary phenomenon, vasoconstriction may impair heat dissipation.

Although the elevated temperature of malignant hyperthermia is clearly secondary to the muscle disorder, hyperthermia *per se* contributes to the mortality of this syndrome. Therapy includes immediate and vigorous physical cooling; ice packs and cool intravenous fluids are the mainstays of cooling, but iced gastric lavage has also been advocated, and in one patient heroic intervention with emergency cardiopulmonary bypass was necessary to control pyrexia (22). In addition to cooling, it is equally important to halt the administration of anesthesia; to hyperventilate the patient with 100% oxygen; and to correct hyperkalemia, acidosis, and hypovolemia. Drugs such as procaine and dantrolene which lower myoplasmic calcium have been therapeutically useful in the porcine model of malignant hyperthermia (3). Even with vigorous therapy, however, mortality exceeds 30%. Clearly the best treatment is prevention. Numerous methods for the identification of susceptible individuals are available (19) but a reliable, simple, and noninvasive screening test is not yet available.

A variety of *hormonal mechanisms* are involved in thermal economy, and various endocrinologic disorders can produce clinical fever (24). Of these, only two can produce extreme pyrexia, and in both excessive heat production is an important mechanism.

Thyroid storm has been aptly called an exaggerated state of hyperthyroidism. Thyroid hormone is calorigenic, probably through stimulation of the membrane-bound sodium-potassium ATPase (sodium pump) (16). Heat intolerance and an elevated basal metabolic rate are common in hyperthyroidism. The incidence of fever in thyrotoxicosis is unknown, but fever may occasionally be the present-ing symptom of hyperthyroidism (24). However, such fever is generally low grade because heat dissipation is increased via cutaneous vasodilatation and increased sweating. In contrast, patients with thyroid storm are all highly febrile, and temperatures in excess of 41°C (106°F) are not rare. The mechanism for the high fever is not entirely clear, since concentrations of thyroid hormone in patients with "storm" do not necessarily exceed hormone levels in patients with ordinary thyrotoxicosis (4). The high fever in thyroid storm may depend on the presence of a concomitant illness and/or a failure of heat-dissipating mechanisms.

Thyroid storm almost always occurs in patients with previously uncontrolled thyrotoxicosis (15). Storm usually begins abruptly and typically follows some major stress such as infection, trauma, or surgery. Clinical features typically include exophthalmos, goiter, and moist fine skin. Tachycardia is universal and arrhythmias and congestive heart failure are common. Other findings may in-clude muscle weakness and wasting and diarrhea. Neurologic abnormalities range from tremor, to confusion or delerium, to coma.

Laboratory findings of thyroid storm include elevated levels of thyroid hor-mone. Treatment must be directed at the thyroid (15) and includes iodine to prevent hormone release and antithyroid drugs to prevent hormone synthesis. The peripheral effects of thyroxin can be blocked with propranolol. Intravenous glucose and therapy with digitalis, diuretics, vitamins, and steroids are often employed. If extreme pyrexia is present, physical cooling should be undertaken and antipyretic drugs should be administered. Even with vigorous therapy the mortality of thyroid storm is about 10%.

Another thyroid disorder in which fever is common is *sabacute thyroiditis.* In this disorder, however, fever is due to inflammation of the thyroid gland rather than to the thermogenic effects of thyroid hormone; thyroid tenderness, elevated erythrocyte sedimentation rates, and responses to anti-inflammatory drugs are characteristic. Temperatures above 40.5°C (105°F) are rare in subacute thyroiditis (13).

Although fever is a common feature of *addisonian crisis,* extreme pyrexia is infrequent in both primary and secondary adrenal insufficiency. Patients with *pheochromocytoma* often have increased basal metabolic rates (29). Catecholamines are important for cold adaptation. Thermogenesis is enhanced, both by nonshivering mechanisms and to a lesser degree by increased muscular shivering. The mechanism of nonshivering thermogenesis is unclear; increased fat mobilization occurs through the activation of hormone-sensitive lipase in adipose tissue (5). Nevertheless, most patients with pheochromocytoma do not have prominent fever, possibly because catecholamines also increase cholinergic sweating mechanisms leading to increased heat dissipation. In occasional patients, however, pheochromocytoma can masquerade as overwhelming sepsis, presenting with high fever and tachycardia (11,20,24). Hypertension may be present initially but shock develops, possibly because of secretion of epinephrine by these tumors. Abdominal pain is common in this syndrome. In the absence of typical antecedent symptoms (paroxysmal hypertension, headache, tachycardia, sweating, nervousness, tremor, congestive heart failure, and glucose intolerance), the diagnosis of pheochromocytoma can be extremely difficult.

A final situation in which excessive heat production may lead to elevations of body temperature is *exercise hyperthermia.* The muscular activity of intensive exercise such as competitive long-distance running generates tremendous heat, often 15 to 18 times above the basal metabolic rate (21). However, in conditioned athletes heat dissipating mechanisms are extremely efficient. Cutaneous vasodilatation and especially sweating increase to match heat production. The steady state which results generally maintains constant core temperatures above 38°C, and temperatures between 39°C and 40°C are common in marathon runners (28). No deleterious effects result from exercise hyperthermia, and body temperature returns rapidly to baseline following cessation of exercise. However, if heat dissipating mechanisms are impaired (dehydration, lack of conditioning, or high ambient temperature or humidity), a very dangerous situation exists, and heatstroke may result.

Decreased Heat Dissipation

Heat stroke is by far the most important disorder resulting from impaired heat dissipation (7,8). Heatstroke represents a dramatic failure of thermoregulation. A prerequisite is high ambient temperature which prevents heat loss by radiation, and high humidity which inhibits cooling by evaporation. Direct sun exposure is not necessary. The elderly or debilitated are most often affected, but healthy young individuals may develop heatstroke following exercise, especially if fluid intake is diminished and the patient has not had an opportunity to acclimate to hot climates.

The onset of symptoms is usually abrupt. A diminution or cessation of sweating is commonly observed shortly before the onset of symptoms. Altered consciousness is an early symptom and rapidly progresses to coma; seizures may occur. Prostration and collapse are typical. Physical findings include flushed, hot, dry skin, tachycardia, and dehydration. Blood pressure is often well maintained early, but without therapy, shock develops. The increased circulatory load may precipitate congestive heart failure in the elderly. Renal failure may develop.

In heatstroke body temperature is markedly elevated; temperatures above 41.1°C (106°F) are common and elevations above 43.3°C (110°F) are well known. The prognosis is worse with higher temperatures.

Laboratory studies may be unrevealing or may include hemoconcentration and leukocytosis, azotemia, acidosis, and abnormal liver function tests and muscle enzymes. Disseminated intravascular coagulation may occur.

The pathogenesis of heatstroke is not fully understood. Most of the clinical and laboratory abnormalities have been atributed to cell damage caused by the hyperthermia itself, but the reason for thermoregulatory failure is uncertain. Failure of sweating and, hence, of heat loss, seems important. Exercise-induced increased heat production is a contributing factor in some patients.

Heatstroke is a medical emergency. The mainstay of therapy is active cooling. An ice water bath is ideal for this, but in less extreme cases a cooling mattress and ice packs may suffice. When the temperature declines to about 39°C, cooling should be stopped, for there is a danger of overshoot. The remainder of therapy is supportive: careful attention to fluid and electrolyte balance, correction of acidosis, treatment of arrhythmias, and circulatory and respiratory support. Heparin may have a role if disseminated intravascular coagulation is present. Even with maximal therapy, mortality is high.

Impaired heat dissipation can lead to hyperthermia in a variety of other conditions. For example, *dehydration* with significant volume depletion can interfere with both cutaneous vasodilatation and sweating, whereas *atropine intoxication* impedes sweating. Patients with *autonomic dysfunction* (Guillain-Barré syndrome, quadra- and paraplegics, etc.) may also have impaired thermoregulation due to their inability to control cutaneous blood flow and sweating, and these individuals are notoriously thermolabile. Finally, *occlusive dressings,* such as those required for major burn victims, can impair heat loss by radiation and evaporation. Extreme pyrexia is common in those patients, but infection is usually present as well (23).

Hypothalamic Disorders

Because thermoregulation requires the interplay of so many homeostatic mechanisms, it is not surprising that disorders of the hypothalamic "thermostat" can lead to clinical fever. A firm diagnosis of "central" fever requires detailed thermal balance studies, and these are not usually available in the clinical setting. Nevertheless, it is likely that abnormalities of the anterior hypothalamus contribute to the extreme pyrexia which may be observed following intracranial hemorrhages, cerebral infarction, or major head trauma. Less commonly, tumors, granulomatous processes, or encephalitis may affect hypothalamic integrity and result in fever. In rare instances, primary or idiopathic hypothalamic disorders may lead to spectacular neuroendocrine dysfunction and fever (27). Finally, phenothiazines have complex effects on hypothalamic thermoregulation. In some instances, phenothiazines may be therapeutically useful to treat hyperthermia, usually in conjunction with physical cooling. But these drugs can also predispose to extreme pyrexia through a variety of mechanisms. Phenothiazines may impair the hypothalamic response to high ambient temperatures, thus predisposing to heatstroke (12). In addition, these drugs can lead to muscular rigidity which increases heat production (17), and they can impair sweating and cutaneous vasodilatation because of their anticholinergic properties.

THERMAL TOLERANCE: THE CONSEQUENCES AND MANAGEMENT OF EXTREME PYREXIA

Fever is alarming to both patients and physicians, and in general, the intensity of concern is proportional to the height of the fever. In syndromes such as malignant hyperthermia of anesthesia and heatstroke there is abundant evidence of tissue damage and mortality is high. Rhabdomyolysis, endothelial damage, and neurologic injury are common in these patients. But these appear to be special circumstances in which the tissue injury is due to the underlying disorder rather than to the fever *per se*. In clinical studies of patients with extreme pyrexia of other causes (18,23) there was little evidence of direct tissue damage caused by fever itself, and mortality was related to the underlying disorder rather than to the magnitude of fever. This is in accord with the older experience of fever therapists, who found that most patients could tolerate temperatures of up to 41.7°C (107°F) for hours without tissue damage (10). Whole-body hyperthermia is now being investigated as a possible adjuvant to cancer chemotherapy. In a recent study of 14 patients with advanced malignant disease, repeated hyperthermia to 41.8°C (107°F) for up to 4 hr was generally well tolerated (6). Tachycardia and marked increases in cardiac index occurred in all patients, but there was no cardiac toxicity and blood pressure was well maintained. Laboratory abnormalities in these patients included leukocytosis, respiratory alkalosis, fall in serum magnesium and phosphate levels, and elevations of creatine phosphokinase and liver enzymes. These abnormalities were transient. Adverse symptoms included fatigue, diarrhea, and nausea; but significant toxicity in these 14 patients with widespread malignancies was limited to peripheral neuropathy in 4 patients.

Given the fact that fever itself is generally well tolerated, what is an appropriate therapeutic approach to extreme pyrexia in man? Clearly the diagnosis of and therapy for the underlying disorder are of the utmost importance; all patients must be systematically evaluated for both infections and thermoregulatory disorders which may lead to extreme pyrexia. In addition to appropriate cultures and radiographs, laboratory studies of importance include the hemogram; clotting studies; urinalysis; renal function tests; and electrolyte, muscle and liver enzyme, and arterial blood gas determinations. Studies of thyroid and adrenal function may be indicated.

The fever *per se* also mandates attention. Patients must be closely monitored for their cardiopulmonary and neurologic status. In particular, elderly individuals and those with underlying cardiac, pulmonary, or vascular disease are at risk for angina, congestive heart failure, and arrhythmias. At the other extreme of life, febrile seizures are a risk in children between the ages of 6 months and 6 years, with the highest incidence in boys between 18 months and 3 years of age. It is important to rule out underlying neurologic disorders and bacterial infections, particularly meningitis, in these patients and a lumbar puncture should be part of the evaluation in most cases. Nevertheless, the great majority of febrile seizures are benign and self-limited. Management should involve vigorous physical cooling, antipyretics, and anticonvulsants. The long-term use of prophylactic anticonvulsants in these children is controversial.

Not all febrile patients require antipyretic therapy. Basically healthy individuals with moderate fever may, in fact, be more comfortable with the fever than with its treatment; but fever should be treated in children, in elderly or debilitated patients, in individuals who are symptomatic from fever *per se,* or when body temperature exceeds the 39 to 40°C range. In patients with fever due to infection or inflammation, antipyretic drugs such as aspirin or acetaminophen are the mainstays of treatment. If a rapid reduction in body temperature is required, physical cooling should also be employed using sponging with tepid water or alcohol, hypothermic mattresses, or, in urgent circumstances, ice packs and ice water. These are all uncomfortable treatments, and should be employed only when the fever itself is truly deleterious. More elaborate methods of physical cooling (ice water gastric lavage, ice water enemas, peritoneal dialysis with cooled fluids, or administration of iced intravenous fluids) appear to offer few advantages and pose additional risks. It should be remembered that physical cooling is much more likely to succeed in patients with fever of infection if antipyretic drugs are also administered; otherwise, thermoregulatory mechanisms may be activated to maintain body temperature at the elevated level set by the hypothalamus. In contrast, patients with fever caused by primary thermoregulatory disorders should be more responsive to physical cooling than to drugs which act to lower the hypothalamic thermal set-point. Nevertheless, it would seem prudent to treat these individuals with aspirin or acetaminophen in addition to physical cooling. In all patients with extreme pyrexia, careful monitoring is needed to prevent both hypothermic overshoot and recurrent fever. Although fever may be the most spectacular symptom, meticulous attention to the underlying disorder is of paramount importance in all patients.

REFERENCES

1. Atkins, E., and Bodel, P. (1972): Fever. *N. Engl. J. Med.,* 286:27–34.
2. Britt, B. A. (1974): Malignant hyperthermia: A pharmacogenetic disease of skeletal and cardiac muscle. *N. Engl. J. Med.,* 290:1140–1142.
3. Britt, B. A. (1979): Etiology and pathophysiology of malignant hyperthermia. *Fed. Proc.,* 38:44–48.
4. Brooks, M. H., Waldstein, S. S., Bronsky, D., and Sterling, K. (1975): Serum triiodothyronine concentration in thyroid storm. *J. Clin. Endocrinol. Metab.,* 40:339–341.
5. Brück, K. (1976): Temperature regulation and catecholamines. *Isr. J. Med. Sci.,* 12:924.
6. Bull, J. M., Lees, D., Schuette, W., Whang-Peng, J., Smith, R., Bynum, G., Atkinson, E. R., Gottediener, J. S., Gralnick, H. R., Shawker, T. H., and DeVita, V. T., Jr. (1979): Whole body hyperthermia: A phase-1 trial of a potential adjuvant to chemotherapy. *Ann. Intern. Med.,* 90:317–323.
7. Clowes, G. H. A., and O'Donnell, T. F. (1974): Heat stroke. *N. Engl. J. Med.,* 291:564–567.
8. Costrini, A. M., Pitt, H. A., Gustafson, A. B., and Uddin, D. E. (1979): Cardiovascular and metabolic manifestations of heat stroke and severe heat exhaustion. *Am. J. Med.,* 66:296–302.
9. Dinarello, C. A., and Wolff, S. M. (1978): Pathogenesis of fever in man. *N. Engl. J. Med.,* 298:607–612.
10. DuBois, E. F. (1949): Why are fever temperatures over 106°F rare? *Am. J. Med. Sci.,* 217:361–368.
11. Fred, H. L., Allred, D. P., Garber, H. E., Retiene, K., and Lipscomb, H. (1967): *Am. Heart J.,* 73:149–154.
12. Greenblatt, D. J., and Greenblatt, G. R. (1973): Chlorpromazine and hyperpyrexia: A reminder that this drug affects the mechanisms which regulate body temperature. *Clin. Pediatr.,* 12:504–505.
13. Greene, J. N. (1971): Subacute thyroiditis. *Am. J. Med.,* 51:97–108.
14. Hoeprich, P. D. (1972): Manifestations of infectious diseases. In: *Infectious Diseases,* edited by P. D. Hoeprich, p. 58. Harper & Row, Hagerstown, Md.
15. Ingbar, S. H. (1966): Management of emergencies: Thyrotoxic storm. *N. Engl. J. Med.,* 274:1252–1254.
16. Ismail-Beigi, F., and Edelman, I. S. (1970): The mechanisms of thyroid calorigenesis role of active sodium transport. *Proc. Natl. Acad. Sci. U.S.A.,* 67:1071.
17. McAllister, R. G. (1978): Fever, tachycardia, and hypertension with acute catatonic schizophrenia. *Arch. Intern. Med.,* 138:1154–1156.
18. McCarthy, P. L., and Dolan, T. F. (1976): Hyperpyrexia in children. *Am. J. Dis. Child.,* 130:849–851.
19. Moulds, R. F. W., and Denborough, M. A. (1974): Identification of susceptibility to malignant hyperpyrexia. *Br. Med. J.,* 1:245–247.
20. Myers, M. G., and Arshinoff, S. A. (1977): Infection and pheochromocytoma. *J.A.M.A.,* 237:2095–2096.
21. Nadel, E. R., Wenger, C. B., and Roberts, M. F. (1977): Physiologic defense against hyperthermia of exercise. *Ann. N.Y. Acad. Sci.,* 301:98–109.
22. Ryan, J. F., Donlon, J. V., and Malt, R. A. (1974): Cardiopulmonary bypass in the treatment of malignant hyperthermia. *N. Engl. J. Med.,* 290:1121–1122.
23. Simon, H. B. (1976): Extreme pyrexia. *J.A.M.A.,* 236:2419–2421.
24. Simon, H. B., and Daniels, G. H. (1979): Hormonal hyperthermia: Endocrinologic causes of fever. *Am. J. Med.,* 66:257–263.
25. Stitt, J. T. (1979): Fever versus hyperthermia. *Fed. Proc.,* 38:39–42.
26. Tomlinson, W. A. (1975): High fever. *Am. J. Dis. Child.,* 129:693–696.
27. Wolff, S. M., Adler, R. C., Elsworth, R. B., and Thompson, R. H. (1964): A syndrome of periodic hypothalamic discharge. *Am. J. Med.,* 36:956–967.
28. Wyndham, C. H. (1977): Heat stroke and hyperthermia in marathon runners. *Ann. N.Y. Acad. Sci.,* 301:128–138.
29. Young, J. B., and Landsberg, L. (1977): Catecholamines and intermediary metabolism. *Clin. Endocrinol. Metab.,* 6:199–201.

Fever, edited by James M. Lipton.
Raven Press, New York © 1980.

Management of Fever in Infants and Children

Sumner J. Yaffe

*Departments of Pediatrics and Pharmacology, University of Pennsylvania,
and Division of Clinical Pharmacology, Children's Hospital of
Philadelphia, Philadelphia, Pennsylvania 19104*

Any discussion of fever management must begin with the fundamental question of whether a febrile episode should be managed, and if so, under what circumstances and to what extent. The decision to treat or not and by which methods to treat fever in infants and children is greatly influenced by the background, experience, and point of view of the individual physician. It should be pointed out that there is a fairly broad spectrum of opinion regarding the treatment decision. Obvious initial considerations in determining whether a fever should be lowered include the magnitude of the temperature elevation, the etiology of the fever, the duration of the febrile episode, and the age and general condition of the child. Normal body temperature in infancy and childhood varies from about 36.2 to 38.0°C; a temperature of 38.9°C (102°F) should be lowered provided that the cause is other than a common infection.

Protracted fevers may be associated with serious disorders such as collagen and autoimmune diseases or malignancy. However, most fevers in infants and children are of viral origin, of relatively brief duration, and have limited consequences (24).

The argument for conservative management of fever generally embodies the following points: (a) the belief that fever in children is rarely a serious problem; (b) a concern that the treatment of fever may obliterate a sign which is of value to the physician in monitoring the course of the disease and the effectiveness of primary therapy; (c) reference to the interesting but as yet unsubstantiated possibility that fever may play a role in enhancing body defenses and/or reducing the viability of infecting organisms; and (d) the fact that drug treatment with antipyretics carries with it some risk of adverse reactions.

Counterarguments to the above points, which are cited by advocates of more aggressive fever management, can be summarized as follows: (a) Although it is agreed that fever in itself usually does not constitute a serious medical risk, the probability of febrile convulsions, particularly during the first 3 years of life, can be lessened by lowering of body temperature. (b) The relief of patient discomfort resulting from fever is an important adjunct to patient management. (c) Very high fevers may produce CNS damage and should be treated vigorously. (d) Although fever may indeed be a guide to the efficacy of primary treatment, the availability of culture and other laboratory techniques have reduced its importance as an aid to diagnosis. It should also be noted, however, that the effect of fever management measures, whether drug or non-drug, is of relatively short duration, and treatment must be repeated. It is therefore possible for the therapist to provide a "window" between antipyretic doses through which to observe the temperature pattern before resuming treatment. (e) Although some authors have noted that the replication of some viruses (16) as well as the growth of certain organisms such as gonococcus and *Treponema* are temperature sensitive (24), this sensitivity has not been found with the most common pneumococci or viruses. Conversely, the possibility of activation of herpesvirus from a latent state by febrile illness has been raised (24). To quote from the well-known publication of Atkins and Bodel (2), "Clearly, under normal circumstances of infection, the raised body temperature does not destroy the microorganisms directly." Whether any more subtle defense mechanism associated with fever can be elucidated remains to be seen, however, and although it has not been clinically obvious to this point, we would certainly agree with Atkins and Bodel that continued research is worthwhile. (f) With regard to adverse effects of fever management, it is fair to say that the risks associated with antipyretic therapy are not large, provided the proper dosage instructions are followed and other factors such as adequate hydration and nutrition are attended to. It must be pointed out that there are also potential risks and disadvantages, as well as benefits, associated with non-drug fever management techniques. Finally, it is important to note that the risk associated with drug therapy is not the same for all antipyretics.

ENVIRONMENTAL MANAGEMENT

Environmental methods of temperature lowering are based on loss of body heat through the principles of conduction, convection, radiation, and evaporation at the body surface. A number of such measures have been utilized to treat fever, including bed rest; exposure; ice packs; cold saline or water enemas; circulating fans; cooling blankets; gentle massage; and sponging with tepid water, ice water, or water/alcohol mixtures.

Bed rest is ineffective (12); also, exposure, although recommended in order to avoid further increase in temperature associated with heat-retaining clothing, is not in itself an effective temperature-lowering measure (40).

The effectiveness of sponging has been moderate in studies by two investigators. Hunter (15) found sponging with tepid water to be more effective than exposure alone, but less effective than drug treatment. Steele et al. (40) also found tepid sponging to be effective in lowering temperature, but only to about 39°C. Sponging with ice water or water/alcohol mixtures may be somewhat more effective than tepid water sponging, but there is considerable discomfort associated with both treatments (40), and there is an additional risk of acute poisoning with alcohol if adequate ventilation and close observation are not maintained (10, 25,37). It is also important to consider that the shivering which frequently results from cold applications to the skin will probably contribute to an initial rise of body core temperature from increased muscle activity (16). Water intoxication has been associated with cool enemas (44), and the enemas can be legitimately characterized, in the words of R. J. Roberts *(personal communication),* as "cruel and unusual punishment." Periodic gentle massage is a logical component of fever management, since the consequent cutaneous vasodilatation brings heat to the surface where radiative and evaporative heat loss mechanisms can operate (16).

PHARMACOLOGIC MANAGEMENT

A substantial number of compounds have been examined in animals and in man for their capacity to reduce elevated temperature, and many have demonstrated antipyretic activity. In addition, drugs which are not specifically antipyretics have been utilized adjunctly in fever management. Chlorpromazine, for example, has been administered to suppress shivering and provide some peripheral vasodilatation when ice blankets are used (16).

Consistent with the direct knowledge and experience of the author, this discussion of antipyretics is limited to single-entity drugs which have both primary antipyretic activity and a history of substantial use in this country, recognizing, of course, that the pattern of drug use for antipyresis differs throughout the world. A number of the more common agents with known antipyretic activity are listed by pharmacologic class in Table 1.

The pyrazoles are generally not considered useful as antipyretics because of the risk of toxicity, specifically, agranulocytosis and aplastic anemia. Phenylbutazone is widely used in adults for the short-term management of acute inflammation, but has no role in the treatment of fever in children.

The closely related compounds aminopyrine and dipyrone have a very checkered history (14). Aminopyrine was widely used throughout the world, including

TABLE 1. *Selected antipyretic agents*

Phenylpyrazoles	Newer nonsteroidal anti-inflammatory drugs	Others
Phenylbutazone (Butazolidin®)	Anthranilic acids Mefanamic acid (Ponstel®)	Salicylamide (Liquiprin[b])
Aminopyrine (amidopyrine) (Pyramidon[a])	Phenylproprionic acids Ibuprofen (Motrin®) Fenoprofen (Nalfon®) Naproxen (Naprosyn®)	Aspirin
Dipyrone (methampyrone) (Pyrilgin[a])	Indoleacetic acids Indomethacin (Indocin®)	Acetaminophen (Tylenol®)
	Pyrroleacetic acids Tolmetin (Tolectin®)	

[a] No longer marketed in the United States.
[b] Product has been reformulated.

the United States, during the 1920s and 1930s. Its use dropped sharply after a large number of cases of agranulocytosis were reported in 1935 (17), and little if any significant use of aminopyrine is known in this country today. Dipyrone was utilized, primarily in the parenteral form, until its removal from the U.S. market by the Food and Drug Administration in 1977.

Nonsteroidal anti-inflammatory agents have generally been shown to have antipyretic as well as analgesic and anti-inflammatory activity. Most drugs in this class fit into one of four basic groups: anthranilic, indoleacetic, phenylpropionic, and pyrroleacetic acids. Of the drugs listed under these headings in Table 1, only tolmetin is presently approved for use in children, in this case for the limited indication of juvenile rheumatoid arthritis. Further, the relative antipyretic effectiveness of most drugs in this class has not been rigorously compared with that of standard antipyretics, and there is no rational basis to recommend their use in the treatment of routine febrile illness.

Salicylamide had been commonly used as a liquid suspension for the treatment of fever in children. However, its use declined rapidly after the most widely distributed product was reformulated with an alternative antipyretic. The significant facts regarding salicylamide are, first, that although it is often perceived as a "liquid aspirin" by parents and some physicians, it is, in fact, not related pharmacologically to the salicylates (6); secondly, salicylamide is relatively ineffective and unreliable as an antipyretic (9). Although the relative ineffectiveness of salicylamide has not been fully explained, variable differences in salicylamide metabolism during pyrogen-induced febrile episodes have been noted (39).

This leaves us with the two agents most commonly utilized for the treatment of fever in children, aspirin and acetaminophen. In my view, the practical choice of therapy is really between these two drugs, and a full discussion of their respective characteristics is warranted.

PHARMACOKINETIC CONSIDERATIONS

Aspirin

The clinical pharmacokinetic profile of aspirin is relatively complex and subject to rather wide interpatient variability (18). Orally administered aspirin is rapidly absorbed (35) and hydrolyzed to salicylic acid. The biologic half-life for salicylate elimination from the body is approximately 3 hr (8). Anti-inflammatory and toxic effects are primarily associated with the salicylate moiety, whereas aspirin *per se* is responsible for inhibition of platelet aggregation and may be a more efficacious analgesic (18).

As indicated in Fig. 1, salicylic acid, the hydrolysis product of aspirin, is eliminated from the body via a number of pathways, including conjugation with glycine, conjugation with glucuronic acid, hydroxylation to gentisic acid, and renal excretion by glomerular filtration and tubular excretion (18,42). Elimination kinetics are complicated by the fact that the two most important metabolic pathways (1a and 2a in Fig. 1) are easily saturated at subtherapeutic aspirin

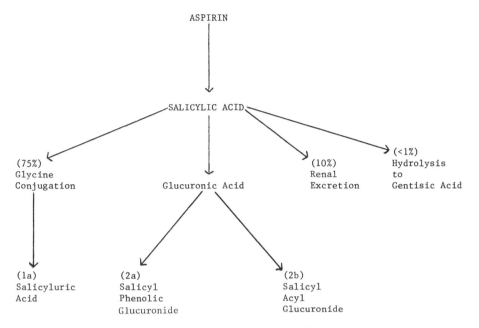

FIG. 1. Aspirin biotransformation pathways.

dosage levels (23). It has been noted that the administration of any drug at dosing intervals congruent with its half-life will produce a doubling of drug concentrations at steady-state levels. In the case of aspirin, the half-life itself, the steady-state plateau level, and the plasma levels of free (non-protein-bound) salicylate all increase as doses exceed the relatively low saturation level, and an exponential increase in circulating blood levels (and amount in the body) may result (8,18). This phenomenon may be further exaggerated by changes in urine pH (4,21,22), acidosis (5), age (19), or dehydration (7). Thus the net result of too frequent or excessive dosing can be therapeutic aspirin poisoning.

Therapeutic misuse of aspirin is not an uncommon event, and although acute aspirin poisonings from accidental ingestion have declined substantially since the introduction of safety closures, therapeutic poisonings have become more prominent (7). One review indicated that approximately 50% of pediatric aspirin poisonings and over 80% of the resultant deaths were due to therapeutic overdosage rather than acute accidental ingestion (41).

Acetaminophen

The other important drug in the management of fever, acetaminophen, has a pharmacokinetic profile somewhat less complex than that of aspirin. Peak plasma levels occur within 30 to 60 min following oral administration in children (43). The plasma half-life is in the range of 1 to 3.5 hr in children and somewhat longer in neonates (33).

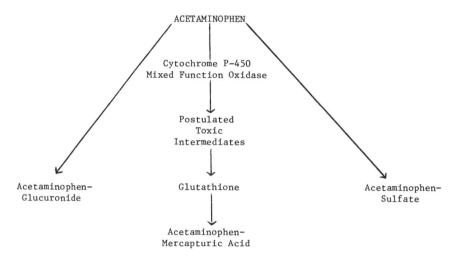

FIG. 2. Acetaminophen biotransformation pathways. (Adapted from Mitchell et al., ref. 30.)

The acetaminophen biotransformation pathways which have been proposed for adults (30,33) are shown in Fig. 2. Studies indicate that the glucuronide metabolite may predominate in adults (1,20,27), whereas the sulfate metabolite is more prominent in infants and children (20,27); however, there appears to be no difference in total elimination rate across age groups (33). Plasma protein binding does not occur at therapeutic dosage levels (11). In adults, hepatic toxicity following substantial intentional acetaminophen overdosage has been reported; however, toxic ingestion in children has been relatively rare. Adult toxicity is believed to be associated with a minor metabolite, mediated by a cytochrome P-450 mixed-function oxidase (29,33). This metabolite is normally conjugated with glutathione and eliminated without serious consequence. However, when massive amounts of acetaminophen are ingested, e.g., for suicidal purposes by adults, glutathione is depleted, and the arylating metabolite binds covalently to liver protein, producing hepatic necrosis (29). It is possible that the rarity of pediatric toxicity is due to a difference in the formation of this metabolite in the young age group.

Finally, very recent work with human isolated fetal liver cells suggests that the fetal liver has the ability to oxidize acetaminophen to an active metabolite at about one-tenth the rate of the adult liver, as well as to detoxify acetaminophen by conjugation (34). The clinical significance of this metabolic capability by the fetus is unknown.

Comparative Clinical Efficacy and Safety of Aspirin and Acetaminophen

Both aspirin and acetaminophen lower temperature by altering the response of the hypothalamus to pyrogens. Possible antipyretic mechansims include inhibition of the synthesis of pyrogenic prostaglandins (28) and suppression of the release of pyrogens from leukocytes (2,24).

Acetaminophen and aspirin have both demonstrated significant antipyretic effects in controlled trials in children, and there has been no marked difference in antipyretic effectiveness in most investigations. In general, studies have indicated a slightly greater maximum temperature change with acetaminophen, a similar time of maximum effect, and a somewhat longer duration of effect with aspirin (24).

With regard to safety, acetaminophen has an extremely low toxic potential, and adverse effects at therapeutic dosages are quite rare. The risk of serious hepatic injury following massive overdosage of acetaminophen is real and should be of concern to the physician, although the data suggest that children are less vulnerable to the effects of acetaminophen overdose. There has been only one documented pediatric fatality due to acetaminophen overdosage alone in this country over the entire history of its medical use (31,36), and this occurred following administration of 11 times the recommended dose over a 24-hr period.

Aspirin, on the other hand, remains a leading cause of childhood poisoning deaths (7) and has a number of additional undesirable characteristics including effects on the hemostatic mechanism (26,32) and the potential for producing gastric mucosal injury (3,13). This does not negate the efficacy of aspirin as an antipyretic; it does, however, emphasize the need for physician and parent awareness of the potential for salicylate toxicity.

The toxic potential of aspirin has prompted some investigators to evaluate a combination of aspirin and acetaminophen in the treatment of febrile children. In one study, concurrent administration of full doses of aspirin and acetaminophen resulted in a more sustained but not greater reduction in temperature (40). In a second study the combination was more effective than either drug alone (38). The efficacy of alternate dosing with aspirin and acetaminophen has not yet been documented. While there is a rational basis for the use of this approach, the potential for parent confusion and resultant dosing errors poses a practical problem which must be considered.

On balance, acetaminophen should probably be the drug of choice for antipyresis, particularly in infants, except where the anti-inflammatory effect of aspirin is clearly required in the management of the patient.

REFERENCES

1. Alam, S. N., Roberts, R. J., and Fischer, L. J. (1977): Age-related differences in salicylamide and acetaminophen conjugation in man. *J. Pediatr.,* 90:130–135.
2. Atkins, E., and Bodel, P. (1972): Fever. *Physiol. Med.,* 286:27–34.
3. Bergman, G. E., Phillipidis, P., and Naiman, J. L. (1976): Severe gastrointestinal hemorrhage and anemia after therapeutic doses of aspirin in normal children. *J. Pediatr.,* 88:501–503.
4. Davison, C. (1971): Salicylate metabolism in man. *Ann. N.Y. Acad. Sci.,* 179:249–268.
5. Done, A. K. (1968): Treatment of salicylate poisoning: Review of personal and published experiences. *Clin. Toxicol.,* 1:451–467.
6. Done, A. K. (1972): Antipyretics. *Pediatr. Clin. North Am.,* 19:167–177.

7. Done, A. K. (1978): Aspirin overdosage: Incidence, diagnosis, and management. *Pediatrics,* [*Suppl.*], 62:890–897.
8. Done, A. K., Yaffe, S. J., and Clayton, J. M. (1979): Aspirin dosage for infants and children. *J. Pediatr. (in press).*
9. Eden, A. N., and Kaufman, A. (1967): Clinical comparison of three antipyretic agents. *Am. J. Dis. Child.,* 114:284–287.
10. Garrison, R. F. (1953): Acute poisoning from use of isopropyl alcohol in tepid sponging. *J.A.M.A.,* 152:317–318.
11. Gazzard, B. G., Ford-Hutchinson, A. W., and Smith, M. J. H. (1973): The binding of paracetamol to plasma of man and pig. *J. Pharm. Pharmacol.,* 25:964–967.
12. Gibson, J. P. (1956): How much bed rest is necessary for children with fever? *J. Pediatr.,* 49:256–261.
13. Haslam, R. R., Ekert, H., and Gillam, G. L. (1974): Hemorrhage in a neonate possibly due to maternal ingestion of salicylate. *J. Pediatr.,* 84:556–557.
14. Huguley, C. M. (1964): Agranulocytosis induced by dipyrone, a hazardous antipyretic and analgesic. *J.A.M.A.,* 189:938–941.
15. Hunter, J. (1973): Study of antipyretic therapy in current use. *Arch. Dis. Child.,* 48:313–315.
16. Keusch, G. T. (1976): Fever. To be or not to be. *N.Y. State J. Med.,* 76:1998–2001.
17. Kracke, R. R., and Parker, F. P. (1935): Relationship of drug therapy to agranulocytosis. *J.A.M.A.,* 105:960–966.
18. Levy, G. (1978): Clinical pharmacokinetics of aspirin. *Pediatrics* [*Suppl.*], 62:867–872.
19. Levy, G., and Garrettson, L. K. (1974): Kinetics of salicylate elimination by newborn infants of mothers who ingested aspirin before delivery. *Pediatrics,* 53:201–210.
20. Levy, G., Khanna, N. N., Soda, D. M., Tsuzuki, O., and Stein, L. (1975): Pharmacokinetics of acetaminophen in the human neonate: Formation of acetaminophen glucuronide and sulfate in relation to plasma bilirubin concentration and *d*-glucaric acid excretion. *Pediatrics,* 55:818–825.
21. Levy, G., Lampman, T., and Kamath, B. L. (1975): Decreased serum salicylate concentrations in children with rheumatic fever treated with antacid. *N. Engl. J. Med.,* 293:323–325.
22. Levy, G., and Leonards, J. R. (1971): Urine pH and salicylate therapy. *J.A.M.A.,* 217:81.
23. Levy, G., Tsuchiya, T., and Amsel, L. P. (1972): Limited capacity for salicyl phenolic glucuronide formation and its effects on the kinetics of salicylate elimination in man. *Clin. Pharmacol. Ther.,* 13:258–268.
24. Lovejoy, F. H., Jr. (1978): Aspirin and acetaminophen: A comparative view of their antipyretic and analgesic activity. *Pediatrics* [*Suppl.*], 62:904–909.
25. McFadden, S. W., and Haddow, J. E. (1969): Coma produced by topical application of isopropanol. *Pediatrics,* 43:622–623.
26. Mielke, C. H., Heiden, D., Britten, A. F., Ramos, J., and Flavell, P. (1976): Hemostasis, antipyretics and mild analgesics: Acetaminophen vs. aspirin. *J.A.M.A.,* 235:613–616.
27. Miller, R. P., Roberts, R. J., and Fischer, L. J. (1976): Kinetics of acetaminophen elimination in newborns, children, and adults. *Clin. Pharmacol. Ther.,* 19:284–294.
28. Milton, A. S., and Wendlandt, S. (1971): Effects on body temperature of prostaglandins of the S, E and F series on injection into the third ventricle of unanesthetized cats and rabbits. *J. Physiol. (Lond.),* 218:325–336.
29. Mitchell, J. R., Jollow, D. J., Potter, W. Z., Gillette, J. R., and Brodie, B. B. (1973): Acetaminophen-induced hepatic necrosis: I. Role of drug metabolism. *J. Pharmacol. Exp. Ther.,* 187:211–217.
30. Mitchell, J. R., Thorgeirsson, S. S., Potter, W. Z., Jollow, D. J., and Keiser, H. (1974): Acetaminophen-induced hepatic injury: Protective role of glutathione in man and rationale for therapy. *Clin. Pharmacol. Ther.,* 16:676–684.
31. Nogen, A. G., and Brenner, J. E. (1978): Fatal acetaminophen overdosage in a young child. *J. Pediatr.,* 92:832–833.
32. Pearson, H. A. (1978): Comparative effects of aspirin and acetaminophen on hemostasis. *Pediatrics,* [*Suppl.*], 62:926–929.
33. Peterson, R. G., and Rumack, B. H. (1978): Pharmacokinetics of acetaminophen in children. *Pediatrics* [*Suppl.*], 62:877–879.
34. Rollins, D. E., von Bahr, C., Glaumann, H., Moldeus, P., and Rane, A. (1979): Acetaminophen: Potentially toxic metabolite formation by human fetal and adult liver microsomes and isolated human fetal liver cells. *Manuscript in preparation.*

35. Rowland, M., Riegelman, S., Harris, P. A., and Sholkoff, S. D., (1972): Absorption kinetics of aspirin in man following oral administration of an aqueous solution. *J. Pharm. Sci.,* 61:379–385.
36. Rumack, B. H. (1978): Aspirin versus acetaminophen: A comparative view. *Pediatrics [Suppl.],* 62:943–946.
37. Senz, E. H., and Goldfarb, D. K. (1958): Coma in a child following use of isopropyl alcohol in sponging. *J. Pediatr.,* 53:323.
38. Similia, S., Keinanen, S., and Kouvalainen, K. (1975): Oral antipyretic therapy: Evaluation of Benorylate, an ester of acetylsalicylic acid and acetaminophen. *Eur. J. Pediatr.,* 121:15–20.
39. Song, C. S., Gelb, N. A., and Wolff, S. M. (1972): The influence of pyrogen-induced fever on salicylamide metabolism in man. *J. Clin. Invest.,* 51:2959–2966.
40. Steele, R. W., Tanaka, P. T., Lara, R. P., and Bass, J. W. (1970): Evaluation of sponging and of oral antipyretic therapy to reduce fever. *J. Pediatr.* 77:824–829.
41. Tainter, M. L., and Ferris, A. J. (1969): *Aspirin in Modern Therapy: A Review.* Sterling Drug, New York.
42. Williams, R. T. (1959): *Detoxification Mechanisms, 2nd ed.* Chapman and Hall, London.
43. Windorfer, A., and Vogel, C. (1976): Projective clinical study on the bioavailability of therapeutic doses of acetaminophen in children. *Klin. Paediatr.,* 188:430–434.
44. Ziskind, A. D., and Gellis, S. S. (1958): Water intoxication following tap water enemas. *Am. J. Dis. Child.,* 96:699–704.

Fever, edited by James M. Lipton.
Raven Press, New York © 1980.

Studies on Fever in Neoplastic Disease

Charles W. Young

Memorial Sloan-Kettering Cancer Center, New York, New York 10021

Fever is a common occurrence in patients with cancer; in some it may be the presenting or even the principal manifestation of the disease process. Although this fever often derives from an infectious complication of the neoplastic process, in many patients, particularly individuals with Hodgkin's disease, kidney cancer, or metastatic neoplasms in the liver, an infectious organism is not detectable. In these instances the fever appears to derive from a tumor product that either acts directly on the central nervous system to produce fever or induces the host's reticuloendothelial cells to produce an endogenous pyrogen. This chapter will review briefly the relationship between fever and causation in various neoplastic disorders. More extensive discussion will be devoted to studies from several laboratories on the mechanisms of pyrogen elaboration and on the changes that chronic pyrexia produces in body fluids of febrile patients with cancer.

INCIDENCE OF FEVER IN PATIENTS WITH CANCER, ITS RELATIONSHIP TO BACTERIAL OR VIRAL INFECTION

Data from serveral studies on fever and infection in cancer patients are summarized in Table 1; they are in accord with the experience of knowledgeable oncologists. At initial presentation the majority of febrile adults with acute leukemia have evidence of an infection. Although fever in chronic lymphocytic leukemia almost invariably is associated with an infectious process, chronic myelogenous leukemia may be associated with a fever of unknown origin. Patients with lymphosarcoma, a term that may include nodular lymphocytic lymphoma and diffuse well-differentiated lymphocytic lymphoma, do not usually have fever in the early phase of the disease. Febrile episodes in the patients are generally associated with infection. Although fever in Hodgkin's disease may be manifest for months or years in the absence of significant infection, in the later phases of the disorder, as the patient's immune functions deteriorate, superimposed bacterial infection is common (20). Fever is rather less common in hypernephroma than in Hodgkin's disease; it is only rarely associated with bacterial infection. In contrast, lung cancer, which produces endobronchial obstruction and pneumonia distal to the obstruction, commonly manifests with fever of infection. Patients with

TABLE 1. *Frequency of fever in patients with neoplasms and fever of unknown origin (FUO)*

Diagnosis	No. of patients	No. of episodes of fever	No. with fever of infection	No. with FUO
Acute leukemia				
Children	71	215	110 (51%)	105 (49%)
Adults	43	87	68 (78%)	19 (22%)
Chronic leukemia				
Lymphoid	10	15	15 (100%)	0
Myeloid	11	11	3 (27%)	8 (73%)
Lymphosarcoma	13	12	8 (67%)	4 (33%)
Hodgkin's disease	72	147	29 (20%)	118 (80%)
Hypernephroma	373	64	0	64 (100%)
Lung cancer	30	21	12 (56%)	9 (44%)

Compiled from data in refs. 4, 8, 9, 13, 20, 21, and 27.

cancer metastatic in the liver may become febrile only after clinically significant liver involvement is present (13).

MECHANISMS PRODUCING NONINFECTIOUS OR NONBACTERIAL FEVER IN PATIENTS WITH NEOPLASTIC DISORDERS

In all probability, the fever of neoplastic disease derives from the release in the periphery of an endogenous pyrogen similar, if not identical, to the endogenous pyrogen released by granulocytes and monocytes in fevers caused by microorganisms. Three mechanisms will be considered for such a release. (a) The endogenous pyrogen may be synthesized and released from the neoplastic cells themselves. This could represent the derepressed release of a normal protein if the neoplasm arose from phagocytic of reticuloendothelial system. The phenomenon would be analogous to the synthesis and release of insulin by islet cell neoplasms. (b) Endogenous pyrogen could arise from granulocytes and monocytes or histiocytes infiltrating a local tumor. Such inflammatory reactions are commonplace; they may be particularly prominent in renal cell carcinoma and malignant melanoma. This concept could also explain the fever associated with hepatic metastases; in this circumstance the tumor has invaded the major reticuloendothelial organ of the body. (c) Phagocytosis of antigen–antibody complexes by inflammatory cells could lead to the release of endogenous pyrogen and the occurrence of fever. It is possible that fever could arise from reaction of the reticuloendothelial system to cancer-related circulating antigen–antibody complexes. Although an attractive idea, this suggestion founders on the commonplace nature of circulating antigen-antibody complexes. They occur much more frequently than does significant pyrexia in patients with neoplastic disease (10).

ENDOGENOUS PYROGEN IN AND FROM NEOPLASMS— *IN VITRO* STUDIES

Rawlins and colleagues reported an "endogenous" pyrogen in renal cancer extracts (22). Subsequently, the late Phyllis Bodel (5,6) demonstrated the *in vitro* release of an endogenous pyrogen that produced fever in rabbits by cultures of human hypernephromas and of lymph nodes and spleen cells from patients with Hodgkin's disease. This elaboration did not require stimulation by phagocytosis of the heat-killed staphylococci. Bodel extended this work into tumor cell lines and obtained pyrogen production by three mouse histiocytic lymphoma lines, one myelomonocytic line, and two lymphoma-derived lines (7). In each case pyrogen was released spontaneously into the culture medium during growth of all cell lines with macrophage or myeloid characteristics. She concluded that these tumor cells retained the capability of producing pyrogen that is characteristic of their nonmalignant cells of origin, but that they had acquired an altered mechanism for production of pyrogen since they apparently required no initiating stimulus. Perhaps inversely, they had lost a control mechanism by which the production of pyrogen is turned off or controlled (23). Since neoplastic cells have, in considerable measure, become refractory to the mechanisms which commonly control the rate of growth, it is not surprising that the control mechanisms governing other macromolecular synthetic events could be lost as well.

When Bodel studied tumor lines of carcinomas or of viral-transformed fibroblasts, she failed to detect pyrogen in culture supernatents. She concluded that fever in patients associated with growth of carcinoma is possibly the result of host cell interactions with the tumor and with the production of pyrogen by host granulocytes, monocytes, or macrophages rather than with the release of pyrogens by the tumor cells themselves (7).

RELATION OF FEVER OF NEOPLASTIC DISEASE TO SYNTHESIS OF PROTEIN

Young and Dowling (33) demonstrated that the infusion of cycloheximide, an antibiotic known to inhibit synthesis of protein, reliably caused lysis of fever in chronically febrile patients with Hodgkin's disease and other neoplastic disorders who did not have detectable bacterial, fungal, or viral infection (Table 2). At the drug infusion rates used in the study, the drug apparently caused an acute alteration of protein metabolism in patients; plasma amino acid nitrogen rose acutely and plasma levels of muramidase and ribonuclease fell during the period of infusion. The data seemed most consistent with the prevention or production or release of an endogenous pyrogen from peripheral tissues. Subsequently, this issue has become considerably clouded by the observation of several laboratories that cycloheximide may block fever produced by exogenous administration of endogenous pyrogen (11).

TABLE 2. *Antipyretic effectiveness of cycloheximide in febrile patients with neoplastic disease*

Diagnosis	Total no. of patients	Defer- vescence	Failure	Technically inadequate
Hodgkin's disease	20	15	0	5[a]
Reticulum cell sarcoma	3	2[b]	1	0
Lymphosarcoma	3	1[b]	2[b]	0
Histiocytic medullary reticulosis	1	1	0	0
Plasma cell myeloma	1	1	0	0
Acute lymphoblastic leukemia	2	2	0	0
Miscellaneous carcinoma	5	3	2	0
Melanoma	2	0	2	0
Neuroblastoma	1	1	0	0
Spindle cell sarcoma	1	0	1	0

[a] Fever became nonpredictable in four patients; three defervesced but remained afebrile, and a fourth with staphylococcal bacteremia did not defervesce acutely but did so within 8 hr. One patient received only cycloheximide p.o., failing to respond to 0.2 mg/kg p.o. four times a day, and refused i.v. medication.
[b] Bacterial infection clinically evident in these patients only.
From Young and Dowling, ref. 33, with permission.

SERUM PROTEIN ALTERATIONS IN CHRONICALLY FEBRILE PATIENTS WITH NEOPLASTIC DISEASE

Young and colleagues (31,32,34) have demonstrated that plasma or serum from chronically febrile individuals, particularly patients febrile from Hodgkin's disease, contain trace proteins not detectable in afebrile individuals. These proteins could be demonstrated by cationic disc electrophoreses in 6 M urea-containing polyacrylamide gels (PAGE) (Fig. 1). The proteins were quantitated by densitometric scanning of stained gels. In these studies, the quantity of trace proteins present in plasma correlated well with the overall severity of Hodgkin's pyrexia, but not with the spontaneous hour-to-hour fluctuations in fever.

In further analyses of these trace proteins, Young et al. (31) demonstrated that under nondissociating conditions four of the trace protein bands appeared to circulate in physical interaction with one another and with normal serum proteins.

Preliminary studies carried out by Young, Hodas, and Franklin *(unpublished observations)* suggest a relationship between the "febrile" serum proteins as monitored by PAGE in urea and the serum precursor of amyloid A (SAA). SAA, an acute phase protein, is believed to be the precursor to tissue amyloid A deposits which characteristically occur in patients with chronic inflammatory disorders and some neoplastic conditions, particularly Hodgkin's disease (17,24). In an experimentally induced model of amyloidosis, SAA appeared to have an immunosuppressive effect, implying that the physiologic role of the material may relate to immunomodulation (3).

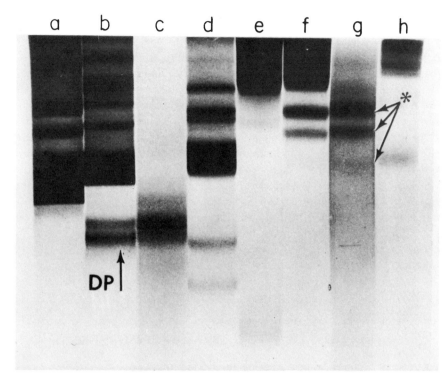

FIG. 1. Polyacrylamide gel electropherograms of: normal serum (**a, e**); febrile serum (**b, f**); partially purified fever proteins (**c, g**); cerebrospinal fluid (**d, h**). Analytical conditions, cationic polyacrylamide electrophoreses in urea-containing gels at pH 3.8 (**a–d**) and pH 6.0 (**e–h**). The sample quantities were serum, 5 μl in pH 3.8 assay and 20 μl in pH 6.0 assay; CSF, 150 μl. Coomassie blue. *, position of individual "febrile" protein bands. (Adapted from Young et al., ref. 31).

All sera which were positive in the PAGE assay showed a positive reaction with anti-AA antisera; furthermore, highly purified fractions of the PAGE febrile proteins gave a precipitin line with anti-AA. In nondissociating media at 4°C, both SAA and the PAGE-urea febrile proteins have a molecular weight of 160,000 daltons; they both interact with serum lipids (2,25,28,31). In the presence of 10% formic acid (1,28,31) they both chromatograph at a molecular weight of 12,000 daltons in gel filtration. They differ significantly in that some sera from afebrile individuals with Hodgkin's disease which had high SAA content by immunoassay did not display a low-molecular weight fragment in the PAGE-urea assay, implying the existence of a non-urea-dissociable form of SAA in afebrile individuals. A possible resolution to this apparent contradiction may reside in the observations of Linke (19), who found that when SAA-containing sera is chromatographed at 40 to 42°C (an *in vitro* equivalent of fever?) all SAA antigenic reactivity exists with an apparent 12,000 MW.

URINARY PROTEINS IN FEBRILE INDIVIDUALS

Endogenous pyrogen is a low-molecular weight protein (12) that may enter the glomerular filtrate. In a group of chronically febrile Hodgkin's patients, Sokal and Shimaoka (29) have reported urinary secretion of a pyrogenic substance with characteristics similar to those of endogenous pyrogens. Although this work has not been duplicated, the physiologic resemblance between the glomerular ultrafiltrate and the entry of protein into the extracellular spaces of the central nervous system suggests that further study in this area might be fruitful. Chronically febrile individuals develop significant proteinuria consisting of low-molecular weight proteins (34); it resembles that of tubular proteinuria seen in cadmium toxicity. Changes of lesser magnitude have recently been demonstrated in acute studies (16). Since the size of endogenous pyrogen is similar to that of proteins, such as muramidase and β_2 microglobulin, that are extensively filtered and excreted in the urine in individuals with tubular proteinurias, it is at least conceivable that in chronically febrile patients with a similar defect in tubular reabsorption of protein, the urine may provide a source for purification of human endogenous pyrogen.

OBSERVATIONS ON PROSTAGLANDIN METABOLISM IN FEBRILE INDIVIDUALS WITH NEOPLASTIC DISORDERS

The work of many laboratories has implicated arachidonic acid metabolites— either endoperoxides, prostaglandins (PG), thromboxanes, or prostacyclin—in the generation of fever following administration of pyrogenic materials (11). This concept is based on (a) the general observation that inhibitors of arachidonic acid release or of the cyclo-oxygenase system which generates endoperoxides from arachidonic acid are clinically useful antipyretics (11,15,30); (b) observation of elevated PGE_2 levels in cerebrospinal fluid of pyrogen-treated cats; and (c) pyrogenic effects of PGE derivatives when injected into thermoregulatory centers of the central nervous system (11). Clinical confirmation for this concept has not yet been forthcoming. Landaw and Young (18) examined levels of PGE and $PGF_{2\alpha}$ in the cerebrospinal fluid of febrile individuals with advanced cancer. No PGE was detectable using methods sensitive to PGE_1 concentrations of 60 pg/ml and PGE_2 concentrations of 375 pg/ml. The studies failed to demonstrate a correlation between elevated levels of $PGF_{2\alpha}$ in cerebrospinal fluid and any pathophysiologic condition including fever.

Phospholipase A_2 (PLA_2) is considered to be the controlling enzyme that releases arachidonic acid from a bound form in membrane phospholipids, thereby "triggering" the cascade that leads to formation of biologically active metabolites. A variety of substances may activate membrane-bound PLA_2 (15,26,30), possibly including endogenous pyrogen (35). Although usually membrane bound, PLA_2 has been detected in some inflammatory exudates (14).

Young and Korngold *(unpublished observations)* have initiated studies attempting to detect increased PLA_2 or PLA_2-activating substances in plasma, urine, and CSF of febrile individuals. The initial studies with ^{14}C-arachidonic acid-labeled erythrocytes have been negative.

ACKNOWLEDGMENTS

This work was supported in part by grants from the Bodman Foundation, DeDombrowski Fund, and by Grants CA 08748 and CA 15928 from the National Cancer Institute.

REFERENCES

1. Anders, R. F., Natvig, J. B., Michaelson, T. E., and Husby, G. (1975): Isolation and characterization of amyloid-related serum protein SAA as a low molecular weight protein. *Scand. J. Immunol.,* 4:397–401.
2. Benditt, E. P., and Eriksen, N. (1977): Amyloid protein SAA is associated with high density lipoprotein from human serum. *Proc. Natl. Acad. Sci. U.S.A.,* 74:4025–4028.
3. Benson, M. D., Aldo-Benson, M. A., Shirahama, T., Borel, Y., and Cohen, A. S. (1975): Suppression of an in vitro antibody response by a serum factor (SAA) in experimentally induced amyloidosis. *J. Exp. Med.,* 142:236–241.
4. Berger, L., and Sinkoff, M. W. (1957): Systemic manifestations of hypernephroma—A review of 273 cases. *Am. J. Med.,* 22:791–796.
5. Bodel, P. (1974): Pyrogen release in vitro by lymphoid tissues from patients with Hodgkin's disease. *Yale J. Biol. Med.,* 47:101.
6. Bodel, P. (1974): Tumors and fever. *Ann. N.Y. Acad. Sci.,* 230:6–13.
7. Bodel, P. (1978): Spontaneous pyrogen production by mouse histiocytic myelomonocytic tumor cell lines in vitro. *J. Exp. Med.,* 147:1503–1516.
8. Boettiger, L. E. (1977): Fever of unknown origin IV. Fever and carcinoma of the kidney. *Acta Med. Scand.,* 156:477–485.
9. Boggs, D. R., and Frei, E. III (1960): Clinical studies of fever and infection in cancer. *Cancer,* 13:1240–1253.
10. Brandeis, W. E., Helsen, L., Wang, Y., Good, R. A., and Day, N. K. (1978): Circulating immune complexes in sera of children with neuroblastoma, correlation with stage of disease. *J. Clin. Invest.,* 62:1201–1209.
11. Cranston, W. I. (1979): Central mechanisms of fever. *Fed. Proc.,* 38:49–51.
12. Dinarello, C. A. (1979): Production of endogenous pyrogen. *Fed. Proc.,* 38:52–56.
13. Fenster, L. F., and Klatskin, G. (1961): Manifestations of metastatic tumors of the liver. *Am. J. Med.,* 31:238–248.
14. Franson, R., Dobrow, R., Weiss, J., Elsbach, P., and Weglicki, W. B. (1978): Isolation and characterization of a phospholipase A_2 from an inflammatory exudate. *J. Lipid Res.,* 19:18–23.
15. Hassid, A., and Levine, L. (1977): Stimulation of phospholipase activity in prostaglandin biosynthesis by melittin in cell culture and in vivo. *Res. Commun. Chem. Pharmacol.,* 18:507–517.
16. Hemmingsen, L., and Skaarup, P. (1977): Urinary excretion of 10 plasma proteins in patients with febrile diseases. *Acta Med. Scand.,* 201:359–364.
17. Ignaczak, T. F., Sipe, J. D., Linke, R. P., and Glenner, G. G. (1977): Immunochemical studies on the nature of the serum component (SAA) related to secondary amyloidosis. *J. Lab. Clin. Med.,* 89:1092–1104.
18. Landaw, I. S., and Young, C. W. (1977): Measurement of prostaglandin $F_{2\alpha}$ levels in cerebrospinal fluid of febrile and afebrile patients with advanced cancer. *Prostaglandins,* 14:343–353.
19. Linke, R. P. (1979): Temperature-induced dissociation of serum amyloid protein SAA. *Z. Immunitaetsforsch.,* 155:255–261.
20. Lobell, M., Boggs, D. R., and Wintrobe, M. M. (1966): The clinical significance of fever in Hodgkin's disease. *Arch. Intern. Med.,* 117:335–342.

21. Raab, S. O., Hoeprich, P. D., Wintrobe, M. M., and Cartwright, G. E. (1960): The clinical significance of fever in acute leukemia. *Blood*, 16:1609–1628.
22. Rawlins, M. D., Luff, R. H., and Cranston, W. I. (1970): Pyrexia in renal carcinoma. *Lancet*, 1:1371–1373.
23. Root, R. K., Nordlund, J. J., and Wolff, S. M. (1970): Factors affecting the quantitative production and assay of human leukocytic pyrogen. *J. Lab. Clin. Med.*, 75:679–693.
24. Rosenthal, C. J., and Franklin, E. C. (1975): Variation with age and disease of an amyloid A protein-related serum component. *J. Clin. Invest.*, 55:746–753.
25. Segrest, J. P., Pownall, H. J., Jackson, R. L., Glenner, G. G., and Pollock, P. S. (1976): Amyloid A: Amphipathic helixes and lipid binding. *Biochemistry*, 15:3187–3190.
26. Shier, W. T. (1979): Activation of high levels of endogenous phospholipase A_2 in cultured cells. *Proc. Natl. Acad. Sci. U.S.A.*, 76:195–199.
27. Silver, R. T., Utz, J. P., Frei, E., III, and McCullough, N. B. (1958): Fever, infection and host resistance in aucte leukemia. *Am. J. Med.*, 24:25–39.
28. Sipe, J. B., Ignaczak, T. F., Pollock, P. S., and Glenner, G. G. (1976): Amyloid fibril protein: Purification and properties of the antigenically-related serum component as determined by solid phase radioimmunoassay. *J. Immunol.*, 16:1151–1156.
29. Sokal, J., and Shimaoka, K. (1967): Pyrogen in the urine of febrile patients with Hodgkin's disease. *Nature*, 215:1183–1185.
30. Tam, S., Hong, S. L., and Levine, L. (1977) Relationships among the steroids of anti-inflammatory properties and inhibition of formed mouse fibroblasts. *J. Pharmacol. Exp. Ther.*, 203:162–168.
31. Young, C. W., Dessources, W., and Hodas, W. (1977): Interactions between "fever" proteins and normal serum proteins in febrile cancer patients. *Cancer Res.*, 37:1356–1359.
32. Young, C. W., Dessources, W., Hodas, S., and Bittar, E. S. (1975): Use of cationic disc electrophoresis near neutral pH in the evaluation of trace proteins in human plasma. *Cancer Res.*, 35:1991–1995.
33. Young, C. W., and Dowling, M. D. (1975): Antipyretic effect of cycloheximide, an inhibitor of protein synthesis, in patients with Hodgkin's disease or other malignant neoplasms. *Cancer Res.*, 35:1218–1224.
34. Young, C. W., Hodas, S., Dessources, W., and Korngold, L. (1975): Observations on trace proteins in plasma of febrile patients by cationic disc electrophoresis in acrylamide gel at pH 3.8. *Cancer Res.*, 35:1985–1990.
35. Ziel, R., and Krupp, P. (1976): Influence of endogenous pyrogen-cerebrosprostaglandin synthetase system. *Experientia*, 32:1451–1453.

Fever, edited by James M. Lipton.
Raven Press, New York © 1980.

Hypothalamic Fever in a Human

B. Massonnet, *M. Pont, and M. Cabanac

*Laboratory of Physiology, Claude Bernard University, Faculty of Medicine of South Lyon, 69600 Oullins, France; and *Department of Internal Medicine, Faculty of Medicine of North Lyon, 69373 Lyon Cédex 2, France*

A number of cases of human "dysthermia" and "hyperthermia" due to brain disease and lesions in the hypothalamus have been reported (1,3,4,12,23). Unfortunately, knowledge of temperature regulation was not well developed at the time of these early studies, and most of the authors slanted their work toward the study of the anatomical site of hypothalamic lesions and limited their exploration of physiological responses to temperature measurement. Modern physiologists make a clear distinction between fever and hyperthermia (22). Although heat storage and the elevation of body temperature may evolve identically in both fever and hyperthermia, during fever the organism defends a high setpoint of body temperature whereas during hyperthermia the organism does its best to return to normal body temperature. Only the simultaneous measurement of deep body temperature and of thermoregulatory responses permits differentiation between fever and hyperthermia. From measurement of rectal or oral temperature alone, it is therefore not possible to differentiate between fever and hyperthermia. In addition, disesases which produce hypothalamic lesions may also be the direct cause of fever.

Atkins and Bodel (2) have recently reviewed the usual etiologies of fever. Three processes are the main sources of fever: phagocytosis, inflammation, and tumors. Most cases of dysthermia reported in the literature came under this pathology: tumoral (1,12,23,24), viral (4), and inflamatory (9,17,18). It is therefore difficult to sort out hyperthermia and fever, and, in the latter case to know whether its cause is systemic, localized, or both. The physician may be faced with a situation in which the patient defends his high body temperature and in which all possible general etiologies for this fever have been ruled out. In this case, he concludes that the patient suffers from "essential" or "central" or "hypothalamic" fever, or fever of unknown origin.

The present chapter reports the case of one patient with high body temperature, still alive. His long survival in good condition has permitted the measurement of his thermoregulatory autonomic responses, in addition to rectal temperature. The body temperature in this man appears to be regulated at a high level and we believe it to be a true hypothalamic fever.

CASE REPORT

The patient, a 40-year-old male, was admitted to the hospital in July 1973 with lung tuberculosis and alcoholism. For 6 months the patient was given intravenous tuberculosis therapy, but in December 1973 thrombophlebitis appeared in one arm, then in the other, and finally in one leg. In January 1974 endocarditis with aortic insufficiency developed. Over a year, the aortic insufficiency worsened, and tuberculosis therapy was irregular due to frequent interruptions on the part of the patient.

In December 1974 a rectal temperature of 38°C, associated with polyuria and polydipsia up to 8 liters/day, was recorded during a hospital stay. Temperature remained stable and followed a nycthemeral cycle. Pulse rate was 60 to 80 beats/min. Periodontolysis was discovered, but rectal temperature remained high even after this disease was cured. An iatrogenic fever due to antituberculosis drugs was suspected, but interruption of treatment did not lower rectal temperature. Blood examinations and complementary explorations performed during this period to investigate the permanently high rectal temperature will be found below. None of these examinations afforded an explanation of the high rectal temperature. Polyuria and polydipsia were associated with a deficit in antidiuretic hormone (ADH), and the patient was thought to have partial diabetes insipidus. Four months after second admission the patient was discharged and when he returned for a check-up 2 months later he was in good health, except for aortic insufficiency; he was afebrile and had no signs of diabetes.

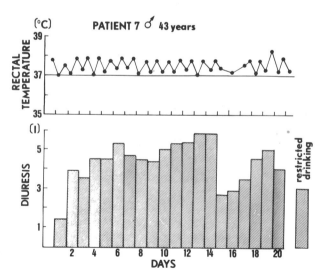

FIG. 1. A sample of rectal temperature and diuresis of the patient during 1 week in February 1976. *Right,* diuresis during a day of restricted drinking.

In October 1975 the patient had surgery to replace an aortic valve with a Lillehei and Caster prosthesis. Records from the cardiac surgery ward show no fever and no diabetes insipidus. The patient was receiving anticoagulant therapy [antivitamin K, then aspirin plus indomethacin (Indocid®)]. Regular check-ups showed that the patient was afebrile until February 1976, when he was hospitalized with disseminated intravascular clotting and brain infarct. Rectal temperature at the time of admission was 38.0°C. The patient was disoriented, aphasic, and had a right motor deficit greater in the face and arm than in the leg. He again showed polyuria and polydipsia consistent with partial diabetes insipidus. The signs of his vascular brain accident gradually faded, but rectal temperature and diuresis remained high (Fig. 1). All tests for infectious disease were negative (see below). Measurement of thermoregulatory responses were performed at this time. In November 1976 the patient left the hospital in good condition, but with moderate fever and diabetes insipidus.

In May 1977 he was hospitalized again for suspected stroke. During his hospitalization his rectal temperature averaged 37 to 38°C; urine output was 1.5 to 5.5 liters/day. When seen in February 1979, his condition was stable.

Laboratory and Radiological Data Obtained During Periods of High Rectal Temperature and Diuresis

Blood

Laboratory studies of blood samples, including sedimentation rate, fasting glucose level, and protein electrophoresis, were normal. No bacteria grew from repeated blood cultures.

Endocrinology and Metabolism

There was no glucosuria at rest and results of glucose tolerance tests were normal. Serum ACTH showed normal circadian changes. Specific gravity of the urine was less than 1.007. Two water restriction tests were done: the first during a period of diuresis averaging 8 liters/day, the second after treatment with carbomagepsine, when urine output was 4 liters/day. On both tests plasma osmolality was 295 to 405 mosmoles with ADH activity present at the 4th hr. Twenty-four hour tests of luteinizing hormone releasing hormone were normal. Thyroid secretions (T3, T4, iodine thyroxinic, TBG) were normal.

Radiography of the skull showed calcifications of the pineal gland and a normal-appearing sella turcica. A brain scan made in August 1978 showed slight distention of the ventricles and a small cyst in the left temporal lobe near the sulcus centralis. Repeated urographies were always normal. The visual field was normal. Electrocardiograms were normal except for evidence of aortic insufficiency. Bronchoscopic examination was normal.

Physiological Data

Thermoregulatory tests were performed in May 1976 at 9 A.M. The patient was immersed in a water bath while autonomic responses were recorded: thermogenetic responses by indirect respiratory calorimetry; vasomotor responses by direct calorimetry of left hand immersed in a glove perfused with water at constant flow and temperature; and evaporative responses by a sweat capsule placed on the subject's forehead. The subject gained or lost heat from or to the bath and his deep body temperature from lower esophagus was continuously recorded.

Figure 2 shows the responses obtained on the patient plotted against deep body temperature. Each response is characterized both by threshold and by slope. The magnitude and slope of the three responses are comparable to those

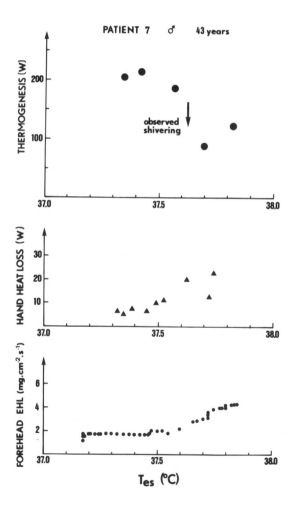

FIG. 2. Autonomic thermoregulatory responses of the patient plotted against his esophageal temperature (May 1976, 9 A.M.). **Top:** Metabolic heat production measured by respiratory calorimetry. **Middle:** Hand vasomotor response measured by direct calorimetry of the heat lost by the left hand to water. **Bottom:** Evaporative water loss in a sweat capsule placed on the forehead. The magnitude of these responses is comparable with that of normal subjects. The only difference is that the threshold for minimal responses, i.e., the set-point, is higher for the patient [between 37.5 and 37.6°C esophageal temperature (T_{es})].

of healthy control subjects. However, the thresholds for these responses (37.5 to 37.6) are higher than in healthy subjects at the same time of day.

DISCUSSION

Figure 2 shows that the internal thermostat of this patient was set, at the time of the measurement, for a body temperature higher (37.6°C) than normal. The high rectal temperature of Fig. 1 is comparable to the thresholds for the three major thermoregulatory responses, and is, therefore, the regulated deep body temperature of this patient. The fever of this patient is not different from clinical (2,10,13,14,19), emotional (15,21), and experimental fevers in humans whether the recorded response is autonomic (5,10,11,16,20) or behavioral (6,7).

Although positive diagnosis of fever is easy with the help of physiological measurements, it is not easy to reach an etiological diagnosis in this patient.

Repeated blood examinations eliminate infection as the cause of fever. The evolution of the fever and its persistence after withdrawal of drug treatment eliminate an iatrogenic genesis. A malignant tumor is also improbable because of the long survival of the patient. The only reliable signs other than the elevated rectal temperature were the ADH deficit and the moderate diabetes insipidus. It is quite striking to observe that both the diabetes insipidus and the fever evolved in parallel as regards both time and amplitude. During the 9 months' remission, both signs disappeared. The close association of fever with diabetes insipidus, a clear sign of hypothalamic disorder, renders it likely that they have a common recurrent origin. This hypothalamic fever is probably pure because in all other explored variables the patient is normal.

Davison (12) and Bauer (3) have reported cases of "dysthermia" or "hyperthermia" with nonmalignant tumors; therefore, presumably, they were nonpyrogenic *per se.*

Cambier et al. (9) observed a patient who remained in the hospital for 7 months with a hypothalamic syndrome characterized by gonadotropic, corticotropic, and ADH deficit and a complete loss of temperature regulation. The patient's temperature passively followed all changes in ambient temperature. During a previous 1-month stay in the hospital, the patient had presented the same sign as our patient: rectal temperature of 38.2°C and an ADH deficit. During his first hospital stay, thorough examinations were all normal. The patient died 1 year later, and histological examination of the brain at that time showed proliferative reticulosis localized in the hypothalamus and having a pseudo-inflammatory appearance. It is remarkable that similar etiology has been associated with thermolability and hypothalamic lesions in other cases (17,18).

ACKNOWLEDGMENTS

This work was supported by the Centre National de la Recherche Scientifique (C.N.R.S./A.T.P. "Habitat Solaire").

REFERENCES

1. Alpers, B. J. (1936): Hyperthermia due to lesions in the hypothalamus. *Arch. Neurol. Psychol.,* 35:30–42.
2. Atkins, E., and Bodel, P. (1979): Clinical fever: Its history, manifestations, and pathogenesis. *Fed. Proc.,* 38:57–63.
3. Bauer, H. G. (1954): Endocrine and other clinical manifestations of hypothalamic disease. *J. Clin. Endocrinol. Metab.,* 14:13–31.
4. Brown, J. A., Baker, A. B., and Cornwell, S. A. (1953): Polyomyelitis. Studies on temperature regulation. *Arch. Neurol. Psychiatry,* 69:332–342.
5. Buskirk, E. R., Thompson, R. H., Rubenstein, M., and Wolff, S. M. (1964): Heat exchange in men and women following intravenous injection of endotoxin. *J. Appl. Physiol.,* 19:907–913.
6. Cabanac, M. (1969): Plaisir ou déplaisir de la sensation thermique et homeothermie. *Physiol. Behav.,* 4:359–364.
7. Cabanac, M., and Massonnet, B. (1974): Temperature regulation during fever: Change of set point or change of gain? A tentative answer from a behavioural study in man. *J. Physiol. (Lond.),* 238:561–568.
8. Cabanac, M., and Massonnet, B. (1977): Thermoregulatory responses as a function of core temperature in humans. *J. Physiol. (Lond.),* 265:587–596.
9. Cambier, J., Masson, M., Urbain, E., Dairou, R., and Henin, D. (1978): Troubles de la régulation thermique et de la régulation hydrique. Processus prolifératif réticulo-granulomateux à détermination hypothalamique. *Rev. Neurol. (Paris),* 134:197–213.
10. Cooper, K. E., Cranston, W. I., and Snell, E. S. (1964): Temperature regulation during fever in man. *Clin. Sci.,* 27:345–356.
11. Cooper, K. E., Johnson, R. H., and Spalding, J. M. K. (1964): Thermoregulatory reactions following intravenous pyrogens in a subject with complete transection of the cervical cord. *J. Physiol. (Lond.),* 171:55–56P.
12. Davison, C. (1940): Disturbances of temperature regulation in man. *Proc. Assoc. Res. Nerv. Ment. Dis.,* 20:774–823.
13. Du Bois, E. F. (1948): *Fever and the regulation of body temperature.* Charles C Thomas, Springfield, Ill.
14. Fox, R. H., and Mac Pherson, R. K. (1954): The regulation of body temperature during fever. *J. Physiol. (Lond.),* 125:21P.
15. Gotsev, T., and Ivanov A. (1962): Psychogenic elevation of body temperature. *Proc. Int. Union Physiol. Sci.,* 2:501.
16. Grimby, G. (1962): Exercise in man during pyrogen-induced fever. *Scand. J. Clin. Lab. Invest.,* 14:1–112.
17. Lipton, J. M., Kirkpatrick, J., and Rosenberg, R. N. (1977): Hypothermia and persisting capacity to develop fever. *Arch. Neurol.,* 34:498–504.
18. Lipton, J. M., Payne, H., Garza, H. R., and Rosenberg, R. N. (1978): Thermolability in Wernicke's encephalopathy. *Arch. Neurol.,* 35:750–753.
19. Mac Pherson, R. K. (1959): The effect of fever on temperature regulation in man. *Clin. Sci.,* 18:281–287.
20. Park, C. R., and Palmes, E. D. (1948): The regulation of body temperature during fever. Project N°1 6 64 12 06. U.S. Army Medical Research Laboratories, Fort Knox, Ky.
21. Renbourn, E. T. (1960): Body temperature and the emotions. *Lancet,* 2:475–476.
22. Stitt, J. (1979): Fever versus hyperthermia. *Fed. Proc.,* 38:39–43.
23. Strauss, I., and Globus, J. H. (1931): Tumor of the brain with disturbance in temperature regulation. *Arch. Neurol. Psychiatry,* 25:506–522.
24. Zimmerman, H. M. (1940): Temperature disturbances and the hypothalamus. *Proc. Assoc. Res. Nerv. Ment. Dis.,* 20:824.

Fever, edited by James M. Lipton.
Raven Press, New York © 1980.

Fever of Unknown Origin

Sheldon M. Wolff and Charles A. Dinarello

*Division of Experimental Medicine, Department of Medicine, Tufts University School of
Medicine, New England Medical Center Hospital, Boston, Massachusetts 02111*

Since antiquity, physicians have described in detail the signs and symptoms
of febrile diseases. Many old descriptions of common febrile illnesses remain
accurate, and modern technology has done little to improve on these old writings.
Although accurate histories and thorough physical examinations can lead to a
diagnosis in some patients with fever, many cases require careful and thorough
investigations. When confronted with the problem of determining the cause of
a prolonged fever, one must consider the spectrum of febrile diseases which,
through the years, has changed considerably. Many factors, such as age, socioeco-
nomic factors, and geography, are important determinants of the causes of prolonged fevers. In the overwhelming majority of febrile patients, an underlying
cause is discovered or the patient recovers spontaneously. When fever continues
for 2 or 3 weeks, during which time a complete physical examination, chest
X-ray, routine blood tests, and cultures do not reveal the cause of fever, a
provisional diagnosis of fever of unknown origin (FUO) is made.

The evaluation of a patient with an FUO requires an organized, detailed
approach. Such an evaluation presupposes an awareness of the multiple causes
of fever. There have been many retrospective analyses of large groups of patients
with FUO. If three representative papers (1–3) describing FUOs in children
are analyzed, it is apparent that over one-third of all FUOs in the pediatric
age group are due to infectious diseases. Such infections in children are often
viral in origin and involve the respiratory tract. Bacterial infections are likewise
common, and the genitourinary tract is often the site of infection. Neoplastic
diseases account for approximately 10% of childhood FUOs and these often
are lymphomas or hematologic malignancies (e.g., leukemias) or tumors such
as neuroblastomas. A significant percentage (close to 20%) of children with
FUOs will have collagen vascular disease as the etiology, the most common
being juvenile rheumatoid arthritis, particularly the Still's variety. Inflammatory
bowel disease is likewise a common cause of fever of unknown origin in teenagers.
It is of note that the incidence of rheumatic fever as a cause of FUO in the
United States has decreased sharply in the last 30 years. Similarly, in most
centers tuberculosis is less commonly seen in febrile children than it previously
was.

In adults, infections are also the most common cause of FUO, representing from 35 to 40% of cases (4–8). Even today, despite the availability of antibiotics, infection predominates as the most frequently diagnosed source of persistent fever. After infections, malignant tumors are the most frequent source of FUOs in adults (about 20%). The next most common underlying cause of FUO in adults is collagen vascular disease. The incidence of such diseases in adults is approximately 15%. Thus, approximately 70% of all FUO patients will have an underlying diagnosis that falls under three categories: infectious, neoplastic, or hypersensitivity diseases. In most published series, about 20% of FUO patients will have a variety of miscellaneous causes for their fever. Such things as factitious fever or self-induced diseases (9), inherited diseases such as familial Mediterranean fever (10), disorders of thermoregulation (11), and granulomatous diseases of unknown etiology (12) all fall into the "miscellaneous" category.

In any large series of FUO patients, approximately 10% will defy extensive evaluation and continue to have fevers without a diagnosis forthcoming. Such patients require close observation and follow-up. Work-up of such patients may have to be repeated. The interval between reinvestigation of such patients is dictated by the course of illness. Thus a patient with an ongoing active debilitating illness requires earlier reevaluation than the patient with a chronic, slowly progressive course. Reevaluation of patients with chronic, long-standing (approximately 1 year) FUO can lead to a diagnosis in approximately 7 out of 10 (13). Patients with such chronic long-standing FUOs have a different spectrum of diagnosis than the usual FUO patient (12). It is to be noted that the longer the patient has an FUO, the less likely is he to have an infectious or neoplastic disease as the etiology.

During the last 20 years we have had the opportunity to see and evaluate more than 500 patients with chronic FUO. The mean duration of illness was approximately 1 year. Infections were responsible for about 6% and neoplastic diseases for about 11% of these illnesses. Granulomatous hepatitis (14) was implicated as a cause for 8% and collagen vascular disease for about 10%. In the latter group, a large number of both adults (15) and children had Still's disease. Of our patients, 9% had factitious illness (9), and a large number had an exaggerated circadian rhythm of body temperature. Any patient, particularly the young, with a "low-grade fever" and no other symptoms or signs of illness should be considered as being a normal variant (16) and only be observed for the development of some abnormality; that is to say, fever is never the only sign of disease.

A patient who has a persistent FUO despite a thorough evaluation presents a therapeutic dilemma for the attending physician. Empiric antibiotic or cytotoxic chemotherapy is not indicated. If the patient is uncomfortable and the fever is having debilitating effects, then empiric antipyretic therapy may have to be employed. We use nonsteroidal anti-inflammatory agents in such patients. We begin with high dosages of aspirin and increase them to the point at which the patient experiences relief or toxicity ensues. If such therapy fails, then we try indomethacin at dosages of up to 150 mg/day. In some patients we find it necessary to use adrenal corticosteroids. Obviously, these are used only when we are confident that there is not an infectious etiology to the fever. We begin therapy, usually with prednisone, on an around-the-clock dosage schedule. Once the symptoms are under control, the steroid dosage is rapidly tapered to an every-other-day schedule.

Many other factors are important in determining the causes of FUO, such as the type of institution in which the patient is evaluated. A tertiary care facility may see more exotic illnesses because of the nature of their referral patterns. Inner city hospitals may have a much higher incidence of infectious diseases. In the same type of hospital, patients may be elderly and more likely to have a malignancy as a cause of their FUO. Therefore, other factors such as economics, race, and geography may determine the distribution of diagnoses.

CAUSES OF FEVER OF UNKNOWN ORIGIN

Infections

It is readily apparent that any infectious agent can be the cause of a febrile illness. Although most will be obvious, self-limited, or responsive to therapy, other infectious diseases may still present as FUO. In particular, certain sites such as bone, the sinuses, heart valves, the subphrenic area, and the biliary and urinary tracts can all provide areas for infections that may not provide localizing signs. Certain types of infectious agents, such as mycobacteria, fungi (particularly the systemic mycoses), and certain parasites, may be more likely than others to present as FUO.

Malignant Neoplasms

Many patients will have fever as a manifestation of an underlying malignant tumor. It is imperative in all cancer patients to define whether an infection is the cause of the fever in these patients. Once infection has been ruled out as the primary cause of the fever, then one may be dealing with a fever as a manifestation of the underlying tumor. In some patients fever can be a prominent manifestation of progression of the disease, such as a "blast crisis" in a leukemic patient, or can occur as a secondary event, such as the fever accompanying thrombophlebitis seen more frequently in patients with certain types of cancer, e.g., of the pancreas. However, it must be emphasized that fever may be a manifestation of a malignancy long before the underlying tumor may become apparent, as occurs with malignant lymphomas. Furthermore, almost all types of tumors of any origin may produce fever even in the absence of metastases. However, some tumors are much more likely to be associated with fever and present as an FUO. Examples of the latter are both Hodgkin's and non-Hodgkin's lymphoma, hypernephroma, atrial myxoma, and hepatoma. The etiology of the fever in these conditions is unknown, although it is intriguing to speculate that these tumors are producing an endogenous pyrogen; in hypernephromas, in fact, such is probably the case (17).

Hypersensitivity Diseases

Almost all collagen vascular diseases can present as FUOs. However, systemic lupus erythematosus, Still's disease, and certain of the disseminated vasculitides are more likely to induce a febrile state. Hypersensitivity states, in particular where drugs are the allergen, may have fever as a major clinical finding. Scleroderma is one of the collagen vascular diseases that rarely, if ever, has fever as a manifestation. In fact, when we are confronted with a patient with manifestations of scleroderma and an FUO, we immediately consider that the patient has a high likelihood of having mixed connective tissue disease. Women in their sixth or seventh decades of life with an FUO, myalgias, arthralgias, and headache often have temporal arteritis. Such patients usually have an elevated blood sedimentation rate and anemia. In fact, in patients with a clinical picture compatible with polymyalgia rheumatica we often blindly biopsy a temporal artery even in the absence of clinical abnormalities of the vessel.

Granulomatous Diseases

Three major granulomatous diseases of unknown etiology often present as FUO. The most common of these is sarcoidosis. Most, but not all, sarcoid patients who present with an FUO have extrapulmonary disease, usually involving the liver. In regional enteritis, fever can sometimes be much more prominent than any gastrointestinal signs or symptoms. In our experience, granulomatous hepatitis of unknown etiology can be a relatively frequent cause of FUO. It is true that many of the well-known causes of granulomatous hepatitis (18), such as tuberculosis, sarcoidosis, and systemic fungal infections, can present as FUO. However, there is a group of patients with granulomatous hepatitis of unknown cause and FUO (14). Thus any FUO patient whose symptoms persist despite thorough noninvasive work-up should also have a liver biopsy.

Inherited Diseases

At least four inherited diseases present as FUO. The most common of these is familial Mediterranean fever (FMF), which is inherited as an autosomal recessive disorder. FMF is most common in Armenians, Sephardic Jews, and Arabs. However, it can occur in almost any ethnic group. In the latter group the diagnosis is most often missed and the patient is considered to have an FUO. In addition to fever, the patient must have serositis (usually peritonitis) during their short-lived episodes. Sometimes clinically mistaken for having FMF are patients with an inherited hyperlipoproteinemia (type 1), which is characterized by recurrent bouts of fever, abdominal pain, a family history of a similar illness, and elevated serum levels of triglyceride. In patients with Fabry's disease, an X-linked inherited error of glycosphingolipid metabolism characterized by telangiectases and lancinating pain, fever may be a prominent sign. A fourth inherited syndrome which may present as FUO is associated with deafness, urticaria, and amyloidosis (19). It should be noted that cyclic neutropenia often presents as FUO, and a small percentage of patients with this disease seem to have a familial form.

Factitious Diseases

All major hospitals, particularly tertiary care facilities, have a small number of patients each year who present with FUO and are found to have a factitious or self-induced illness. In general, these patients are young female adults in the health-related professions (9). These patients can be roughly separated into two groups. The first group are patients who feign illness by manipulating thermometers and often have a bona fide febrile illness prior to the onset of their so-called FUO. They often are seeking attention or attempting to avoid difficult or demanding situations either at home, school, or work. The second group are predominantly in the third and fourth decade of life and have more profound psychiatric problems (many are of the "borderline" type). These patients often induce disease and, in fact, can do themselves considerable harm. Such patients are in obvious need of psychiatric help, and the sooner the cause of their FUO is uncovered and they can enter a psychotherapeutic setting, the better the chance of recovery (9).

EVALUATION OF THE FUO PATIENT

The approach to the patient with FUO requires an awareness of all the potential causes of fever and a willingness to demonstrate a thoroughness and patience in the work-up that few other situations in medicine demand. Needless to say, observation of the temperature pattern can have diagnostic significance (e.g., Pel-Ebstein fever in Hodgkin's disease, the extraordinarily high fever of the thermometer manipulator). Careful attention to the history is required. Has there been any exposure to infectious agents? Any unusual travel? These and many other questions must be asked; if the answers are positive, then follow-up laboratory procedures will be required. A thorough and complete physical examination is mandatory. Furthermore, repeated attention must be paid to any changes, such as the appearance of septic phenomena in the skin, fundi, and nailbeds.

The laboratory evaluation of the patient with FUO should be logical and complete. Knowledge of the causes of fever should direct the physician towards appropriate laboratory tests. Certain tests are mandatory, such as skin tests, liver function tests, and complete blood count. However, too often things are done for the sake of completeness which have little or no chance of providing useful information. Appropriate cultures must be made, but again reason should prevail. For example, we regularly see patients who have 20 to 30 blood cultures when it is well known that the chances of finding a positive culture after 4 to 6 attempts are almost nonexistent.

Radiographic studies must include the chest, sinuses (if headache or pain is present), the entire gastrointestinal and biliary tracts, and the urinary tract. Radionuclide scanning should be employed after the appropriate X-rays have been obtained. CAT scans and ultrasonography are newer but very useful techniques.

Once all of the above noninvasive procedures have been performed and a diagnosis has not been made, then invasive procedures must be employed. Bone marrow and liver biopsies should be done. Other biopsies (e.g., biopsy of a skin lesion, biopsy of an enlarged node, temporal artery biopsy) may prove useful in selected patients. The availability of needle biopsy techniques and the use of scanning methods and, when indicated, peritoneoscopy, make exploratory laparotomy no longer indicated in the evaluation of FUO patients.

SUMMARY

The work-up of patients with fever of unknown origin is not only demanding and difficult, but also interesting and often rewarding. The approach to such patients requires care, patience, and recognition of all the potential causes of fever. This chapter summarizes the various possible etiologies and evaluation of patients with fever of unknown origin.

REFERENCES

1. McClung, H. J. (1972): Prolonged fever of unknown origin in children. *Am. J. Dis. Child.,* 124:544–550.
2. Lohr, J. A., and Hendley, J. O. (1977): Prolonged fever of unknown origin: A record of experiences with 54 childhood patients. *Clin. Pediatr.,* 16:768–773.
3. Pizzo, P. A., Lovejoy, F. H., and Smith, D. H. (1975): Prolonged fever in children: Review of 100 cases. *Pediatrics,* 55:486–491.
4. Sheon, R. P., and Van Ommen, R. A. (1963): Fever of obscure origin. *Am. J. Med.,* 34:486–499.
5. Petersdorf, R. G., and Beeson, P. B. (1961): Fever of unexplained origin. *Medicine (Baltimore),* 40:1–30.
6. Deal, W. B. (1971): Fever of unknown origin. *Postgrad. Med.,* 50:182–188.
7. Frayha, R., and Uwaydah, M. (1973): Fever of unknown origin. *Leb. Med. J.,* 26:49–58.
8. Howard, P., Jr., Hahn, H. H., Palmer, P. L., and Hardin, W. J. (1977): Fever of unknown origin: A prospective study of 100 patients. *Tex. Med.,* 73:56–59.
9. Aduan, R. P., Fauci, A. S., Dale, D. C., Herzberg, J. H., and Wolff, S. M. (1979): Factitious fever and self-induced infections. *Ann. Intern. Med.,* 90:230–242.
10. Wolff, S. M. (1977): Familial Mediterranean fever. In: *Harrison's Principles of Internal Medicine, 8th ed.,* edited by G. W. Thorn, R. D. Adams, E. Braunwald, K. J. Isselbacher, and R. G. Petersdorf, pp. 1124–1126. McGraw-Hill, New York.
11. Wolff, S. M., Adler, R. C., Buskirk, E. R., and Thompson, R. H. (1964): A syndrome of periodic hypothalamic discharge. *Am. J. Med.,* 36:956–967.
12. Wolff, S. M., Fauci, A. S., and Dale, D. C. (1975): Unusual etiologies of fever and their evaluation. *Annu. Rev. Med.,* 26:277–281.

13. Aduan, R. P., Fauci, A. S., Dale, D. C., and Wolff, S. M. (1978): Prolonged fever of unknown origin. *Clin. Res.,* 26:558A.
14. Simon, H. B., and Wolff, S. M. (1973): Granulomatous hepatitis and prolonged fever of unknown origin: A study of 13 patients. *Medicine (Baltimore),* 52:1–21.
15. Bujak, J. S., Aptekar, R. G., Decker, J. L., and Wolff, S. M. (1973): Juvenile rheumatoid arthritis presenting in the adult as fever of unknown origin. *Medicine (Baltimore),* 52:431–444.
16. Dinarello, C. A., and Wolff, S. M. (1978): Pathogenesis of fever in man. *N. Engl. J. Med.,* 298:607–612.
17. Cranston, W. I., Luff, R. H., Owen, D., and Rawlins, M. D. (1973): Studies on the pathogenesis of fever in renal carcinoma. *Clin. Sci. Mol. Med.,* 45:459–467.
18. Fauci, A. S., and Wolff, S. M. (1976): Granulomatous hepatitis. In: *Progress in Liver Diseases, Vol. 5,* edited by H. Popper and F. Schaffner, pp. 609–622. Grune & Stratton, New York.
19. Muckle, T. J., and Wells, M. (1962): Urticaria, deafness and amyloidosis. A new heredo-familial syndrome. *Q. J. Med.,* 31:235–243.

Subject Index

A

Acetaminophen
    efficacy and safety of, 230–231
    pharmacokinetics in, 229–230
Adaptive role of fever, 31–32
Addisonian crisis, 220
Ag–Ab complexes, 16–19
Alanine formation, 41
Albumin
    decontamination of, 24
    fever, 23–29
        pyrogenic action in, 27–28
Ambient temperature and neuro-
        genic hyperthermia, 168–169
Aminopyrine, 227–228
Andogenous pyrogen-activating
        factor, 12
Anesthesia, malignant hyperthermia
        of, 218–219
Anisomycin, 106–108
Antipyresis
    endogenous, 184, 189–196
    transport processes in, 78–79
Antipyretics
    hypothermic responses to, 133
    mechanisms of actions of, 131–140
    neurogenic hyperthermia and, 167
    normal temperature and, 131–
        133
Aquatic ectotherms, fever in
    behaviorally-mediated, 197–205
    pharmacology of, 209–210
    prostaglandins in, 209–210
Arachidonate hyperthermia,
        151–152
Arachidonic acid, 240–241
    intraventricular, rectal tempera-
        ture and, 162
    metabolic pathways of degrada-
        tion process of, 159
    neurochemistry of, 149–151
Arginine vasopressin, 192–194

B

B cells, fever with cell-mediated
        immunity and, 15–16
Behaviorally-mediated fever
    aquatic ectotherms and, 207–212
    rabbit pups and, 197–205
BGG and rabbit antiserum, 17

C

Calcium ions as thermogenic inter-
        mediary, 102–106
Cancer; see also Neoplastic disorders
    cycloheximide and, 115–116
    fever incidence in, 235–236
Catecholamines, 62
Cell-mediated immunity, fever in,
        11–16
    in endogenous pyrogen produc-
        tion during, 11–12
    T and B cells and, 15–16
Central nervous system, pyrogens,
        fever and, 92
Cerebral trauma
    direct or secondary injury to
        thermoregulatory pathways
        in, 166–172
    fever and, 165–175
Cerebrospinal fluid, blood in,
        172–174

Aspirin

Aspirin
    efficacy and safety of, 230–231
    endotoxin and, 155–156
    pharmacokinetics of, 228–229
Atropine intoxication, 221
Augmentation of fever
    iodipamide and, 77–78
    transport inhibitors and, 77–78
Autonomic dysfunction, 221
Autonomic shift, 53